IMPROVING HEALTH CARE MANAGEMENT

Organization Development and Organization Change

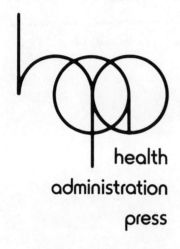

health
administration
press

IMPROVING HEALTH CARE MANAGEMENT

Organization Development and Organization Change

Edited by
George F. Wieland

Health Administration Press
Ann Arbor, Michigan
1981

Library of Congress Cataloging in Publication Data
Main entry under title:

Improving health care management.

    Bibliography: p.
    Includes index.
    1. Hospitals—Administration—Addresses, essays,
lectures. 2. Health services administration—
Addresses, essays, lectures. 3. Organizational
change—Addresses, essays, lectures. I. Wieland,
George F. [DNLM: 1. Health facilities—Organ.
2. Psychology, Applied. WX150 I34]
RA971.I43   362.1'1'068   80-21283
ISBN 0-914904-49-3

Health Administration Press
School of Public Health
The University of Michigan
Ann Arbor, Michigan 48109
313-764-1380

Contents

I. THE SPECIAL CHARACTER OF
HEALTH CARE ORGANIZATIONS AND
THEIR MANAGEMENT

II. MANAGERIAL ACTIONS TO
IMPLEMENT STRUCTURAL CHANGES

III. PSYCHOLOGICAL CHANGES AND ORGANIZATION DEVELOPMENT: THE BEHAVIORAL APPROACH TO IMPROVING ORGANIZATIONS

List of Figures

Preface

This book is addressed to managers of change, to those who would take an organization in hand and steer it in new directions. In contrast to the "administrator" (a term long in vogue in the nonprofit sector), the manager must be prepared to be fully responsible, to take authority for making changes and altering health care organizations in major ways. The times require more than merely administering the dictates legislated by others. Such managers of change include not only hospital administrators but also nurses and doctors and others in the health care system who are responsible for its great progress to date, but also for its apparent shortcomings.

Paramount among the changes the manager must institute are organizational changes that will promote greater efficiency—changes in the organizational structures, practices, and human factors that contribute to improved productivity. Pressures from the government and the public generally are requiring that spiraling health care costs be controlled, that waste and unnecessary services be eliminated. Here we shall emphasize the management of organizational changes that contribute to greater patient care efficiency, to the patient's getting out of the hospital and home more quickly than in the past.

To this end we shall also emphasize findings from research, rather than simply the current fads in management practice. Experiments that are the subject of evaluation research are much more valuable, even if the experiments fail, than accounts of organizational changes that have nothing more to recommend them than their being "new."

There has not been a great deal of systematic research on methods of organizational change in health care organizations. But the evidence that has emerged suggests that there are two general approaches to change. One is structural, in which managers take action to solve problems by altering and improving the formal arrangements of the organization: job descriptions, authority relationships, communications and reporting channels, policies, routines, control systems, or even physical and architectural arrangements. The other approach is psychological, in which managers work with organizational members in developing the psychological or interpersonal aspects of the organization: motivations, attitudes, patterns of informal relations, and, ideally, the human culture of the organization. Readings have been selected to illustrate both approaches.

Many managers as well as management consultants seem to advocate and emphasize only one of these two ways of changing and improving organizations. Some of the research reported here suggests that each strategy of change has its place, depending in part on the nature of the organizational subsystems involved. The later chapters of the book will introduce "action" and "understanding" systems and will show how these help us see when one or the other approach to change might be more appropriate.

Introduction

A major thrust of this book is the presentation of two basic and different approaches to organizational change, arising out of two basic conceptions of management. First, there is the traditional structural approach to change in which the manager treats people as objects. The manager acts impersonally to change the structure of the work of the situations around the worker, which will in turn change the worker's behavior. Secondly, the manager can take a psychological approach to change in which such factors as human emotions, motivations, and attitudes are taken into account. The manager makes changes by motivating the people involved to want to make the changes themselves. Behavioral change comes not from external structural changes, but from within the person.

Origins of Different Approaches to Organizational Change

The traditional structural approach to change grew out of notions of management as expertise in organizing people and things. When Frederick Taylor (1947) devised scientific management he took the view that the manager was the expert on organization. In Taylor's famous experiment, he gave laborers expert direction about what shovel to use and just how to use it, and the men tripled their output with this new managerial direction. Taylor also told the laborers with whom to work, and where; he organized the schedules and the groupings of the workers. In general, Taylor as manager structured the job and, when opportunities or problems arose, he changed the structures—the routines, the procedures, the equipment, the role relationships, and so on. Here changes in these structural matters will be termed "managerial action."

Managerial action is the traditional approach to change in which the manager is faced with a problem, for example, inefficiency in an employee. The manager considers various changes in the work or organizational arrangements in which the problem employee is involved, and after making a considered judgment, the manager uses his or her authority to implement the solution, for example, from now on the subordinate will refer certain difficult problems upward in the hierarchy, or, the subordinate will perform tasks giving priority to B instead of A.

The second major approach to change is a psychological one. As jobs and organizations have become increasingly complex, superiors cannot know everything about the work of their subordinates. In fact, some organizations have come to be composed mainly of highly trained professionals, and these organizations make relatively little use of traditional authority. One professional cannot make decisions about the minutiae of the work of another; one cannot order another to change this or that behavior. If change is to occur in the professionalized organization, the manager must use a psychological (or "understanding") approach, which induces those who must be changed to make the changes themselves.

In this psychological approach to change, the problem is not often so apparent as is the case with managerial action. There may be symptoms of work inefficiency, but the basic problem may be a matter of distrust and poor informal communication between interdependent members of a team. Or there may be good understanding of team members' expectations of one another, while the problem is one of different basic goals in the work (e.g., research or learning versus dedication to human service). Perhaps there are interpersonal tensions because of work overload (sometimes self-imposed) or because of "personality" conflicts. The psychological approach to change gets "inside of peoples' heads." The root source of the problem is assumed to be psychological, and the changes are matters for discussion, for the exchange of opinions and deeply held attitudes and feelings, as well as "facts." From these exchanges, learning and attitude change occur, workers commit themselves to working differently and to supporting one another in new efforts, they experiment with new behavior, and gradually a new social system evolves.

The modern manager has been exhorted to make use of psychology, to study "organization behavior," and to employ "human relations." But often when the "crunch" comes, the manager must act, and must make the best decision that will get quick results—often a decision that involves changing structures. There is no time for the long-term effort, and uncertain benefits, of a psychological approach.

When it comes to planning major changes, however, there is more time; there has to be, for much more is at stake. The strategy for change must be a considered one, and the question addressed in this book is whether, or when, the manager should take the more traditional structural approach to change and when the manager should consider the newer psychological approaches, such as organization development (OD).

Further, when one does use a structural appoach, how does one take into account resistance to change by subordinates? If one turns to a psychological approach, how does one choose among the wealth of techniques offered by OD, such as team building, survey feedback, and management by objectives? How much do the different techniques matter, or is the important thing how the techniques are used? Most importantly, can OD actually eliminate organizational inefficiency and save money? Finally, where do the physicians fit in? They control such a large share of health care costs, and yet have great power to resist major changes. Why do some of these change techniques seem to be effective in getting physicians to change their behavior?

ORGANIZATION OF THE BOOK

The book is divided into five sections. Part I briefly introduces the basic nature of the hospital and other health care organizations and the problems involved in their management. These organizations have highly complex and heterogeneous technologies, they must usually deal with extremely variable patient inputs, and there are enormous problems of coordinating very specialized knowledge and care around an individual patient. The informal social system is an important concern in effective management. The role of the administrator is a particularly difficult one, given the increasing outside pressures for cost control and improved efficiency, with at the same time the need to cope with an almost chaotic organizational structure.

Part II examines the traditional approach to the management of change. The manager in a pyramidal, hierarchical organization is charged with responsibility for organizing the work of his or her subordinates, for giving them direction, and, when problems intervene, for dealing with these problems, often by making new structural arrangements. Planned major change occurs in a process much like everyday management: problems are perceived and a solution is devised, implemented, and if successful, incorporated into the organization routine. If a management consultant is employed, the same process is used. The new structural design is first developed, then the manager uses his or her power to implement that new design, and to get acceptance by the people involved.

The unfortunate situation the manager faces in trying to improve efficiency will be described. There is little real power for administrators to implement changes in many of the important cost-generating sectors of the hospital—the medical sectors. Nevertheless, there have been successes in this direction, and we shall briefly describe what is possible if physicians themselves can be persuaded to begin acting like managers.

Administrators' implementation of several new structures will also be explored, not so much for intrinsic value, but more to exemplify how the traditional structural implementation process can be facilitated by the use of psychological and organizational knowledge. Two experiments, one a success, one a failure, in instituting admissions-scheduling systems and a survey of the factors differentiating between successful and unsuccessful implementation of service unit manager structures will illustrate this point. These studies will detail the importance of conflict and tension, of influence and participation, of training and psychological support, and, finally, of diffusing changes into more distant parts of the oganization.

THE PSYCHOLOGICAL APPROACH TO ORGANIZATIONAL CHANGE

In Part III we examine the psychological approach to improving organizations. Highly professional staff, such as doctors, coordinate their activities by internal controls, or by the orientations, motivations, attitudes, and values they have internalized as part of their long training and apprenticeship. The psychological approach to change operates on these internalized factors. The behavior of physicians cannot be readily changed by structural changes, by simply assigning them a new role, by ordering a new policy, by instituting new routines and physical arrangements, or in general, by making changes that are not closely compatible with their internal psychology. One must first seek psychological acceptance; then changes in behavior, together with structural changes, may be feasible.

Organization development, or OD, is a psychological approach to change which emphasizes the development of new attitudes, motivations, values, etc., in individuals and new forms of open, more trusting, and collaborative behavior between individuals. The aim is a new organizational culture which enables people to harness their latent and blocked energies, to be creative and to collaborate in constructive ways, ultimately making for more efficient and more effective organizations.

In describing a whole host of intervention and change techniques used in OD, we shall emphasize that what makes these techniques organization development is how they are used—as a collaborative process of developing change from within individuals. OD is not being practiced, for example, if the results of a survey are fed back, and then supervisors order subordinates to make changes. Rather, the OD practitioner will use the survey data to elicit discussions about the problems emerging from the survey as well as about new problems, and also to initiate discussions about how problem solving typically occurs in the organization and in the discussion group at hand.

The OD change agent is not much interested in the "facts" of the data, but in using the discussions about the data as a vehicle to develop the group and the individuals in the group. The OD change agent hopes to get individuals to look at the psychological and interpersonal factors operating in the work environment, and he or she hopes to develop new norms or patterns of behavior in which these factors are used to build a better functioning social organization. The new norms created in OD often include trying to understand better what the other person wants, expressing better one's own needs, and being ready to discuss basic purposes and also shortcomings, difficulties, and conflicts.

A CONTINGENCY MODEL BASED ON ACTION AND UNDERSTANDING SYSTEMS

In Part IV we shall review a research project covering 10 different hospitals and some 40 different projects, of which some have implemented structural changes and some psychological changes to improve organizational efficiency. The average length of patient stay did decrease for many patients and in most of the hospitals, and this information indicates which change processes were more effective.

Building on the experiments presented in Part III, which shows that OD worked in some organizational settings but not in others, Part IV develops a contingency model of organization change. OD, or psychological change generally, seems to be most effective in what are termed "understanding" systems. These are organizations or organizational subsystems in which goals of learning are very important, in which the technology is complex (requiring considerable exchange of information), and the structure is organic (or decentralized and informal). On the other hand, the traditional structural approach to change seems to be most appropriate in "action" systems, which have action or production in quantity as a goal with relatively simple technologies, and centralized and bureaucratic structures.

We shall contrast action and understanding systems by the differences one finds between surgical and internal medicine wards, respectively. We shall see that an important aspect of action and understanding systems is that the people involved in such systems seem to be psychologically compatible with system requirements. Surgeons, for example, seem to view organizations as if they are based on the principle of external or structural control. They are action-oriented, they think in terms of physical or structural change, and they are authoritarian in demeanor. Internists, on the other hand, seem to view organizations as based on the principle of internal or psychological control. They are eager to understand how a person feels and what he or she wants. They think in terms of psychological commitment and change, and they value exchanging information and learning from others.

The success of the ten-hospital project, and especially its success in getting doctors, as well as nurses and administrators, to initiate effective organizational changes, lay in recognizing these psychological differences. Structural approaches to change, or "managerial action," tend to be more acceptable to those in action systems, while psychological approaches are more acceptable to those in understanding systems. The manager (or the outside management consultant) advocating one or the other approach to change is not likely to receive uniform acceptance throughout the organization. The differentiating factors will be the nature of the subsystems involved and, especially, the personal predilections, whether toward action or understanding, of certain key, powerful figures, such as doctors.

Part V is a summary of this information, which can help the manager of change avoid some major sources of resistance. It will also point the way to important resources that can facilitate organizational change.

REFERENCE

Taylor, Frederick Winslow. *Scientific management*. New York: Harper & Brothers, 1947.

I

The Special Character of Health Care Organizations and Their Management

Introduction

This initial section of the book provides some perspectives on the settings with which health services managers are concerned: the nature of health services organizations and managerial roles within them, and the problems which are now pending—especially the improvement of organizational efficiency.

ELEMENTS OF THE ORGANIZATION

The diagram in Figure I-1 is most useful in thinking about an organization and where in that organization the manager is to focus his or her efforts at change and improvement. Analytically, one may view the organization as comprising four elements—goals, structures, technologies, and the people, with a fifth element, the environment, surrounding the organization and its components.

The primary goal of the health services organization is to provide various patient services. To this end, the several elements are marshalled and coordinated, producing outcomes of varying quality with varying degrees of efficiency.

Formal structures, such as hierarchies and role descriptions, are used to make the behaviors within the organization dependable. Structures also include regulations and procedure manuals, management information and control systems, budgets and plans. They are all tangible mechanisms which can be likened to an organizational skeleton.

Technology refers to the physical devices as well as the problem-solving techniques used in getting the work done. Scientific theories and artistic "rules of thumb" are thus technologies, too. These technologies might be likened to the physiological mechanisms by which the body functions.

The people, or human elements, are provided in the form of motivations, attitudes, propensities to communicate, and the like. To complete the analogy, they are like the mind, they determine whether or not, or how, the skeleton and the physiological mechanisms are used. They make the structure and technology "work."

Finally, as indicated above, the organization is in an environment. It is an open system, relying on patients and workers coming from the community, as well as being dependent on other organizations for referrals and funds. The community and governmental expectations regarding cost containment, and the threat of new regulations in this area, provide examples of the organization-environment relationship.

In this first section of the book, we shall be concerned with the overall picture portrayed in Figure I-1, the health services organization composed of

FIGURE I-1
ANALYTICAL MODEL OF THE ORGANIZATION

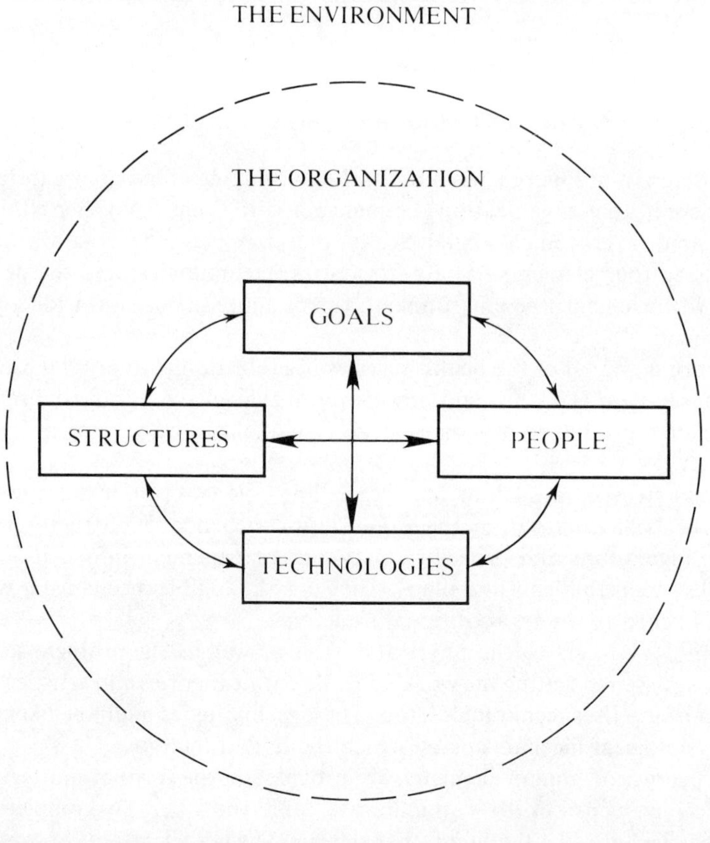

THE ENVIRONMENT

THE ORGANIZATION

GOALS

STRUCTURES

PEOPLE

TECHNOLOGIES

Adapted from Figure 1 in Leavitt, Harold J., "Applied Organizational Change in Industry: Structural, Technological and Humanistic Approaches," in James G. March (ed.) HANDBOOK OF ORGANIZATIONS, Copyright © 1965 by Rand McNally College Publishing Company.

goals, structures, technologies, and people, and with the organization in relation to its environment. This section provides an introduction to the specific concerns in the rest of the book—the ways in which the manager can change structure and technology (Part II), people (Part III), or combinations of these (Part IV).

THE READINGS

In the first reading Basil Georgopoulos articulates the key elements of hospitals and other similar health services organizations. He sees these elements as including professionalization and specialization, with consequent high interdependence of subunits, all of which makes for a human, organic kind of system. Paradoxically, there are also important authoritarian elements—a great reliance on authority and formal directions. Coordination is achieved by both such formal controls, but also by complementary and common norms and values. In addition, special problems occur because of the existence of multiple lines of authority, the independence of physicians, and the overall dependence of the hospital on the outside world—on the community and on patient inputs and outputs.

In the next reading (Chapter 2), Peter Drucker takes a look at the role of the hospital manager, specifically the administrator. The advice from this famous management consultant is that the administrator should free his time from reacting to day-to-day problems and that he should focus on the patient. "Results are with the patients. . .and the major hope of the patient is to get out of the hospital as fast as possible."

In the final reading (Chapter 3) in this section, Robert Allison and his colleagues take a look at the nature of organizations, and from this, the nature of the manager's role. They provide an introduction to the "contingency" theory of organizations and to types of control systems, both of which will be discussed further in the introduction to Part II.

Allison and his colleagues present an empirical study describing differences in the roles of effective chief executives of four different kinds of health care organizations—hospitals, long-term care facilities, multispecialty group practice clinics, and health maintenance organizations. In the last part of their study, the researchers try to ascertain how these successful chief executives developed their competencies in the different role requirements, whether by learning by doing, from other managers, or from formal training and education. That learning by doing seems potent to these effective managers finds some corroboration in Part IV, where a successful experiment in learning by doing is described.

1 | Distinguishing Organizational Features of Hospitals

Basil S. Georgopoulos

The basic system properties of organizations discussed above are complexly interrelated, affect behavior within the system, and have important implications for the problems that organizations face, both internally and in relation to the environment. An important task of modern organization research and theory is to deal adequately and explicitly with these properties, their interrelationships, and their consequences for organizational behavior. Of particular importance in this connection, for both hospitals and other organizations, would be research efforts to relate these properties to the structural, social-psychological, and informational complexities of the system, and to the major problems which the system encounters along its characteristic input-transformation-output work cycle.

But with reference to specific types of organizations such as hospitals, which are likely to present relatively distinctive organizational problem and system property profiles, the major problems and basic properties of the organization could be more adequately understood if the more peculiar, specific, and unique characteristics of the system were also taken into account. In common with other complex social organizations, hospitals exhibit to some degree all of the above system properties. But at the same time, and unlike a great many other organizations, they also have distinguishing organizational features of their own—features not unrelated to the basic system properties described above, or to the major problems to be discussed subsequently, but sufficiently characteristic of the hospital as an organization to warrant special attention. Before discussing the major organizational

From Basil S. Georgopoulos (Ed.), *Organization Research on Health Institutions*, Chapter 2, "The Hospital as an Organization and Problem-Solving System," pp. 16-26. Copyright 1972 by the University of Michigan; reprinted by permission of the publisher, the Survey Research Center of the Institute for Social Research.

problems of hospitals, therefore, we shall briefly deal with some of the distinctive characteristics of hospital organization (for more detailed accounts and related research findings, see Georgopoulos and Mann, 1962; Georgopoulos and Wieland, 1964; Georgopoulos, 1966; Georgopoulos and Matejko, 1967; and Georgopoulos and Christman, 1970; and the various contributions in Georgopoulos, 1972).

First, the main objective of the general hospital, though currently under redefinition, is still to render personalized care and professional treatment to individual patients. This treatment is provided according to their particular problems and needs and is based upon what is considered medically appropriate within the constraints of facilities and medical-nursing skills available, and in the context of organizational and financial limitations which society deems proper or prevailing circumstances dictate. This objective has not been modified to any substantial degree by the current trends toward hospital-based but out-reaching community health medicine with comprehensive coverage, toward more home care and outpatient treatment and minimal in-hospital stay in place of the traditional emphasis on in-patient hospitalization arrangements, and toward health care, preventive medicine (or preventi-care) rather than conventional patient care. However, it is virtually certain that such progress will be seen in the future (see Zald and Hair, 1972; Pellegrino, 1972; Kovner, 1972). In the future, the community's wishes will undoubtedly be taken into account much more fully than is now the case for the vast majority of hospitals.

Until very recently there was little ambiguity about the primary organizational objective of the hospital, about society's acceptance and support of it, or about the legitimacy and importance of the institution within the larger community in which it is embedded. Moreover, within the system (which has such additional objectives to attain as research and experimentation, teaching and training, employment), there was relatively high agreement among all concerned about the principal purpose of the organization (Georgopoulos and Mann, 1962; and Georgopoulos and Matejko, 1967). Conflicts and disagreements concerning means were, of course, not lacking. Nor did the harmony extend to encompass all of the objectives of the institution, either in terms of emphasis and priority or in terms of commitment by the various participants. Now, however, this picture is changing, moving from consensus and becoming considerably more ambiguous even in relation to the overall objectives of the organization.

Because the main objective of the hospital is professional individualized care and treatment rendered directly to the client by medical, nursing, and other specialists, according to the needs and requirements of each case, much of the work in the system cannot be mechanized, standardized, or preplanned. Thus the work problems of the organization and its members tend to be more variable and more uneven than is the case for industrial and other complex organizations whose principal output is a physical product, with the result that the hospital has relatively little control over the volume or makeup of its work load at any given time. In addition, the demands of work are frequently of an emergency nature and nondeferrable, and this demands readiness which places a heavy burden of both functional and moral responsibility upon the organization and its members.

Moreover, the nondeferrable character of work and the relative inability to anticipate some of its demands often lead administrators and supervisors to adopt a management-by-crisis, instead of management-by-objectives, approach in running the organization. Similarly, the emergency nature of the work invites certain exploitation of ambiguity by physicians, some of whom do not hesitate to make unreasonable demands upon organizational facilities and resources on the grounds of "emergency" which they alone so define (see chapters by Guest, 1972; Straus, 1972; Pellegrino, 1972). Except for a few hospitals having a salaried staff, the organization has little effective control over its most influential group, the medical staff which—by controlling the clinical decision-making process—affects the functioning of the total organization to a degree far larger than patient care requirements necessitate (see Pellegrino, 1972). Thus, it is not difficult to explain some of the intergroup tensions and friction in the system.

Because of the nature of its work, moreover, the hospital shows great concern for favorable outcomes and for clarity of responsibility and accountability, with little tolerance for ambiguity or errors. Correspondingly, even at the risk of dysfunctional rigidity, it frowns upon deviation from existing rules and procedures. The familiar emphasis on traditionally close supervision in nursing, leading to frequent "checking and correcting" of the work of subordinates, for example, is not accidental. These organizational concerns often result not only in exacting performance expectations and associated pressures upon many of the members, but also in organizational inflexibility, aversion toward social and organization innovation, and even economic inefficiency, while failing to reduce the very social-psychological uncertainty and informational complexity that the organization attempts to combat and make manageable for its members.

In the hosptial, people with extremely different skills and abilities and very unlike backgrounds are in frequent interaction, within a work structure whose requirements for functional interdependence and close cooperation are unmatched when compared to the great majority of complex human organizations of similar size. Work in the sysem is highly specialized and divided among a great variety of roles and numerous members with heterogeneous attitudes, needs, orientations, and values. When compared with organizations of similar size, the hospital has a remarkable division of labor; specialization of roles and functions therein reach extremely high levels both in intensity and extensiveness. In an organization such as this, the sources and possibilities of stress, friction, and misunderstanding are numerous, while the impact of errors and difficulties can readily generalize throughout the entire system. The fact that the system can contain and resolve conflicts and contradictions to the extent that it does is an important result of member adjustment, voluntary cooperation, and involvement, more than it is an outcome of formal authority sanctions, high professional standards, or monetary rewards to complying participants.

As unlike as they may be in their organizational roles and professional-occupational skills and characteristics, the numerous participants do not merely perform as separate individuals who carry out their respective roles independently of one another, in a parallel or unilateral fashion. On the contrary, they can only work interdependently, because their inputs and outputs are highly interrelated and the performance of each is always contingent on the performance of others. No single group or individual in the hospital can escape for long the pervasive interdependence of activities in which members engage. One's tasks, role performance requirements, and the problems to whose solutions one contributes are all contingent upon those of other organizational groups and members. The efforts and contributions of all the participants, therefore, would be ineffective if not coordinated and made to converge toward the solution of organizational problems and system outcomes which promote the collective objectives of patient care and service to the public. But convergence presupposes adequate coordination and requires partial subordination of personal interests to collective concerns, mutual trust and understanding, and continuous voluntary cooperation, adjustment, and readjustment by all involved.

As an organization, the hospital formally defines the roles of its members, constrained only by its own sociotechnical limitations and limitations associated with prevailing societal definitions of the major professional roles of physicians and nurses. It sets limits to the amount and kinds of interaction, communication, responsibility, and discretion that are appropriate for different role incumbents. To a certain extent it also constrains the work and performances of participants by insisting upon particular approaches and not others. For example, it may favor the "team approach" in preference to "functional assignment" in nursing, or it may support an individual practice approach as against various forms of group practice for its medical staff. It may resist or promote the introduction of computer aids not only for its administrative, personnel, financial, and record-keeping functions, but also for computer-assisted medical and nursing practice. It may actively foster an interdisciplinary approach to solving problems of all kinds and at all levels, or continue the older separation-of-disciplines, divide-and-rule philosophy. It may foster professional collaboration among physicians, nurses, and others, consistent with the requirements of their work interdependence, and irrespective of authority considerations or traditional status distinctions, or may reinforce the conventional dependence of other groups upon medicine. It may emphasize group problem-solving or individual problem-solving confined to superior-subordinate channels and mechanisms. Behavior in the system is, in turn, correspondingly affected and constrained, with certain patterns of relationships being more likely or prominent and others absent.

Hospitals typically tend to prescribe and expect of their members relationships which are task-relevant, impersonal, and authority-oriented, i.e. contractual or secondary relations. Yet patient care, which is both the main objective of the organization and the principal product of medicine and nursing, presumably must be individualized and personalized, rendered according to the specific requirements of the patient and his condition rather than on the basis of generally applied organizational rules and standards. In effect, members are likely to refrain from innovative and spontaneous behavior. They participate in the system primarily in terms of fragmented and impersonal relationships, rather than on the basis of a more encompassing psychological involvement which is possible only where a substantial volume of primary relations and informal interchange among the participants occurs. Patient participation in the care process is similarly constrained, partly for the same reasons and partly as a result of traditional medical and nursing practices, possibly prolonging the patient's health impairment. Observers of the health scene are beginning to suggest the introduction of the concept of "patient's advocates" (see Straus, 1972; Pellegrino, 1972), pointing out that the patient should have someone in the system to represent all of his interests so long as doctors, nurses, and others continue to relate to him not only with professional detachment but also in highly specialized, partial, and discontinuous ways. More generally, for most people it is the primary kind of social relations that is psychologically most gratifying.

Still, a hospital in its present organizational form cannot function effectively without a good deal of compliance by members with existing rules, regulations, and prescriptions for role performance that result in regimentation of behavior. In turn, members cannot satisfy important personal needs and goals that are met through work without subjecting themselves to such organizational regimentation and behavioral constraints. At the same time, however, some of the more important psychological needs of the participants, including the need for primary relations, are so potent that when the organization fails to meet them the members may create an informal organization with which to offset or attenuate some of the work requirements imposed by the formal system.

Moreover, professionals, including physicians and nurses, have strong needs for personal independence, prefer maximum freedom and autonomy in their work, and are averse to the regimentation to which organizational prescriptions tend to lead (see Scott, 1972; Guest, 1972). On the other hand, even though organizational regimentation and constraints could be minimized through more prudent management and administration, they could not be eliminated altogether. This would not be possible because of the specialization of work and the high functional interdependence among organizational groups and members, and also because current trends are in the direction of greater involvement in decision making by nonphysicians and broadening of the base of the control-influence structure of the organization (see Pellegrino, 1972). However, organizational regimentation and administratively imposed requirements can be minimized as doctors, nurses, and others learn to accept their interdependence and function both according to the demands of their respective roles and according to each other's work problems and needs.

Effective role performance in the hospital seems to require a balance between primary and secondary relations (in most cases at the expense of the latter). This can be brought about only by system-wide efforts which minimize unneeded organizational requirements and constraints, on the one hand, and maximize opportunities for sufficient professional autonomy and self-expression for all participants (not just doctors), on the other. Yet these efforts must be consistent with the patterns of functional interdependence which characterize work in the system. It is basically the responsibility of organizational leadership, both administrative and medical, to achieve and maintain such a balance, provided, however, that members accept their interdependence and behave accordingly, and provided also that the distribution of influence and rewards among organization groups and members in the system itself is generally acceptable to all concerned. Authoritarian leadership does not promote excellent and reliable role performance in the hospital, just as the pure human-relations approach with its one-sided emphasis on primary and informal relations is unworkable. The best solution is to be found in a combined emphasis on broad member participation in the decision-making processes of the system at all levels, in the context of a structured yet not rigid work framework, and upon task-oriented behavior which does not disregard the personal needs and goals of members (see e.g. Searles, 1961; Georgopoulos and Mann, 1962; and Georgopoulos, 1966).

The fact that the principal workers in the hospital—physicians and nurses—are professional specialists raises additional issues, which are further complicated by the coexistence of multiple authority lines in the system. These authority lines are the administrative line, extending from the patient's physician, and the quasi-professional, quasi-administrative line encountered in the nursing service. Specialists and professionals tend to be committed to their profession more than to the organization where they work, and this generates both administrative and motivational difficulties. For example, research by the author shows that nurses in general hospitals are more strongly identified with their profession than with the team which treats the patients, and only then with the hospital and with the outside community, in that order (Georgopoulos and Matejko, 1967). Other obvious reasons for the complex personnel and management problems that a hospital faces include: (1) the professional nursing shortages experienced in recent years, (2) approximately forty percent of hospital-employed registered nurses are working only part-time, (3) nurses constitute both the largest and the most unstable organizational group in the system. It should be noted that this instability is in terms of length of employment, turnover, mobility, extraorganizational female role obligations, and other characteristics.

Furthermore, specialists and professionals presumably have the expert knowledge and technical competence required to perform their roles relatively autonomously, but many organizational decisions which affect them and their work often are made by administrators who have legitimate organizational authority to do so. The latter ordinarily have good knowledge of hospital organization, but very limited technical, medical, or nursing expertise; the former usually are organizationally naive, having a very narrow conception of the total system and its problems and needs. These circumstances can readily lead to serious conflicts, or at least raise important authority issues revolving around the question of right balance between power and knowledge for the various groups of organizational participants (see Kovner, 1972; Guest, 1972; Pellegrino, 1972). As the "explosion of knowledge" continues and specialization increases further in all fields, hospitals and other complex organizations will be forced to devise and use more satisfactory mechanisms than they now employ for handling this problem.

A certain degree of specialization among and within organizations, and professions and occupations, is indispensable to efficient role performance, individual adaptiveness, and organizational effectiveness. In the hospital field, over the years medical and nursing specialization have undoubtedly led to improved patient care, just as administrative professionalization has led to improved hospital functioning. The basic advantage of specialization is that it makes possible the utilization and assimilation of available human knowledge as well as the generation of new knowledge, while itself being the most powerful social invention available with which to handle the great complexity engendered by man's vast and growing knowledge. But increased specialization also makes it more difficult for the individual to relate effectively to his coworkers or to understand satisfactorily the relationship between his activity and the organization's total effort. Specialization makes interaction more demanding for all involved, frequently leading to excessive fragmentation of organizational tasks and member functions with the result that a great many of the members find their work uninteresting and psychologically meaningless or unrewarding.

Increasing specialization, moreover, results in higher interdependence at work among the paticipants, and excessive specialization tends to engender problems of professional allegiance and organizational identification, and even problems of competition and conflict. The disadvantages of specialization can be minimized, but only through elaborate coordination, effective communication, and member cooperativeness in all parts of the system. At optimal levels, specialization (particularly professional specialization and specialization by skill rather than by task) makes for efficiency and adaptability. Underspecialization and overspecialization may be equally detrimental (the former by impeding efficiency, and the latter by generating unnecessary complexity and conflicts in the system) to an organization and its members. Regrettably, research to date has not provided satisfactory answers as to the levels of specialization that would be optimal for hospitals and other organizations. What is clear, however, is that properly regulated specialization in organizations with high internal social integration need not be dysfunctional (Georgopoulos and Christman, 1970; Georgopoulos and Jackson, 1970; Georgopoulos and Sana, 1971).

In any case, the nature of work in the hospital, along with the high levels of professionalization and specialization among its members, and accompanying functional interdependence for all involved, necessitates the development and maintenance of complementary expectations and mutual understanding among the participants about one another's roles and work problems and needs. Member compliance with formal rules and requirements is not enough if members are to perform their roles effectively. The same conditions necessitate elaborate provisions for adequate coordination of work efforts throughout the organization, and particularly at points where diverse and specialized activities converge, e.g. the patient. Good coordination is essential because it is a necessary though not sufficient condition for work efficiency and good patient care. But, again, much of the required coordination must be achieved directly by human means and through voluntary efforts and spontaneous adjustments by the members; it cannot be effected through departmental routines, work schedules, and work plans alone. This entails further difficulties.

The issue of balance between the performance of clinical and coordinative functions by nurses, for example, continues to be a thorny one in hospitals. Nurses are the only major professional group whose members are present at work at all times, thus being capable of ensuring continuity of effort. But the more nurses assume coordinative functions, the less time and energy they have to devote to patient care functions. Traditionally, nursing has served as repository of residual and supportive functions in the system—functions that are essential to coordination but not necessarily to professional nursing practice. As nursing specializes further (very likely in the manner and pattern of medicine), however, it will no longer be willing or able to carry out coordinative activities and still discharge its professional responsibilities to the patient and the organization. New ways of handling coordination problems will have to be sought out, for such problems will become even more acute rather than diminish.

It must also be pointed out that both nursing and medicine today face a twofold and somewhat paradoxical problem, which is also a hospital problem. On the one hand, the supply of adequately trained professional manpower to meet existing and future health needs and demands is deemed insufficient and unsatisfactory by all concerned (although in significant part the problem may be one of proper manpower utilization). On the other hand, as in most other fields, the amount of relevant knowledge and expertise available to the health professions is constantly growing through research, and growing much faster than utilized to raise the levels of clinical competence and professional excellence in actual practice. Moreover, all available evidence and discernible trends indicate that the needs for more and better trained doctors and nurses, and also administrators and technical personnel, in the years to come will increase further, becoming even more pressing than at present.

Among the major factors and trends which are combining to assure even higher levels of need for well-trained physicians, nurses, and allied health professionals in clinical, administrative, teaching, and research roles in the field of health are:

1. population increases, longevity, rising living standards, higher public aspirations and expectations (in part brought about by improvements in medicine), and staggeringly rising hospital, medical, and health care costs;
2. the nationwide emphasis on comprehensive planning and far-reaching national and regional organization (e.g. Medicare, Regional Medical Programs, Community Health Planning, Health Maintenance Organization programs) for comprehensive and high-quality health care for all;
3. continuing improvements in medicine, nursing, and other health-related fields, as well as better management and organizational knowledge based on social-psychological and behavioral research;
4. the ever more rapid obsolescence of scientific, technical and professional knowledge transmitted to medical, nursing, and other

professional students in formal education settings, with accompanying greater needs and demands for continuing education and training throughout one's professional career; and

5. the increasing specialization and interdependence among all health workers inside and outside the hospital.

The preceding characteristics of hospital organization make it clear that in a social system such as they portray no organizational work plan, however rational, can be mechanistically or routinely implemented. Even a perfect work plan could not be effectively implemented without consideration for the social efficiency of the system (including both social-pscyhological and "political" efficiency), or without taking into account the complex human factors and powerful social-psychological forces at work, in addition to economic and technological efficiency.

For hospitals, organizational effectiveness depends upon social efficiency more than it does upon technical-economic efficiency, and the same may be said of reliable and high-level performance on the part of the members. Stated differently, a high level of commitment, loyalty, and involvement, as well as a genuine sense of satisfaction on the part of its numerous groups and members, are critical to the functioning of this organization (Dalton, 1970; Georgopoulos, 1971). In general, social efficiency entails personal goal-attainment for the participants at all levels, and this includes meaningful participation in the decision-making process, identification with the organization, opportunities for expressive behavior and satisfaction of intrinsic motives, and psychological rewards. The social-psychological efficiency of an organization, of course, in the short run may be low while its technical-economic efficiency is high, and vice versa. In the long run, however, high technical-economic efficiency in the absence of substantial social efficiency would be extremely unlikely for hospitals in this country. At any rate, organizational effectiveness in the case of the hospital requires a high level of both.

Economy of operation is obviously a critical factor in hospital effectiveness (see Kovner, 1972). Technological efficiency is likewise critical, not only from the standpoint of having and using up-to-date equipment, but also and more significantly, from the standpoint of how the work technology, broadly defined (for example as treated by Scott, 1972, rather than in the more narrow sense used by Woodward, 1970), is perceived and used by the participants. The importance of work technology for organizational behavior and hospital effectiveness has been emphasized by Perrow (1965), and is insightfully elaborated by Scott (1972) in relation to the work of professionals in hospitals.

Less obvious, perhaps, may be the critical role of social efficiency in hospital effectiveness. This is further clarified and more convincingly shown in another place (Georgopoulos, 1972). Here, we shall confine ourselves to only a few further observations. To reiterate, the organizational effectiveness of the hospital depends both upon technical and social efficiency. For its social efficiency, the hospital must rely on its members and their behaviors and contributions. Formal authority principles and hierarchical arrangements have their place in the hospital, as in any complex large-scale organization, and the same is true of formal work plans, rules, regulations, and procedures. These serve to minimize uncertainty, to enable the participants to cope with complexity, to ensure certain continuity and uniformity of action and its outcomes, and to maximize reliability and predictability of role performance and organizational functioning along the entire input-transformation-output cycle of the system. But concerted effort and organizational effectiveness cannot be attained by means of impersonal controls, standardized work routines, explicitly detailed job prescriptions, and rational activity programs alone.

Adequate organizational coordination, which is a necessary condition for effective functioning by the total system, for example, cannot be achieved and maintained on the basis of hierarchical authority and rational controls, or on the principle of planned means and programmed activity for all involved. It also depends very greatly, according to much recent research (Georgopoulos and Mann, 1962, especially chapters 6 and 7; Heydebrand, 1965; Wieland, 1965) upon the voluntary and spontaneous adjustments which organizational groups and members are able and willing to make in order to accommodate one another and mutually facilitate their role performance in the daily work. A great deal depends upon the extent to which the various groups and members understand each other's work problems and needs; the degree to which the work-relevant expectations, attitudes, motivations, and values of members in related jobs are congruent or complementary; the degree to which interacting groups and individuals are guided by informal norms of reciprocity, trust, and mutual helpfulness; the degree to which members can satisfy important personal needs and goals within the system rather than outside; and the extent to which the participants, regardless of their professional role and formal status, are willing to cooperate and promote organizationally relevant behavior on the basis of self-discipline, professional self-control, self-regulation of individualistic activity, and internalized altruistic motivation.

It is these and other similar social-psychological forces which make possible not only the coordination of diverse and specialized efforts of numerous members of the hospital, but also the integration of members into the organization and the social integration of the system itself. Concepts such as those of hierarchical authority, formal executive power, delegation and decentralization, administrative discretion, work standardization and simplification, industrial engineering, task control, and cost accounting are useful, but inadequate from the standpoint of total system effectiveness. The same may be said of technological innovations, including improvements in equipment design, work techniques and procedures, automation of routine activities, and other technological innovations which are frequently introduced in hospitals. Even sophisticated PPBS ("planning, programming, budgeting 'systems'") are not exempt from serious limitations, and the same may be expected regarding the much talked about computer-assisted professional practice by the medical and nursing staffs of hospitals in the foreseeable future. These improvements and innovations are all very useful work means to the modern hospital, but of themselves they cannot ensure high organizational effectiveness if not accompanied by commensurate levels of social efficiency. As stated earlier, for its social efficiency, the hospital depends upon its human assets and resources.

References

Dalton, G. W., Influence and organizational change. In A. R. Negandhi and J. P. Schwitter (Eds.) *Organizational behavior models.* Kent, Ohio: Kent State University, 1970.
Georgopoulos, B. S., The hospital system and nursing: some basic problems and issues. *Nursing Forum*, 1966, *5*, 8–35.
Georgopoulos, B. S., Individual performance and job satisfaction differences explained with instrumentality theory and expectancy models as a function of path-goal relationships. In E. L. Abt and B. F. Riess (Eds.) *Clinical psychology in industrial organization.* New York: Grune and Stratton, 1971.
Georgopoulos, B. S., (Ed.) *Organizational research on health institutions.* Ann Arbor: Survey Research Center of the Institute for Social Research, University of Michigan 1972.
Georgopoulos, B. S., and Christman, L. The clinical nurse specialist: a role model. *American Journal of Nursing*, 1970, *70*, 1030–1039.
Georgopoulos, B. S., and Jackson, M. M. Nursing kardex behavior in an experimental study of patient units with and without clinical nurse specialists. *Nursing Research*, 1970, *9*, 196–218.
Georgopoulos, B. S. and Mann, F. C. *The community general hospital.* New York: Macmillan, 1962.
Georgopoulos, B. S., and Matejko, A. The American general hospital as a complex social system. *Health Services Research*, 1967, *2*, 76–112.
Georgopoulos, B. S., and Sana, J. M. Clinical nursing specialization and intershift report behavior. *American Journal of Nursing*, 1971, *71*, 538–545.
Georgopoulos, B. S., and Wieland, G. F. *Nationwide study of coordination and patient care in voluntary hospitals.* Ann Arbor, Mich.: Institute for Social Research, 1964.
Guest, R. H. The role of the doctor in institutional management. In Georgopoulos, *Organizational research on health institutions.*
Heydebrand, W. V. Bureaucracy in hospitals: an analysis of complexity and coordination in formal organizations. Doctoral dissertation, University of Chicago, 1965.

Kovner, A. R. The hospital administrator and organizational effectiveness. In Georgopoulos, *Organizational research on health institutions.*

Pellegrino, E. D. The changing matrix of clinical decision-making in the hospital. In Georgopoulos, *Organizational research on health institutions.*

Perrow, C. Hospitals: technology, structure, and goals. In J. G. March (Ed.) *Handbook of organizations.* Chicago: Rand McNally, 1965.

Scott, W. R. Professionals in hospitals: technology and the organization of work. In Georgopoulos, *Organizational research on health institutions.*

Searles, R. E. The relation between communication and social integration in the community hospital. Doctoral dissertation, University of Michigan, 1961.

Straus, R. Hospital organization from the viewpoint of patient-centered goals. In Georgopoulos, *Organizational research on health institutions.*

Wieland, G. F. Complexity and coordination in organizations. Doctoral dissertation, University of Michigan, 1965.

Woodward, J. Technology, material control, and organizational behavior. In A. R. Negandhi and J. P. Schwitter (Eds.) *Organizational behavior models.* Kent, Ohio: Kent State University, 1970.

2 | The Effective Executive

Peter F. Drucker

"What is it the effective people in executive and administrative policy-making positions do that the rest of us do not do and what is it they do not do that the rest of us do?"

The first thing I would like to say is that there is no effective type. Effective executives come lean and fat, tall and short, outgoing and morbidly shy, broad-minded and narrow-minded; they are indistinguishable from any other assortment of the human race by personality type. Further, it is not an ability, it is a set of habits that they have. In other words, effectiveness is essentially a practice and like all practices, it is unbelievably simple. There is no practice that a nine-year-old child cannot understand but, on the other hand, every practice is very hard to acquire because there is only one way of acquiring it—and that is by continual practice.

Now, as an example, everybody has learned the multiplication tables not just by being bright, not by being mathematically talented, but by drilling with them until they came quite naturally. This is the only way one can acquire knowledge of the multiplication tables or, on the other hand, one can learn to play musical scales, or tennis, or anything else.

Therefore, effectiveness is a practice that has to be practiced until it becomes, in effect, second nature, until it becomes an automatic habit. Those who are successful have all discovered that effectiveness is an acquired habit. I don't think anybody is particularly born with it. Of course, some people take to it more kindly than others, but everybody has to acquire it by practicing it. To illustrate this fact, I would like to report on some very simple practices.

Notes on a talk presented as the 1967 Arthur C. Bachmeyer Memorial Address at the Tenth Congress on Administration of the American College of Hospital Administrators in Chicago, February 10, 1967. Reprinted with permission from the quarterly journal of the American College of Hospital Administrators, *Hospital Administration* (retitled in 1976 *Hospital & Health Services Administration)* Summer, 1967 (Volume 12, Number 3) pp. 7–20.

Every book and every article I've read on the subject of how to get work done starts with the injunction: plan. Well, the effective executives do not start this way—they know better. They know, for example, if you start with a plan, it ends up in the bottom drawer; six months later you then draw up another futile one and throw the first one away!

EFFECTIVE EXECUTIVE DEVELOPS TIME LOG

Therefore, the effective executive does not start out with planning his work. He starts out by determining how he's spending his time. He develops a time log on himself. Now, when you consider this, you realize it makes sense. After all, time is a very peculiar resource. Everything takes time; in fact, most of our work takes not only time but a substantial amount of it in a lump sum—or we get nothing done, whether it is writing a report, making a major personnel decision, etc.

All of you who have written reports know that when you initially sit down to write a report, you estimate it will take about six hours. In the final analysis, it often may actually take twelve. However, if you work on it for twenty minutes each of the twenty working days of a full month, you will not have progressed much beyond a blank sheet of paper embroidered with some doodles. You will have wasted six and one-half hours. At that point, you realize that if you really want to get the job done, you must disconnect the phone, lock the door, wrap a wet towel around your forehead and work uninterruptedly for six hours. At the end of that time, you may produce what I call a "zero draft." This is the copy that comes before the first draft! I have been a professional writer for almost forty years and I have yet to produce a first draft the first time. However, once you have the zero draft, you can then work ten, twenty minutes at a time, straighten out a sentence here and a paragraph there, refine and complete it.

Everything the administrator does takes time—especially the personnel decisions. In my consulting work I see a great many poor personnel decisions. Unfortunately, I also usually see them very late, often a couple of years after they have been made. Without a single exception, they reflect undue haste.

The two best executives I have had the experience of observing in action were both unbelievably impatient men. One of these was General George Marshall, Chief of Staff of the United States Army during World War II. The other was Alfred P. Sloan, Jr., of General Motors. Both of these people had a notoriously short fuse and terrible impatience. Yet, when it came to decisions about personnel, they took their time: as long as from six to twelve hours, in four specific instances that I can recall. The worst personnel mistake made by General Marshall resulted from the fact that President Roosevelt had ordered him to prepare a name for major command by four o'clock in the afternoon of the same day he received the request. The General, his biographer tells us, never ceased to regret that particular appointment.

Time, you see, is a unique resource: no matter how great the demand, there is no more to supply—it is totally inelastic. And time cannot be stored. For example, the time you spend here in Chicago is going by the second and you either get something out of it or you don't. However, you cannot regain it. Time is totally perishable, and so it is always in very scarce supply.

TIME IS NOT YOUR OWN

Now, in this sense, as an executive most of your time is not your own. By and large, you have control over very little of your time. Most of it, in fact, is taken up by everyone else, superior and subordinate alike, and there is very little you can do about it. For example, if you are the marketing vice president of a company and your best customer calls on the telephone and spends three hours talking about his golf game or about the difficulty of getting his daughter into the college of her choice, there's little you can do about it. You might suspect that he has some job in front of him he doesn't want to begin! However, you cannot tell him this. All you can do is hope that next time you have a job you don't want to tackle, he will return the compliment. So it goes.

Everybody in your executive position has the same problem. This applies to both the heads of large and small organizations. Here let me say that there are no "small" hospitals. A hospital, even if it has only a small number of beds, is still a very complex organization. It is probably one of the most complex organizations in our society; there is nothing quite like it. There are only large hospitals in terms of the administrative job to be done—there are no small hospitals. They may be small in terms of budget or beds but not in terms of the administrative tasks; their complexity alone makes them most difficult.

WHY MOST WORK PLANS FAIL

The moment you become the head of an organization, you must accept the fact that you are a very good manager of your time if you have as much as one quarter of it available for the things that are really important, the things you really want to do, the things that really contribute. This is why most work plans fail. You see, we start out with the assumption that we have eight hours. But this isn't true in practice. On the average, we only have about one and one-half hours. If we diligently work at getting rid of unnecessary time wasters, we may increase that to two hours and ten minutes. Now, the effective individuals know this, not because they are brighter than we are but because they keep a time sheet on themselves. By so doing, they see what the situation really is and can, in turn, make provisions for the things they wish to do. For example, one is to determine those that do not really contribute but which demand time and which do not actually have to be done at all! You will be surprised at how many of these turn up.

For example, you may have your two most important subordinates coming into your office feuding, so you spend the morning smoothing them down and kicking them hard simultaneously; then, by noon, you have them back on the rails again. This is something that is terribly exhausing and yet you know perfectly well that these same two individuals will, in the not too distant future, be back before you feuding again. Now, there is really little that you can do in this situation because these two persons continually act out this peculiar ritual and so you have to suffer it through. Therefore, you go along with it.

However, in the final analysis, if you find out where your time goes, then you can really start managing it by getting rid of the things that need not be done at all, by eliminating things that somebody else can do just as well as you, and, finally, by making sure that the little discretionary time that is left to you is in large enough chunks to have practical value. This is not only the first step toward effectiveness but the biggest one. This is, however, not easy. That is why the most effective executives watch every minute of their time and, in the end, sometimes are able to double and triple its effectiveness.

Another thing executives consider in their work, especially when they start it, is the contribution it will make. They ask themselves what is the one contribution they can make which, if done superbly well, will really make a difference to the results of their particular institution. Also, when they begin their work, they do not look down but, rather, up. In other words, they know that results do not exist inside an organization; only costs and efforts exist there. Results are with the patients, at least in your case, and the major hope of the patient is to get out of the hospital as fast as possible. Therefore, your main objective is to accommodate him. He represents the outside. Inside the hospital, on the other hand, you have a complexity of efforts and costs which, let me say, would stagger most business managers and all of the governmental managers I know. Nobody is really used to that complexity. You, however, take it for granted.

Focus Should Be on Contribution

Now, all of your activities contribute to the cost and only become effective when they really do something for a patient or when, for your counterpart in business, a customer in the market place is really going to exchange his purchasing power against the company's product. Effective individuals know this and they focus their attention upon contribution and not merely on work. This is considerably more difficult to do in a non-profit organization because money is a much greater tyrant there than it is in a profit-seeking business. In a business you can go out and sell more; you can do something about creating revenue. In a non-profit organization, money is only a limitation, a restraint and, therefore, it is much easier in a non-profit organization to become wrapped up in the inside in the efforts.

START WITH SPECIFIC ACHIEVEMENTS

But even business executives, as a rule, are not contribution, or end-result focused but rather work-effort focused. The effective ones, however, do not start out with the work—they start out with specific achievements.

In every case where I have met an executive who has succeeded in a new job to which he had been promoted, I met a man who asked of himself: what specific achievement can I contribute *now*? And in every case he came up with a new dimension, a new contribution that had never even been mentioned in the job description. The reason for this is that the job description always defines yesterday. One can only codify what has already happened—one cannot define or describe tomorrow—and so the contribution is always beyond what one can put into the job description. Therefore, it is always a new dimension to the job, a new potential that is being released. There is always a new freedom of action that the organization achieves with the results and the effective ones do this as a matter of habit. And when they have finished a job, they go back and say, "All right, what contribution can we make *now*?"

To me, one of the worst wastes we have is the failure rate of promotions in high level positions. It is very high. I know "you can't fire a nun." But it also isn't so easy to fire a vice-president. However, whether it is a business, a research laboratory, or even a government agency, many of them are littered with good people who became casualties when they earned their promotion, particularly to one of the top spots. Why does this happen? It occurs because they assumed that what was their right contribution in the lower job is likewise automatically going to be the right one in the next job. They don't stand back and ask: "What is the right contribution for the higher job?"

Another thing that characterizes effective people is their practice of doing one thing at a time. They do first things first and second things not at all.

I know a few people who seem to do an incredible number of things. However, when one looks a little more closely into precisely what they do, he learns that, without exception, their impressive versatility is based mainly upon doing one thing at a time. This also means they can do it many times as fast as the rest of us who try to do many things at one time. In other words, they concentrate; they set priorities and stick to them.

There are, of course, some people I know who work better doing two things at a time; but nobody I know can do three things at a time and do them well. The most effective individuals are single-minded.

All of us have read about how difficult it is to set priorities. But no one ever has much trouble with priorities. Our trouble is not with the priorities from one to three—it is with the posteriorities from four to infinity. Let me explain. . . .

Posteriorities always involve a risk. Also every project and job has an advocate somewhere. The project, in other words, is on sombody's "must" list. Finally, we don't like to say "no." As a result, we do indeed establish priorities. But then we add "just a little bit" of 85 other things and end up by getting nothing done.

CONCENTRATION AND COURAGE

The worst offenders in this respect, let me suggest, arc research organizations. I have seen research programs with 900 projects for 40 scientists. If you have forty scientists, and you really want to achieve something, you can only have a maximum of fifteen projects because most of them require the skills of more than one man. Also, if you have more than a small number of projects nobody is going to do anything. Everybody is much too busy exchanging memoranda on what should be done. Universities are especially guilty of this—they tend to do a little bit of everything. And, speaking quite bluntly, hospitals are almost as bad. You also are trying to do far too many things. Trying to please everybody, you are eventually going to find, is not compatible with doing anything worthwhile.

One cannot achieve excellence except through concentration. This involves concentration only on a few things. Therefore, one has to say about a proposed project, "This is very nice but it is not our first priority and, therefore, we'll have to let somebody else do it if it has to be done." Effective individuals know this and they take the risk: they make the decision. It is not easy but they stick to it.

Let me add that when these individuals have finished priority task number one, for example, they do not immediately take up priority task number two. Rather, they repeat the same exercise. They respect the fact that nothing becomes more obsolete than a priority list! Timing is an important consideration and they know that what was number two six months or even six weeks ago, may not even belong on the priority list today. This reevaluation isn't time-consuming. In fact, it takes courage and not time, because, as you know, a priority list can be drawn up in no time at all. Also, let me add that people in the same organization usually have very high agreement on top priorities; there is very little dispute over the relative importance of projects. Unless we assess them critically, however, we merely dilute our efforts and, as a result, get nothing done.

CITES CONSULTING EXPERIENCE

Another habit of the effective executive is to build on strength and not on weakness. Let me explain what I mean: as a consultant I did not want to have a large organization. As a result, I have a small practice with a modest staff and I aim to keep it that way. Under these circumstances, you can appreciate, I cannot take a great many assignments. This, in turn, means that when a potential client sits down with me, I have to make up my mind very quickly whether or not I want to work with him.

The reason I have to do this fast is that the executives of the potential client organization will immediately start divulging secrets that they really should not be telling an outsider. As you know, people, particularly those in the upper levels of organizations, are lonely. They just cannot talk freely to subordinates about things that really are troublesome. Everybody comes to the boss and wants something from him; it puts him in a unique position. As a result, he's inclined to unburden himself to an outsider. Often, these people do not even realize they do this. The consultant, under these circumstances, is in a rather embarrassing position. He *must* respect a confidence. If he listens to them for several hours, and then indicates that he will not accept a consulting relationship he certainly has not made friends. Therefore, in my preliminary interviews I have to make up my mind very fast. I quickly have to determine whether it is an assignment to which I am even willing to listen. If this is not the case, then it is easy to deflect the conversation into other channels and to have just a pleasant noncommittal chat.

A SIMPLE DECISION

You may think this is a complex decision to reach speedily. In actual fact, it isn't. Rather, it is very simple, so simple in fact, that when I inquired among my fellow consultants who face comparable situations, I learned that they also had no difficulty with it. Upon examination—what they do and what I did—I found the answer an easy one.

For example, when I listen to an individual with my inner ear and hear him say, "Tom Jones is a good cost accountant but I am afraid I have to let him go because he can't get along with other human beings," then I know I do not have a client. Why? Because these are people who want to build on what an employee doesn't have. They don't want to use strength—they look for the absence or weakness. Now, on the other hand, when I hear somebody say, "Tom Jones is the best tax accountant in the industry and it is my job as his boss to make it possible for him to do his work," then I know that this is a person I can work with. In other words, he is looking for what a man can do and not for what he cannot do!

I learned this lesson years ago when a good friend took his first job— manager of an opera company in England. We held a party for him and during the evening one of the guests asked, "Aren't you scared of all these temperamental prima donnas, with their tantrums?"

My friend looked at her with amazement and said, "Temperamental prima donnas—tantrums—my dear girl, that is what I am being paid for, as long as they bring in the cash customers." This, let me say, epitomizes the effective manager. It is the manager's job to enable people to do what they can do. Organization exists to make strength productive and weaknesses irrelevant. The tax accountant who cannot get along with human beings would be a failure in private practice, regardless of his competence. For there, he would have to associate with human beings. However, a large company can use him advantageously for his strength and let other personnel deal with people.

The small businessman who is very good at manufacturing and knows nothing about marketing and finance will go bankrupt fast. However, he will excel as manufacturing manager in a company. There we can provide the strengths that he lacks in finance and marketing.

EXCELLENCE IS ALWAYS LIMITED

This, then, is the purpose of organization: to use strength. The question is: "What can this person do well?" Unless there are serious weaknesses of character, ignore what he cannot do. If you are looking for people without weaknesses, then you will find the only thing that is in abundant supply: universal incompetence. This, of course, is easy to obtain.

Let me submit that the most broadly gifted people on whom we have any history were 99.9 per cent pure moron, if measured against the whole spectrum of human accomplishment, human knowledge, and human ability. Take, for example, Leonardo da Vinci. People have called him a universal genius. However, there was really only one thing he could do and that was design. And, as we all know, he did it exceedingly well.

Albert Einstein is another example. In your job, he would not have been a great success. However, I don't think many of us would do very well as physicists.

The important point to remember is that excellence is always limited. It is our responsibility to use the areas of excellence and, where possible, ignore the areas of incompetence. The Good Lord has given us a responsibility for utilizing the skills of a person. If he doesn't belong in a hospital, but rather a bank, we must tell him.

WHAT CAN A MAN DO?

To worry about what people cannot do means that you are always going to accept mediocrity in the end. People of strength almost always have visible weaknesses. This is partly an optical illusion; you see their weaknesses the way you see valleys where there are high mountains around. In the person who has no strengths, however, everything is on the same plateau and, therefore, you do not see weaknesses as clearly. But also where there are great strengths there almost always are also real weaknesses. Therefore, effective executives always ask: what can a man do? and what has he done well? Then they ask: what is he likely to do well? They finally ask what he has to learn in order to get the full benefit of his strength. Of course, one can always acquire knowledge and skills but not temperament. Don't delude yourself for a moment about that—temperament is established very early in life. I am the father of three daughters and I suspect that their temperamental personality was set at six hours of age. Of course, in the case of a baby boy, it may be a little later—around six weeks perhaps. But after that, only the Good Lord can change personality and He does this through life's experiences. These are not in our domain, however.

As I've said, one can always acquire knowledge and skills. To some it comes more easily and to others a little harder. But we can always acquire competence in a knowledge or skill, particularly if it thereby enables us to make our strengths more productive.

With all of the thousands of things every one of us cannot do, let us be grateful for a little strength. There is not enough of it around, so let's make sure we put it to work. The effective executives do just that.

Within the lifetime of a good many of us in this room—certainly all those over fifty—our world has changed dramatically from one in which organization did not exist to one in which all major tasks are done in and through highly complex institutions organized for perpetuity. A good friend of mine, a Sister who is the administrator of a hospital not very far from here, once said years ago, "You know, when I joined the Order its members served the neediest and performed the most menial jobs. But today I do not have a single

Sister in the hospital who doesn't have a Master's degree, at least. This is wonderful—but I'm glad I'm about to retire."

HOSPITALS A LEGAL FICTION

I know how she felt. When she started work the hospital was a place where the poor went to die. I'm sure you're aware of the fact that in 1900, apart from a few nurses, employment in the hospital was for menial jobs. In a good general hospital, there were about thirty employees for each hundred patients. I think you know the figures today—250 employees in a general hospital for each hundred patients or thereabouts. Further, the majority of these 250 individuals are health-care professionals of one kind or another. This is quite a change.

The universities have changed similarly. For example, before World War I no universities in the world had as many as 5,000 students. Berlin and Tokyo came close with some 4,500, and everyone acknowledged that they were much too big to be manageable. In fact, there were proposals seriously discussed in both countries to split them. In this connection, let me say parenthetically that I have been either a full- or part-time teacher for some thirty-seven years and I have seen a lot of academic institutions. I have yet to see anything that convinces me those people were wrong in their assessment of the unmanageability of large universities. However, what can you do when there are 8,000,000 students? Obviously, you have to have large universities to accommodate them all.

In 1910, society looked like the Kansas prairie. The individual was the tallest thing on the horizon. There was a little hill on the horizon, "The Government," but it was incredibly small. I don't know whether you realize it, but except for teachers, post office employees, and the military, all employees of the Federal Government in 1912 would have fitted into the smallest governmental building in Washington today and probably left enough room for a luxury hotel.

The Swiss army of today has more fire power than the mighty German Imperial Army of 1914. Our defense budgets just before Viet Nam would have supported that unbelievably big German military establishment of 1914 for a full hundred years. This is the scale to which we have exploded. I am not saying it is good or bad, I am only saying that it has happened. Every social task today is being discharged through an institution which is incredibly big and also incredibly complex and, most of all, an institution comprised of knowledge rather than manual workers.

Admittedly, institutions have no existence by themselves. To say, for example, that Inland Steel has done this, that, or the other thing is nonsense. Inland Steel doesn't do anything. Joseph Block and many other people have done something. The hospital does nothing. The administrator or the nurse does this, that, or the other thing. The hospital is a legal fiction and a building and so is Inland Steel and any other organization. It is people who make decisions; we call them executives. They are the agents, the organs of organizations. And every single social task today depends on their effectiveness, their vision and their knowledge. Our civilization is simply not viable unless the executive is effective.

DR. BACHMEYER A PRIME EXAMPLE

Let me conclude by saying that a lot has been written about the executives of tomorrow. Every time I read one of these articles I'm scared by the fact that we are apparently going to require people who have every talent in the world, from ability to analyze to intuition in human relations and political science. In actual practice all these talents rarely come in one package. We are told that we need people who know equally every area of human knowledge from astronomy to zoölogy, at a time when it is difficult to know a little bit about even one subject. We are not, however, going to breed supermen. We had better expect the next generation to be no brighter, no more talented than have the generations in the past. We have had no demonstration of any improvement in the species for a very long time, at least since we have had any records. Also, biologically at least, there is little possibility of much improvement. In fact, we are at the limit of what the blood pressure and the organic system can stand. If we want a bigger brain then, in turn, we must all be prepared to die of stroke at the age of 17. We simply cannot go any further in the evolutionary direction from which man evolved. We are at the very limits a biological system can take.

Yet the demands on the executive are rising. In view of this, we must look toward making the executive more effective. If the supply of a resource is not capable of being enlarged and yet we have to get more out of it, then we have to increase the yield. There is no other way.

Effectiveness, let me say, was one of the great lessons taught to us by the distinguished man for whom this lecture is named. He saw that the hospital administrator was neither a physician nor a nurse nor a health-care specialist but the agent that makes all this unbelievable knowledge and unbelievable capital investment and unbelievable equipment of the modern hospital effective—the individual who makes it produce, who makes it perform, who focuses it on the end-result. I think that this is something that Dr. Bachmeyer understood long before any of us really thought much about it.

Therefore, let me say that I think I am only repeating in my own words what I know he preached and lived throughout his entire career: that the frontier, the area where a little effort will pay all of us the most, is executive effectiveness—the one thing we can do to improve ourselves and to prepare our successors for the even greater demands of tomorrow.

| 3 | # The Role of the Health Services Administrator and Implications for Educators |

Robert F. Allison
William L. Dowling
Fred C. Munson

The size and growth of an industry currently comprising eight percent of the nation's Gross National Product has generated an interest in effective and efficient delivery of health services. Those who provide much of the money to pay for health services are understandably interested in the stewardship of such funds exercised by executives of health service delivery organizations. Patients, consumer groups, and the general public are equally interested in the social responsibility of leaders in an industry characterized by problems concerning distribution and access of health care. Managers of these delivery organizations who find themselves between the conflicting demands of third parties desiring efficiency and patients desiring effectiveness are likewise interested in how successful executives manage such diverse and conflicting demands. Educators devoted to the preparation of such executives are concerned with understanding the real and ideal roles of management in delivery organizations as well as the educational preparation recommended for such roles. The research conducted in 1973 and reported here was an attempt to provide some answers for these diverse groups interested in the

Reprinted from *Selected Papers of the Commission on Education for Health Administration, Volume II,* "The Role of the Health Services Administrator and Implications for Education," by Robert F. Allison, William L. Dowling, and Fred C. Munson, by permission of the Health Administration Press, © 1975, The University of Michigan.

leadership role in delivery organizations and to extend certain theories of organization to a role study.

Twenty-four chief executive officers completed questionnaires and were given structured interviews. There were six respondents in each of four types of delivery organizations i.e., hospital, long-term care facilities (LTC), multi-specialty group practice clinics, and health maintenance organizations of the prepaid group practice type (HMO's).

Since we were interested in the role of "successful" chief executives, both the research sites and respondents were selected on the basis of meeting certain criteria of success. Principal criteria for organizational excellence included accreditation and licensure where applicable, and reputation among knowledgeable sources within the relevant industry. Criteria for successful executives included membership and offices held within the relevant professional society and reputation among leaders within the relevant industry. The assumption was made that successful executives would be associated with organizations of recognized quality.

Specifically, our study sought to achieve the following objectives: develop a methodology for describing and analyzing executives' roles: develop a more detailed understanding of the administrative role in organizations; identify the key determinants of the roles studied; and identify the sources of obtaining the competence required to perform the roles.

A problem in empirical research is the time-bound nature of the data. That is, considering the rate of change, of what relevance to education of future executives is information about today's executives? One approach is to make prognostications about the future and deduce the future role from such assumptions. Another, nonempirical approach is to conceptualize the ideal role devoid of assumptions about the situational context. In our research, we took a middle course in solving this problem. We identified the leading edge of growth in the field today and chose our organizations accordingly. Because the average size of hospitals is growing, we selected one-half of the hospitals from the over 400 bed size category. The rapid growth in group practice medical clinics led to the inclusion of this type organization. Since HMO's are currently in favor and growing in size and numbers, they too were included. Traditionally, long-term care facilities have been of the owner-operator, "ma and pa" type. Recent growth of corporate chains in this industry led us to choose one-half of our sample of LTC facilities from each of these two subtypes. The relevance of our data depends on the assumptions one makes of the future. If one assumes HMO's are the organizational form of the future, our data on present HMO's may be of value in conceptualizing the future role within that type organization.

A second approach we took to the time limitations of a role study was to address the question of role determinants i.e., cause and effect. If one knows the present causal factors influencing roles, by making assumptions about the future value of causal determinants, predictions of future effects (i.e., roles) is possible. It was necessary, therefore, to specify a theory of role determination. We address now the theoretical perspective guiding this comparative study of executives' roles.

THEORETICAL PERSPECTIVE

There has been no lack of research into the nature of executive roles in delivery organizations, but much of it has suffered from one or more deficiencies. Perhaps the most basic deficiency has been what Bennis described as viewing "organizations without people" or "people without organizations."[1] Studies which have proceeded from a theoretical perspective have commonly used a closed-system or mechanistic view of organizational reality. Such studies assume given organizational goals and view the executive function as determining organizational structure and carrying out "management functions" such as planning, organizing, staffing, directing, and control.[2]

More practical problems arise from the difficulty in interpretation and utilization of the units of analysis recommended by such perspectives. For example, when the unit of analysis is a managerial function such as planning, the usefulness of the data is limited because of lack of information about the nature or object of the planning i.e., "Planning for what?" An approach which utilizes functional departments as the unit of analysis and specifies the proportion of executive time devoted to each fails to indicate the problem or responsibility demanding the executive's time. Coding problems likewise plague such approaches. Ambiguities occur in assigning executive activities to such overlapping categories as planning and control, and various organizations group different functions within departments having similar titles.

In our research, we assume that individual roles are a joint function of environmental, organizational, and individual influences. Such a view is an extension of "contingency" theories of organizations and leadership.[3] The nature of the role is dependent upon the situational context within which it occurs as well as the preferences and power of the role performer.

We view organizations as both a means of individuals using the organization in pursuit of individual goals and as a collectivity using individuals in pursuit of corporate objectives.[4] Exchanges between the organization and elements outside the organization provide part of the resources allocated in a series of internal exchanges to induce contributions from members. The nature of the product exchanged externally by the organization largely defines the character of the other external exchanges necessary for organizational functioning. For example, if the product exchanged is health care, the organization must engage in an intrinsically related series of exchanges concerned with legal status (licensure), professional legitimacy (accreditation, certification), professional expertise (hiring certified health workers), etc. Levine and White list the three main categories of elements typically exchanged by health-related organizations:

1. referral of cases, clients, or patients;
2. giving or receiving of labor services encompassing the use of volunteers, lent personnel, and offering of instruction to personnel of other organizations; and
3. sending or receiving resources other than labor services, including funds, equipment, case and technical information.[5]

As we have said, to accomplish these exchanges, an organization must relate to elements outside itself in the environment. Duncan has divided the organization's external environment into five categories:

- customer component (distributors and users of product)
- supplier component (providers of labor, materials, equipment, and parts)
- competitor component (competitors for customers, suppliers)
- sociopolitical component (government regulators, public attitudes toward industry, organization product, and the relationship with trade unions)
- technological component (meeting new technological requirements of own industry and related industries and improving and developing new products by implementing new technological advances in the industry)[6]

Which of these environmental elements is relevant to an organization depends on how dependent the organization is on valued resources provided by the element, and on the strategies adopted by the organization to handle such dependencies. For example, the fact individuals rather than organizations are licensed to perform functions related to the healing arts makes delivery organizations particularly dependent upon professions and professionals. Faced with a dependency on professionals, an organization such as a hospital might adopt a strategy of employing physicians to alleviate this dependency. The ultimate strategy of managing dependence is to simply choose the product having the environment deemed most benevolent i.e., Weick's notion of chosen and enacted environments.[7]

Being an open system vulnerable to uncontrolled, often unpredictable environmental influences, organizations must assess relevant elements in their environment, predict their future probable states, select objectives, select strategies of controlling organizational activity toward such objectives, and monitor feedback of actual performance. The most general statement of the categories of organizational activities made necessary by the open systems perspective is that offered by Katz and Kahn.[8] These activities, which will be presented and discussed in detail later in the paper, are:

- adaptive subsystem activities to sense the environment and make recommendations for organizational response;
- boundary-spanning, production-supportive subsystem activities to negotiate with the environment, to secure resource inputs, and dispose of outputs;
- production subsystem activities concerned with producing the organization's principal product;
- maintenance subsystem activities concerned with maintaining the human and material resources and providing organizational stability;
- managerial subsystem activities to coordinate and control relations between functional departments and hierarchical levels and optimize relations between the organization and its environment.

The Katz and Kahn typology is useful in identifying the types of organizational activities required by open systems. However, knowing organizational activities is not the same as knowing the activities of a single role within an organization. To provide our explanation of the relationship between environmental and structural influences and executive role activities, we introduce Figure 3–1.

The principal outputs exchanged by delivery organizations are custody, diagnosis, treatment, referral, and sometimes research and education. (Figure 3–1, Box 1) Such outputs recommend appropriate technology, principal among which is medical technology. In one sense, physicians can be seen as being outside delivery organizations, presenting them with demands for certain types of services. Physicians could be viewed as the real "customers" or "salesmen" for such delivery organizations.[9] The nature of the physician's demands depends on the nature of the technology appropriate to his medical speciality. For example, the radiologist presents to hospitals the need for certain expensive equipment and trained personnel that differ from demands presented by the psychiatrist. Hence, our measure of technology is the number of different medical specialties routinely admitting/serving patients in the organization.

What we have referred to as technology, the Aston group terms "operating variability" and Heydebrand terms "complexity of task structure."[10] We recognize that by measuring only the number of physician specialties, we have ignored the range of demands presented by general practice physicians. Since every delivery organization would be associated with at least one general practitioner, this scale item would have added little to the discriminatory power of the measure. Considering that GP's can call forth a wide range of technological responses on the part of a delivery organization, an organization having no specialists associated with it would still be characterized by a

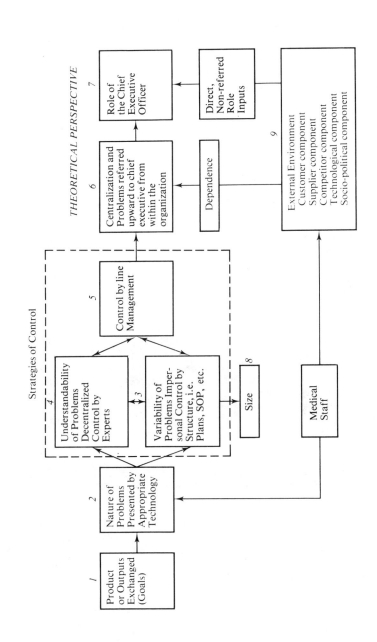

FIGURE 3-1

THEORETICAL PERSPECTIVE

certain minimum level of technical complexity. This in fact is the case with LTC facilities. Due to the loose relationship between physicians and LTC facilities, we were unable to accurately determine the type of physician specialists associated with such organizations. Consequently, our measure produced a zero score rather than a low numerical value for LTC facilities. (Table 3–1, "Technology")

STRATEGIES OF CONTROL

As we have portrayed the concept here, technology exists separately and independently of any one delivery organization. Whether and how an organization responds to the demands of technology is an organizational choice. The essence of management is control of means toward desired ends. Managers choose among three broad "strategies of control" in their efforts to respond to the demands of technology and other external and internal influences. Perrow's model is helpful in identifying these strategies and their association with technology.[11]

TABLE 3–1
STRUCTURAL CHARACTERISTICS of HEALTH ORGANIZATIONS

Variable	Hospitals	Long-Term Care*	Medical Clinics	HMOs
Technology	19.3	0.0	12.5	18.5
Specialization	25.3	7.0	14.8	19.5
Expertise	32%	13%	28%	39%
Formalization	3.77	3.89	2.97	2.98
Dependence	62.8%	57.2%	0.00	2.3%**
Centralization	4.27	5.2	5.3	4.5

*All data for LTC are for individual facilities—excluding headquarters groups for the three facilities that are a part of a corporate chain. This makes a real difference in the matter of "expertise" since the relatively low expertise within the branch facility of a chain is offset considerably by the very high level of expertise available to them from their corporate headquarters. Expertise, using the present method, averages 42% for the three corporate headquarters offices. Specialization for central office only = 10.0.

**Our measure of dependence: the proportion of funds deriving from third parties having ability to influence how the provider operated his facility (i.e., Blue Cross, Government) was inappropriate for HMOs since sometimes almost 100% of their funds derived from an external group having power to constrain, i.e., organized clientele, members.

Rather than deal with the descriptive, literal aspects of a given technology, Perrow takes a more cognitive approach by dealing with the nature of the search process involved in solving problems associated with the technology. Since the problem-solving process is inherently related to the nature of the raw material presenting the problems, he introduces a second variable he terms "variability" of raw materials. The interaction among these two variables in turn heavily influences the nature of the coordinative mechanism characterizing the task structure. Considering organizations as sociotechnical systems seeking predictability and control, each of these three variables may be seen as conscious strategies chosen by management to gain such predictability and control. Management chooses the value of each of these variables. Each strategy is an alternative method of control which is interdependent with the other two. Hence, to increase predictability, management can reduce the variability of the raw materials it processes (i.e., a hospital can choose to treat only one class of illness such as female disorders or tuberculosis). Alternatively, an organization can continue to receive the same raw material inputs but increase predictability and control through increasing its ability to handle that type raw material i.e., increasing the ratio of specialists to primary-care physicians and/or introducing newer, more complex diagnostic-therapeutic equipment. Finally, greater control could be attempted through an increased emphasis on hierarchical control i.e., more, better, or more powerful line managers. The success in handling these strategies of control influences the number of cases or problems that are not handled well and therefore must be referred upward to the chief executive. As we see it, therefore, these three strategies of organizational control operate together to influence the problems and responsibilities referred up to the chief executive in delivery-type organizations. (Boxes 3 through 6 in Figure 3-1)

Control Through Reducing
Variability—(Figure 3-1, Box 3)

The evidence of control is predictable results. It is evident that, *ceteris paribus,* the simpler the problem confronting the individual the greater the possibility of obtaining successful, predictable results in handling the problem. Hence, those management actions taken to reduce the difficulty and variability of problems presented to individuals for solution increase the level of control.

There are several strategies for reducing the variability and increasing the uniformity of raw materials or problems to be handled by individuals. First, the organizations may simply choose to process a simpler class of raw materials or problems to be solved by the organization. When an LTC facility chooses to not admit mental patients, it simplifies its task complexity and avoids task demands that may lessen the predictability of results it presently enjoys. The same would be true of an HMO that chooses not to add psychiatric benefits to its benefits package. Second, an organization can fail to perceive the inherent variability of the raw materials it is already processing. Perrow makes it clear that his model addresses the perceived rather than the real nature of raw materials.[12] For example, behavioral scientists and nurses have long held that hospitals are "curing" physical ailments of bodily organs and processes rather than "caring" for the entire range of psychosocial-physiological problems that could be handled by a more holistic approach to patients as humans.[13] Clearly, the work of health organizations would be significantly more complex, and the level of predictability lower if they addressed all the causes of physical and psychological pathology among their patient populations!

A third strategy for reducing variability of raw material inputs is to reduce the range and difficulty of problems confronting an individual by dividing the task among several positions. Technology presents a solution to a complete problem. It is management's choice as to whether and to what extent that problem shall be solved by individuals or groups. Maytag chooses to let one worker construct an entire washing machine while other manufacturers choose to divide this task among many workers on an assembly line. How to make a machine or solve a patient's problem is a question of "machine technology." How such a solution is implemented within an organization is a managerial decision based on "administrative technology."[14] Machine technology specifies only the complete set of necessary procedures while administrative technology recommends how the set of procedures shall be divided into subsets i.e., functional specialization.

In our study, we measured functional specialization along an ordinal scale of 1 to 39 representing different "functional specialisms" adapted by the research group from a smaller scale developed by the Aston Group.[15] Each scale point is a type of work rather than an occupational title—thus avoiding the problem of having similar titles for dissimilar duties. It could be expected that the more varied the task demands placed on organizations by technology, the greater the functional specialization within organizations to reduce this complexity—a relationship which in fact obtained in the organizations we studied. (Table 3–1)

A fourth method of reducing the variability associated with handling raw materials is through specification of standard procedures and rules. In our research, we operationalized this variable by use of a Guttman-type scale incorporating the extent to which standard procedures have been developed, extent to which such procedures have been officially recognized, and extent to which such official and standard procedures are in fact adhered to in practice. (Table 3-1, "Formalization")

The four methods of reducing variability appear often in the literature under a variety of titles. Three of the dimensions of Bureaucracy specified by Weber and operationalized by Hall serve a similar purpose (i.e., division of labor, rules, and procedures).[16] The first factor extracted in the statistical analysis by the Aston Group and termed "structuring of activities" contains specialization, standardization, formalization, and concentration of authority. This last item is similar to our third strategy of control. Their inclusion of it in the same factor along with items similar to our first strategy is not inconsistent considering the negative loading of the former and the positive loadings of the latter.[17] Reliance on both specialization and formalization is referred to by March and Simon as "coordination by plan."[18] All of these methods relate to externalized, impersonalized means of management control that is sometimes so subtle that it is hardly perceived as such by subordinates.[19] It may be impersonal in nature, but it is nonetheless a quite effective strategy of control. Rules and procedures are more palatable than verbal commands.

CONTROL THROUGH INCREASING UNDERSTANDABILITY— (FIGURE 3-1, BOX 4)

The simplest way to process raw materials is by hiring individuals possessing the skills appropriate to the class of decisions involved in handling that type raw material. Clearly, the predictability of the organization's performance increases as the proportion of individuals with the appropriate expertise increases. Hence, a non-bureaucratic mode of organization control is through self- and collegial control associated with the expertise of employees. A related form of control is the expertise incorporated into machines.

Control through expertise is constrained by the nature of the technological demands placed on the organization. For example, the technology of surgery is much better understood than that of the mind. It would be possible to array the various medical specialties along a continuum of uncertainty.[20] Specialties characterized by relatively high levels of certainty and predictability would *permit* lower levels of expertise although legal barriers and professional self-interest would militate against organizations employing non-professionals to perform such tasks. Hence, there is an inherent relationship between the range and degree of uncertainty characterizing the technology placing demands on the organization and the level of employee expertise needed to properly handle such task demands—a relationship borne out by our measures. (Table 3–1)

In our research, we measured Expertise as the proportion of employees earning as much or more than the entry-level, inexperienced registered nurse in that organization. The assumption was that this position requires a somewhat standard level of professional preparation and expertise which would be reflected in the pay for that position. It was assumed that similar levels of expertise among other positions would be accurately reflected in pay levels for those positions. Hence, employees earning as much or more than the beginning RN were presumed to have as much or more expertise than the RN. A score of 39 percent for HMO's is taken to mean that this proportion of employees has expertise comparable to the RN. (Table 3–1) Since the measure excludes physicians, it undervalues the expertise available to organizations having physicians working for them on a continuing basis. Adding physicians to the expertise measure for clinics raises it from 28 to 39 percent; for HMO's the figure increases from 39 to 47 percent. The presence of such an expert group of employees who, in the case of physicians, is also an organized and powerful group, certainly leads to greater reliance on self- and collegial control and lessened reliance on procedural and hierarchical forms of control—a phenomenon that in fact obtained in clinics and HMO's as we shall discuss later in the paper.

This strategy of control appears in the literature under a variety of titles. It is the third factor extracted in the statistical analysis of the Aston Group and termed "line control of workflow" i.e., control resting in the hands of workflow personnel themselves, and well-developed personnel procedures for selecting employees qualified to make such decisions.[21] Hage and Aiken utilize a similar measure they call "degree of complexity."[22] Building on Litwak's work, Hall found professionalization and bureaucratization to be inversely correlated to each other and related to the degree of routine involved in task performance.[23] Montagna reports in his study of a large accounting firm that where procedures were routinized, computers replaced experts.[24] Note that this merely shifts the source of expertise from humans to equipment rather than from expertise to some alternative strategy of control.[25] Hickson refers to this concept as "knowledge technology."[26] Perrow's concept of "understandability" and most of the other authors cited here refer back to an earlier distinction between "algorithmic" and "heuristic" problems made by Simon et al.[27] Problems solvable through determinate search procedures are intrinsically simpler and capable of being handled through delegation to groups of lesser-trained individuals than the heuristic-type problems requiring problemistic, nondeterminate search procedures i.e., intuition informed by extensive knowledge. Some feel multi-part problems are simpler and lend themselves better to solution by delegation to groups than the more difficult

variables. The theory proved to be very useful in doing this in this exploratory study. In a definitive study involving a larger sample size it would be possible to make explicit use of quantitative measures of each of the variables in the analysis.

Having provided this theoretical background on the perspective guiding the collection and analysis of data, we turn now to an explanation of the variable of interest in the study, the role of the health service administrator.

METHOD

Using a perspective in which it is held that executive activities flow from and are a subject of organizational activities, it becomes necessary to specify first the organization activities and from that derive the role activities of the executive. In the previous section we discussed a theory of how organization activities become role activities. In this section we shall provide a methodology for specifying organizational and role activities.

As we have said, in our approach we view the executive role as flowing primarily from organizational activities. This requires a typology of required organizational activities within delivery organizations as viewed from a social system perspective. Our approach begins with the Katz and Kahn model which specifies the five organization subsystems listed in Table 3–2.[34] Since these categories specify only the broadest of activity types, it was necessary to specify the individual organizational activities within each of the five subsystems. We began with the list of sixteen generic, staff-like organizational "specialisms" the Aston Group developed from an earlier paper by Bakke.[35] To these were added managerial and line-type production activities specific to health service delivery organizations. Some of these activities were from the Aston Group's "centralization" index. The result was a Standard List of 46 Organizational Activities. The items were general enough to be useful with all levels of employees in all types of health service delivery organizations yet specific enough to provide insights into the nature of role activity.

Two scales were used to allow respondents to indicate which of the 46 organizational activities were relevant to their roles. Respondents indicated both their degree and type of personal involvement in each of the activities and the importance of the activity to their role. Combining these importance and involvement scores allowed identification of the approximately 40 percent of the organizational activities which were "crucial" role activities. Those role activities which are crucial to each type executive are marked by an "X" in Table 3–2.

To test our assignment of these activities to the five subsystem categories of Katz and Kahn, six Ph.D. candidates in Organizational Psychology from the

TABLE 3–2

TAXONOMY OF ORGANIZATIONAL ACTIVITIES

I. Adaptive Subsystem Activities:
Oriented toward external environment. Intelligence, research, development, planning activities resulting in *recommendations* to managerial subsystem for purpose of assisting organization in changing, adapting, surviving.

Activity	Hosp.	LTC	Clinic	HMO	Activity
1.	X		X	X	Market research
2.	X		X		Product research
31.	X	X	X	X	Long-range planning
	3	1	3	2	

II. Supportive/Boundary Subsystem Activities:
Carries out two types of exchanges between organization and elements within organization's external environment: (1) securing production-related inputs of materials and manpower and disposing of outputs; (2) legitimating the organization through image building and manipulation of relevant elements in organization's environment.

Activity	Hosp.	LTC	Clinic	HMO	Activity
3.	X	X	X	X	Public relations
4.	X	X		X	Lobbying: influencing rulings of gov't. agencies
7.		X			Determine buying procedures
10.	X			X	Obtaining long-term capital
11.			X		Obtaining working capital; collections
14.		X		X	Labor negotiations
15.	X	X		X	Establish agreements with other health organizations
20.					Decisions re: appointments of physicians
22.	X	X	X	X	Recruiting professionals, physicians
46.	X			X	Negotiating with powerful external org's.
	6	6	3	7	

III. Production Subsystem Activities:
Activities related to accomplishing the most directly goal-related tasks. Throughput activities re: transforming information, materials, people, etc.

Activity	Hosp.	LTC	Clinic	HMO	Activity
6.					Transporting, distributing patients, supplies
19.					Decisions re: patient appointments, routing, etc.
36.					Decisions re: nursing care given
37.		X			Decisions re: dietary services, patient food
38.					Decisions re: laundry and linen
39.					Decisions re: medical-type records
40.				X	Decisions re: housekeeping
41.					Decisions re: diagnosis of patients i.e., x-ray, lab, etc.
42.					Decisions re: treatment of patients i.e., medical and nursing orders, drugs, therapy, P.T., O.T., etc.
	0	1	0	1	

TABLE 3-2, *continued*

IV. Maintenance Subsystem Activities:
   Mediating between demands of the tasks and needs of the members to achieve greater predictability, stability. Concerned with both the human and material "equipment" necessary for work. Socializing members; setting up reward systems and monitoring performance; standardizing and formalizing procedures ("SOP"), etc.

Activity	Hosp.	LTC	Clinic	HMO	Activity
9.	X	X	X	X	Decisions re: professional/managerial salaries
17.		X	X		Devising work procedures for professionals
18.			X		Devising work procedures for nonprofessionals
21.	X	X	X	X	Promoting/rewarding professionals/managers
23.					Routine work assignment scheduling
24.		X	X		Employee/management development and training
25.		X			Disciplining professional/managerial employees
27.		X			Decisions re: maintaining building/equipment
32.	X	X	X	X	Motivating/directing immediate subordinates
35.					Disciplining/dismissing physicians
43.	X	X	X	X	Dealing with personal/interpersonal problems
	4	8	7	4	

V. Managerial Subsystem Activities:

   Though defined as a "sub" system, actually close to a "supra" system having activities that cut across, overlay other four subsystems. Purposes are: (1) control – resolving conflicts between hierarchical levels; (2) coordination = optimizing relations between functional (horizontal) substructures, adjudicating between them; (3) optimizing relations between organization and environment, deciding whether and how to implement recommendations of adaptive subsystem (the implementation being carried out by supportive subsystem, however).

Activity	Hosp.	LTC	Clinic	HMO	Activity
5.		X	X		Decisions re: charges/prices for services etc.
8.					Decisions re: type new equipment needed
12.					Approving exceptions to budget of less than $500
13.					Determine cost-finding system or items to be studied
16.	X	X		X	Developing criteria/systems to control quality
26.	X	X	X	X	Decisions re: new construction
28.			X	X	Creating/changing professional job units
29.	X	X	X	X	Decisions re: changes in decision/authority structure
30.	X	X	X	X	Decisions re: financial/managerial information system
33.	X	X	X	X	Influencing decisions of Board/Owners
34.	X		X	X	Influencing decisions made by Medical Staff
44.			X	X	Arbitrate between internal units, departments
45.	X		X	X	Arbitrate between policy-making groups
	7	6	9	9	

Institute of Social Research at the University of Michigan were asked to replicate our judgments. The Institute is the employing organization of Professors Katz and Kahn. Statistical analysis of the degree of consensus among independent ratings by these individuals produced a "kappa" value indicating overall agreement 40 percent in excess of that which could be expected to have occurred by chance alone. (Standard Error .062)[36] Tests of their agreement with the choices we made as shown in Table 3-2 indicated agreement 59 percent in excess of chance.[37]

Use of the term "standard" list does not imply the activities are in any way standardized or routine. Standard means simply a single or common list of organizational activities developed on an a priori basis. The advantage of this approach is the ability to compare the variation in responses to a single stimulus—a necessity in comparative research. The disadvantage of this approach is the failure to anticipate all relevant activities on an a priori basis. To overcome this deficiency, we developed a complementary set of open-ended questions in which the subsystem category was given to the respondent as a cue or probe. He was asked to volunteer any "crucial responsibilities and problems" he might have that are logically related to that general class of organizational activity. While the results of that approach are not presented here, the analysis presented here did involve reference to such responses. In general, this free response mode produced few types of activities not anticipated in the Standard List, but it did provide the richness of detail missing in the more structured approach. Complementing the field research was an extensive review of the literature in each of the relevant areas of theory and research. Draft copies of the analysis were shared with a subset of the respondents to verify our preliminary conclusions.

Two approaches were used to provide insight into the question of the relationship between these role activities and educational preparation. The first approach involved respondents scoring each item in the Standard List according to the best source of obtaining competence to perform the activity. Nine response categories were provided ranging from inherited attributes to a professional degree program. Responses were aggregated into three categories i.e., "other," "self," and "educational institution." The second approach involved the direct question of indicating which five of the 46 activities respondents feel health administration programs should stress.

RESULTS: THE ROLE OF HEALTH SERVICES ADMINISTRATOR

Of the "crucial" role activities (indicated by an "X" in Table 3-2), 17 are crucial to three or four of the roles. An additional 13 activities are not considered crucial to any of the four roles. These 30 activities comprise the major points of commonality between these four roles. The remaining 16 items are activities that are unique to only one or two of the roles—providing many of the points of difference among the roles. The hospital role is the most generic in that it is characterized by all 17 common core role activities common to three or four of the roles and is not characterized by any activity unique to itself. The LTC role is the least generic of the roles studied in that it is characterized by fewer of the common core activities and contains the most unique activities. The hospital and HMO executive roles are quite similar. The medical group manager role falls between the hospital and HMO roles on the one hand and LTC executives on the other.

Clearly, there is a great deal of commonality among these roles. These similarities occurring as they do among executives within a single sector of the same industry lend some support to the hypothesized relations between technology and organization structure as they ultimately influence role activities. Since chief executives are one or more hierarchical levels removed from activity differences introduced by technology, our focus on a single role at the apex of the organization likewise tended to produce role similarities. That is, a study of the highest-level role removes the differences inherent in the "machine technology" employed at operating levels in the organization and documents the generic nature of the "administrative technology" common across organizations at this hierarchical level. Although the terminology and method of aggregating discrete activities differs, the common core activities identified in our study are quite consistent with those identified by Mintzberg in his recent study. [38] At a certain level of abstraction, there do appear to be certain universal managerial activities.[39] Empirical studies tend to support the following conclusions about managerial roles: (1) an emphasis on planning or structuring the decision environment for others as contrasted to performing or supervising performance; (2) tend to deal with less structured situations and problems having longer, more futuristic time frames; (3) greater orientation toward external environment than internal affairs.[40] Since ours was an exploratory study designed to answer other questions, we cannot go beyond saying our data are consistent with these conclusions from other studies.

Adopting the convention that the common core activities characterizing three or more roles represent a tentative description of the role of the health service administrator, we shall examine that role as it relates to each of the five organizational subsystems (Table 3-2). We shall, of course, also be comparing the four roles studied in the research.

The data reveal a relatively great concern with adaptive type activities such as market and product research, and long-range planning. In an industry characterized by monopoly, one naturally wonders why executives would be motivated to engage in activities focused on organizational flexibility and survival. LTC executives are not concentrating on such activities because their heavy reliance on federal funds creates a dependence on federal guidelines for programs. In effect, LTC executives are reacting to external imperatives more than they are sensing market conditions and initiating change.[41] Chain-type LTC corporations engage in a great deal of forward planning at the corporate level, but it is done by staff specialists more than by the chief operating executives we interviewed. The motivations are presumably similar to those of executives of public utilities where it is necessary to react to edicts of the public utility commission.

It would be erroneous to equate the "research" activities of these executives with the view of research activities advocated in college courses drawn from experiences in profit-oriented, product-type industries. To Procter and Gamble, "market" means the consuming public. While the public is the ultimate consumer of medical services, it is mostly in the "co-op" type HMO's that executives are engaged in anything resembling classic market and product research. In the other types of organizations, executives are vitally concerned with marketing, but they define the market as the "principal sources of resources." Since physicians provide patients to the organizations, physicians are in fact the operational definition of the market for these organizations. "Research" in this case means such activities as: (1) keeping up with trends in medicine and the types of services offered in their size and type of facility, (2) efforts to attract adequate numbers and types of physicians, (3) knowing the competition, and (4) knowing changes in politics of funding and regulatory agencies. Product research may be as casual as emulating the competition or some role-model facility reported in the industry's trade journal, or buying some new technology introduced to the organization by a salesman. Often it is the lay executive who then sells the medical staff on the equipment or service rather than the medical staff selling the administration. An exception is the HMO where the Medical Staff has both the financial incentive and a group structure enabling them to take initiatives in the area of product research. What is clear is that the executives we studied are not researching the health needs of the population as is taught in consumer-oriented research commonly taught in college courses. In contrast to the traditional focus in research on consumer characteristics on the demand side, health service organizations enjoying a relatively high degree of monopoly power tend to focus on research of factors related to providers of care on the supply side.

Everyone "sells," only the definitions differ. As long as social organizations are open systems vulnerable to uncontrolled inputs and constraints from their environment, boundary-spanning transactions with such groups will be necessary. Such exchanges go under names like public relations, negotiations, lobbying, recruiting, contracting, etc. It may be significant that clinics, the organizations with the most monopoly power of those we studied, were the least involved in such activities. By our measures, they scored zero (0) in "dependence" (Table 3-1).

The health service administrator is engaged in seeking legitimization for himself and his organization through speeches and service in various groups in the community. Heavy dependence on federal and state funds and regulations causes all but the clinic manager to engage in influencing legislation and rulings of pertinent agencies of federal and state governments. This may mean literally lobbying in the direct sense, calling one's local legislator, or calling the executive director of their trade association. In the smaller organizations— LTC facilities and clinics—executives were directly involved in relations with the consuming public. Since family members actually make the decision to admit the elderly to LTC facilities, LTC administrators are continually engaged in currying the favor of individuals who have or might admit patients. An announced goal of LTC facilities is to increase the proportion of patients who pay for their own care i.e., private-pay patients. In the early stages of growth where reaching the financial break-even point is crucial, marketing aimed at employed groups is a crucial concern of HMO executives.

Chief executives are quite involved in almost every type of exchange their respective organizations engage in. They are quite attuned to those aspects of their environment crucial to organizational survival and growth. Whether it is making agreements with related health organizations, negotiating with the local planning agency, state regulatory agency, accrediting group, city planner, or labor union, these executives are quite involved. However, their most crucial activity both in terms of importance and time, is probably that of recruiting key professionals and physicians. As we have said, the real market is the physician who admits patients and the real producer is a set of key physicians for whom legally there are no substitutes. Unlike other industries where management's efforts can increase sales and provide adequately trained employees, these decisions are largely uncontrollable by health service executives. Hence, they must recruit. Especially in the larger hospitals, they may try to close the system by entering into contractual arrangements to provide house staff physicians.

To better control the supply of other key professionals, the organization can begin its own training program, encourage the local community college to begin such a program, or substitute lesser-trained individuals.

It is clear from observation of the *Production Subsystem* (Table 3-2) the health service administrator is not directly involved in such activities. Our data match well the conceptualizations of Thompson who sees the "technological core" as the most closed part of the organization and of Simon et al. who view the role of management as closing this part of the organization by structuring the decisional environment. Hence, although executives aren't directly involved in either performing or supervising performance of the highly technical work of providing diagnosis, cure, and custody of patients, they are indirectly working to ensure that such services are routinized and rationalized. Lack of technical expertise by lay executives and legal prohibitions against laymen making medical decisions have given rise to the very real phenomenon of the dual hierarchy in which physicians and other professionals dominate the delivery subsystem within health organizations. However, while this militates against personal involvement and interpersonal forms of influence by the lay executive, it does not preclude the less obvious but no less effective forms of impersonal influence i.e., defining scope of services, programming, standardizing, recruiting, etc. The health service administrator is involved, but more in the sense that the late Henry Ford still influences those who work on the assembly line he popularized over a half century ago. In theoretical terms, control is more by experts and structure and less by hierarchical control.

The most obvious feature of the *Maintenance Subsystem* (Table 3-2) is how emphasis on these types of activities varies inversely with size of organization. Executives in LTC facilities and clincs, both of which organizations average about 100 employees, are more concerned with such activities than executives in the larger hospitals and HMO's. Even so, all these executives are personally involved in decisions concerning salaries and promotions of key individuals, motivating their key subordinates, and handling personal and interpersonal problems of key individuals.

The health service administrator, especially in larger facilities, is normally dealing primarily with his subordinates and others who occupy key positions of influence. Even though executives in the larger organizations are engaged in fewer maintenance-type activities, our research design does not permit the conclusion that this class of activities is less important than activities in other subsystems. It is still true in large organizations that employee-centered, group-process-type activities are necessary concomitants of production or task-centered activities. Whereas task and process leader roles may well be held by different individuals in the larger organizations, in LTC facilities and clinics chief executives must give attention to both roles. Of all the roles studied, the medical group manager is most involved in group maintenance activities. Since his is the task of, in effect, managing his superiors, he must possess either the ability to acquiesce to their desires or superior ability to influence them toward his managerial initiatives. We turn now to an examination of the essence of the managerial role i.e., the managerial subsystem.

With the exception of LTC, the emphasis on *Managerial Subsystem* activities is relatively equal among the organizations studied (Table 3-2). Differences in the LTC role arise from two structural features i.e., monolithic power structure and lack of an organized medical staff. Of course, it is the presence of an organized medical staff in delivery organizations that makes their power structure pluralistic in nature. LTC facilities are typically privately owned and controlled by either the owner or his agent. While LTC facilities are required to have physicians visit patients and perform certain functions required by the government, this provides physicians little leverage over owners of the facilities. Since such physicians serve at the pleasure of the owner of the LTC facility, physicians lack a base of power from which they might effectively countervail the power of the owners. Hence, the LTC executive is not engaged in negotiating between policy-making groups or between semi-autonomous professional departments.

The essence of organization and therefore the principal role of management is control. Organizations seek to order reality toward some idealized state or collective level of aspiration. At the most general level of abstraction, management activities involve prognostication and planning of the ideal or hoped for state of reality, devising of methods and measures of acceptable progress toward the goal, collection of feedback or information about actual performance, and the taking of corrective action. Some of these control activities have already been discussed under the other four subsystems. Three of the activities fall within the managerial subsystem.

First, the health service administrator is engaged in activities concerning the authority structure making the decisions i.e., influencing decisions by the owners or Board of Control. The medical group manager presents an interesting example of the problem presented in these types of activities. He has a task similar to that of leaders in voluntary organizations who must first elicit the consent of the governed before they can govern. He must "manipulate" his superiors to gain the legitimacy and base of authority necessary to "manage" his subordinates.[42] To do this, he influences whether and to what extent the physician-owners organize, who gets appointed to what positions within the resulting structure, what issues are placed on the agenda, and what fact sets they use in deciding. Notice that he is not passively waiting for them to do these things; he is influencing these processes. Contrary to classic management theory, the manager is manipulating the owners through reliance on bases of power other than legitimate authority.[43]

The hospital administrator has a somewhat different problem. Medical staffs in hospitals must organize; therefore the hospital administrator is concerned with managing their exercise of power. He must encourage them to organize yet keep them from using their power to actually run the hospital. As one administrator put it, he must guide their use of power to a position of planned responsibility midway between the extremes of uninvolvement and assertion. Translated, this means manipulating the type and degree of their participation in decision making.

Having influenced whether and how boards and medical staffs organize, the health service administrator influences which matters are brought before such groups for decision (agenda building) and how such issues are decided. The biggest such decision in health service organizations relates to the criteria of quality employed in judging the services provided. In LTC facilities, these criteria originate largely from governmental agencies and are enforced through the monolithic power structure characterizing that type organization. In clinics, the owner-operators are the task group leaders providing the bulk of the services. Therefore, the clinic manager has little role in developing such quality control criteria. Since hospitals are increasingly being made responsible for the quality of care provided by the medical staff, to fulfill this responsibility hospital administrators are increasingly faced with the task of gaining sufficient authority over medical staffs. And, as we have seen, gaining such control in the absence of a sufficient formal base of power requires administrators to resort to manipulative strategies. The more ideal situation among those we studied exists within the HMO.

The structural feature of HMO's whereby both management and the medical staff are committed to a fixed, prospective budget provides a common fate tending to encourage the two groups to assume a problem-solving rather than a negotiating posture toward each other. This non-zero sum distribution of outcomes leads to attitudes and behaviors better characterized as cooperation than as conflict. While pluralistic centers of power remain, the mode of interaction shifts from manipulation and bargaining to sharing of information and reliance on less coercive forms of interpersonal influence. Both the medical staff and administration are equally interested in usage patterns since both are constrained by an unyielding fixed sum of member revenues.

The inability to separate the responsibility of management and medical staff in the HMO leads to an unwillingness and in fact inability to separate their respective spheres of authority. The HMO executive and chief medical officer in effect exercise mutual veto power over each other. They have what Burns and Stalker refer to as a "rationale for non-definition" resulting in a purposive avoidance of clear lines of authority and function.[44] Only one-half the HMO executives had job descriptions and these considered them quite unrealistic representations of reality.

We have to this point discussed such aspects of control as authority structure, decision making, and specification of criteria. We have seen the variety of approaches each of the four executives takes to these common managerial tasks. They are all engaged in decisions concerning the management information system required to monitor performance. While it is true, especially in the larger organizations, that such monitoring is on the basis of a formal and written system of feedback, it is certainly not confined to that means. Executives in even the largest organizations engage in personal, informal monitoring which might be characterized as a sort of inspection tour. A useful metaphor for this approach might be the practice of Air Force pilots in which they search for "targets of opportunity" after they have fulfilled their assigned bombing run. Similarly, the health service adminstrator compares the visual reality about him with his personal and largely intuitive standards of quality. Such a tour might be no more than walking through the building and calling the executive housekeeper to report a dirty hallway, etc. While such is not the stuff of which college courses are made, it is very much a part of the essence of health service administration.

Katz and Kahn include within the managerial subsystem the general function of "optimizing relations between the organization and its environment." The crucial question in this function is the decision criterion used in the optimizing. That is, does the organization act in its own best interest in making a decision or act to optimize the health system? If a hospital is chronically full while neighboring hospitals are well below capacity, does the hospital build or encourage physicians to utilize other hospitals? Stated differently, does optimizing involve global or local rationality?[45] Does the chief executive officer guide policy-making groups toward a set of internal decision criteria or stress a social welfare criterion?

In the sense that the health service administrator tries to get units within his organization to decide issues on the basis of what is good for the whole organization, he is encouraging "global rationality." However, when dealing with issues whereby his organization stands to lose what is gained by other organizations, he exercises a "local rationality." It was clear from the free response questions in the structured interviews that these executives were not overly enamored with comprehensive health planning. Relations with neighboring health facilities of a similar type were perhaps superficially friendly, but the underlying posture was nonetheless that of competition. Optimizing in the case of one clinic faced by an equally powerful clinic nearby and a hospital threatening to enter into ambulatory care meant merger of the clinics to better equip them for facing the threat posed by the hospital. Optimizing for a hospital meant expanding into ambulatory care to counter the threat posed by proliferating group practices. Optimizing for the nursing home chain meant allocating resources among the various branch facilities according to corporate-level global criteria of rationality.

This emphasis on internal, local criteria says more about our theories than it does about these organizations. Theorists can't have it both ways i.e., define groups and organizations on the basis of shared values and goals while advocating they act on behalf of the values and goals of outsiders. These executives acted on behalf of their organizations because they must. If they are to act differently, then these organizations must first be structurally integrated with the organizations with whom it is desired they act cooperatively. An example of this structural means of inducing global rationality would be the integrating function served by the prospective budget in the HMO by which common responsibility induced common authority.

Another means of encouraging decisions that put the system's interests ahead of the organization's would be professional status for executives. The physician can put the patient's interests ahead of the hospital's because only physicians can legally practice medicine and every physician has a medical staff and a profession to back his claims to autonomy. The administrator has no legal protection and no professional group capable of successfully backing him. Consequently, he lacks the base of power necessary to be socially responsible. It is this deficiency that above all defeats the claims of executives to professional status.[46]

Educational Implications

In addition to collecting data on role content, we asked for other information bearing more directly on the question of educational preparation to perform role functions. Rather than directly assessing the knowledge and skills necessary to perform each of the role activities listed in Table 3-2, we asked respondents to indicate for each of these activities the best source of obtaining competence to perform the activity.

It is abundantly clear in Table 3-3 that these successful executives generally prefer "self" as the best source of obtaining requisite skills for their position. We could say this means either they have forgotten where they in fact learned their role skills, or they had poor educational preparation and learned mostly by experience. Or, we could say that the skills necessary for the chief executive are either not teachable or weren't taught to these respondents. One is always on firm ground in taking respondents at their word and assuming they in fact know what they are saying. These respondents are saying experience has been their best teacher.

How can we reconcile a complex role in a highly complex, technical organization with statements from some of the best leaders of such organizations to the effect that for them education is not the best way to prepare to perform their role? A possible answer might be that technical knowledge and discrete job skills—the emphasis of all graduate educational programs—simply are not the crucial variables for this role. It may well be as C. Wright Mills says, more a question of personal values and who you know than specialized knowledge such as middle-level managers must possess.[47] If it is a matter of values, whose values? The chief executive probably must conform to the values of those who are "significant" to him either in terms of granting or withholding personal rewards or in being instrumental in aiding or blocking

TABLE 3–3
SOURCE OF COMPETENCE

Activity No.	Others	Self	Education	Activity No.	Others	Self	Education
1.	33%	43%	24%	24.	26%	37%	37%
2.	45%	41%	14%	25.	21%	71%	8%
3.	6%	71%	23%	26.	33%	54%	13%
4.	18%	64%	18%	27.	31%	57%	12%
5.	33%	78%	9%	28.	30%	44%	26%
6.	36%	52%	12%	29.	24%	46%	30%
7.	31%	49%	21%	30.	25%	42%	33%
8.	42%	52%	6%	31.	20%	54%	26%
9.	33%	57%	10%	32.	6%	73%	21%
10.	30%	46%	24%	33.	9%	71%	20%
11.	32%	45%	23%	34.	25%	57%	18%
12.	34%	64%	2%	35.	23%	69%	8%
13.	32%	38%	30%	36.	39%	42%	19%
14.	23%	48%	29%	37.	40%	40%	20%
15.	13%	63%	24%	38.	36%	45%	19%
16.	39%	22%	39%	39.	39%	33%	28%
17.	30%	44%	26%	40.	31%	50%	19%
18.	27%	44%	29%	41.	46%	27%	27%
19.	31%	48%	21%	42.	46%	29%	25%
20.	24%	65%	11%	43.	12%	76%	12%
21.	23%	67%	10%	44.	12%	78%	10%
22.	26%	61%	13%	45.	16%	61%	23%
23.	32%	57%	11%	46.	7%	71%	22%

Each respondent indicated both a first and a second choice for each of the activities in the Standard List of Activities, choices indicating the best and next best sources of obtaining the competence required to perform the activity. The above data are an average of both choices combined for the entire sample of respondents (N=48 Max.)

Others: 1. Rely on others i.e., consult with other managers, staff experts, M.D.'s, etc.
Self: 2. Personality, charm, persuasive and interpersonal skills.
  3. Basic inherited intelligence; common sense.
  4. Experience.
  5. Self-instruction, and read books, journal articles, etc.
Education: 6. A course, workshop, institute, etc., on a specific subject; continuing education.
  7. Well-rounded, broad, general, or liberal education.
  8. Professional, specialized education.

the decision process. As we have seen, he is most concerned with managing environmental dependence and internal decision making. Hence, the health service administrator could be expected to adopt the values of the power elites with whom he works, in and outside the organization. Tagiuri's study of executives, scientists, and research managers revealed research managers had value orientations consistent with their organizational positions.[48] That is, research managers were the "men in the middle" between scientists and executives. Research managers were found to have value sets representing an amalgam of the two groups with whom they worked. It is unlikely that it could be otherwise, for prolonged interaction between individuals with incompatible values and attitudes should result in either continual psychological or social conflict or changes in the conflicting values.

We did not directly assess executive values and attitudes or attempt to document the individuals and groups who would constitute the set of significant others for these executives. A study incorporating these objectives is now underway. It is clear, however, that role incorporates these psychological attributes as well as role behaviors.[49] When executives indicate that experience, other forms of self-preparation, and relying on others are more crucial than classroom instruction, they may well be telling us that these are the relevant arenas in which to gain personal attributes such as values, contacts with influential people, etc.

We also cannot ignore what these executives said about education as a preferred source of competence for certain activities. In Table 3–4 we have presented the activities in an array based on the scores for education only.

TABLE 3–4

RELATIVE EMPHASIS ON EDUCATIONAL INSTITUTIONS AS
SOURCE OF COMPETENCE TO PERFORM ACTIVITIES

(Percentage of respondents who name some type of educational method as their first or second choice of gaining competence to perform executive activity. Question number given in parentheses at end of activity.)

%	Activity
39%	Decisions re: Quality control system procedures. (16)
37%	Employee/Management development, training. (24)
33%	Decisions re: Management information system. (30)
30%	Decisions re: Cost finding. (13)
30%	Decisions re: Organization structure. (29)
29%	Labor negotiations. (14)
29%	Devising work procedures for nonprofessionals. (18)
28%	Decisions re: Medical-type records. (39)
27%	Decisions re: Diagnosis, i.e., Lab., EKG, X-ray, etc. (41)
26%	Devising work procedures for professionals. (17)
26%	Creating/changing professional jobs/units. (28)
26%	Long-range planning. (31)
25%	Decisions re: Treatment, i.e., medical, drugs, etc. (42)
24%	Market research. (1)
24%	Obtaining long-term capital. (10)
24%	Establishing agreements with other health organizations. (15)
23%	Public Relations. (3)
23%	Obtaining working capital; collections. (11)
23%	Arbitrate between policy-making groups (Boards, Staff, Administration). (45)
22%	Negotiating with powerful external organizations. (46)

TABLE 3-4, *continued*

%	Activity
21%	Determine buying procedures. (7)
21%	Scheduling, routing throughputs (patients). (19)
21%	Motivating immediate subordinates. (32)
20%	Influence decisions made by Board/Owners. (33)
20%	Decisions re: Dietary. (37)
19%	Decisions re: Nursing care. (36)
19%	Decisions re: Laundry and linen. (38)
19%	Decisions re: Housekeeping. (40)
18%	Lobbying and influencing government agency rulings. (4)
18%	Influence decisions made by the medical staff. (34)
14%	Project research. (2)
13%	Recruiting professionals, physicians. (22)
13%	Decisions re: new construction. (26)
12%	Transporting, distributing throughputs (patients). (6)
12%	Decisions re: maintaining building and equipment. (27)
12%	Dealing with personal and interpersonal problems. (43)
11%	Decisions re: appointments of physicians. (20)
11%	Routine work assignment scheduling. (23)
10%	Decisions re: professional and managerial salaries. (9)
10%	Rewarding professional and managerial employees. (21)
10%	Arbitrate between internal units, divisions. (44)
9%	Decisions re: charges/prices for services and products. (5)
8%	Disciplining professional/managerial employees. (25)
8%	Disciplining physicians. (35)
6%	New equipment decisions. (8)
2%	Approving exceptions to the budget of less than $500. (12)

While all the scores are low, it is instructive to examine their relative rankings. Two conclusions seem justified from the data. First, items with the highest scores, activities they think educators could help them with, are almost exclusively technical in nature. Second, items with low scores are role activities that are either inconsequential to the role or very crucial role activities requiring essentially political and human relations skills. Clearly, these executives see educators as technically oriented and ill-prepared to impart the skill these executives have already indicated in Table 3-3 that they see are best gained in the arena of life.

We used a second approach to gain information about educational preparation. Each respondent was asked to select five of the items in the standard list which he felt educators should stress in health service administration programs. (Table 3-5) There is a moderate correlation between the data in Tables 3-4 and 3-5—a correlation which should occur if respondents were consistent.

TABLE 3–5

ITEMS EDUCATORS SHOULD STRESS

Activity Number	Item	(f)
31(a)	Long-range planning for the organization.	15
32(a)	Motivating and directing immediate subordinates.	14
24(b)	Systematic development of employees i.e., mgt. development, empl. training.	13
3(c)	Influence public knowledge, opinion, or attitude.	12
30(a)	Decisions concerning financial and managerial type information.	12
16(d)	Developing criteria and systems to control quality of patient services.	11
33(e)	Influencing decisions made by Board/Owners.	9
43(a)	Dealing with personal and interpersonal problems.	8
45	Arbitrating, negotiating differences between medical staff, Board or owner, and administration.	6
29	Decide on changes in the authority structure i.e., who reports to whom, committee membership, who is involved in decisions, etc.	5
34	Influencing decisions made by the Medical Staff.	5
14	Represent the organization in labor negotiations or disputes.	5
44	Arbitrating, negotiating differences between departments/units within organization.	4
46	Arbitrating, negotiating differences between us and influential coalitions and organizations outside our organization.	4
10	Obtaining long-term capital financing (stocks, bonds, loans, appropriations).	3
18	Devising or approving work procedures used by professionals.	3
22	Recruiting professional employees, physicians.	3

Notes:
(a)   Mentioned by respondents from all four types of organizations.
(b)   Mentioned chiefly by long-term care and clinics.
(c)   Mentioned equally by all types of organizations except clinics. This is possibly clear difference between type i.e., the "market" for clinic manager is his captive M.D. panel, not "public" per se.
(d)   Mentioned by only hospitals and long-term care—the two types most dependent on external financing from payors who can constrain!
(e)   Mentioned by only hospitals and clinics.

Perhaps the two most important conclusions which might be made from these data are: (1) although the health services administrator emphasizes the external environment, he generally does not see educators as able to provide him with much help in this area; and (2) although he feels interpersonal skills are best learned through experience or self-learning methods, he is wanting educators to stress influence processes. Considering the pluralistic structure within which the health service administrator must create bases of power, it is understandable why he would thus advocate the teaching of same. In a situation where one is first given responsibility and usually not granted sufficient authority and power to fulfill it properly, it is understandable that he would denigrate the normative-type management course he may have had in which it was taught that one was first given authority and subsequently expected to be held accountable for only those matters over which he was granted sufficient authority. While it may not be palatable for educators to be confronted with such data from practitioners, in cases where theory and practice diverge, it is theory that must yield to the reality it purports to represent. It would appear, therefore, that educators should consider these findings when making curriculum decisions.

We began our paper with a discussion of our theoretical perspective. The purpose was to indicate the issues we were sensitive to in our investigation rather than to set the stage for testing the theory or certain hypotheses. In retrospect, it appears the theory was both useful in developing a methodology for studying roles and in identifying key aspects of managerial function. Clearly, differences and commonalities among the four roles can be isolated and explained on the basis of the variables presented within the theory. Only a study involving larger numbers and random sampling techniques would permit definitive judgments about either the theory or the data. However, at the risk of being accused of seeing what we sought to see, it does appear that the open systems approach to organization structure and the decision theory or political models of decision making are closer approximations of reality than competing perspectives. In addition, it is clear these executives needed interpersonal and group process skills of the human relations type. It was less clear they needed to learn descriptive details of technical matters occurring in the production subsystems of their organizations. Generally speaking, they opt for either relying on experts or learning these details by experience.

Finally, this study raises even broader questions of knowledge versus values and training versus placement. Although we had no systematic method of collecting and analyzing our observations of such matters, we did become sensitized to the issue of certain personal characteristics and values that may be as important to success as the possession of discrete skills and knowledge. For example, it appears that to be hired and to remain as a medical group manager, one must hold values supportive to entrepreneurial medicine. Hence, one would be better advised to come to clinic management from the business school than through the public health school. Likewise, the consumer advocate might have problems in a foundation-type HMO but be quite at home in a prepaid group practice, consumer-oriented HMO such as the Group Health Cooperative of Puget Sound.

If values are as important as knowledge and skills, and self-instruction is a better source of competence than preparation in an educational institution, it follows logically that placement may be as important or more so than training. While we don't advocate such, we do feel it worthwhile for educators to be aware of these data and give these matters due consideration. For example, should values be a selection criterion in HSA programs and/or an explicit part of the curriculum? Should HSA programs reconsider their role in placement? Should HSA programs re-think the relative importance of on-campus and continuing education? Considering the priority practitioners place on "live action," current information as contrasted to dated/written information, should HSA programs re-think the definition of their product i.e., "education"? If education is to become increasingly the on-line type knowledge of the external and internal organizational environments, then educators may well need to expand their domains into collecting and disseminating such information.

We don't maintain that our study offers data to answer such fundamental questions. It is sufficient that the study has raised what may be the right questions.

NOTES

1. Warren G. Bennis. "Leadership Theory and Administrative Behavior: The Problem of Authority," *Administrative Science Quarterly*, December 1959. Vol. 4. pp. 259–301.
2. Ralph T. Murray, Paul R. Donnelly, and Margaret Threadgould. "How Administrators Spend Their Time." *Hospital Progress*, September 1968. pp. 49–58. Edward J. Connors and Joseph C. Hutts. "How Administrators Spend Their Day." *Hospitals*, February 1967. Vol. 41. pp. 45–50, 141. Donald E. Saathoff and Richard A. Kurtz. "What Administrators of Small Hospitals Do." *Modern Hospital*, August 1962. Vol. 99, No. 2. pp. 85–87, 142–147.
3. Paul R. Lawrence and Jay W. Lorsch. *Organization and Environment: Managing Differentiation and Integration.* Homewood, Illinois: Richard D. Irwin, Inc., 1969. Charles Perrow. "A Framework for the Comparative Analysis of Organizations." *American Sociological Review*, April 1967. Vol. 32, No. 2. pp. 194–208. Fred E. Fiedler. "A Contingency Model of Leadership Effectiveness." In L. Berkowitz, ed. *Advances in Experimental Social Psychology.* Vol. 1. pp. 149–190. D. S. Pugh, D. J. Hickson, C. R. Hinings, K. M. Macdonald, C. Turner, and T. Lupton. "A Conceptual Scheme for Organizational Analysis." *Administrative Science Quarterly*, December 1963. Vol. 8, No. 3. pp. 289–315.
4. Chester I. Barnard. *The Functions of the Executive.* Cambridge: Harvard University Press, 1938. Herbert A. Simon. *Administrative Behavior*, 2nd ed. New York: The Free Press, 1957. Richard M. Cyert and James G. March. *A Behavioral Theory of the Firm.* Englewood Cliffs, NJ: Prentice-Hall, Inc., 1963. Jeffery Pfeffer and Gerald R. Salancik. "Organizational Decision Making as a Political Process: The Case of a University Budget." *Administrative Science Quarterly*, June 1974. Vol. 19, No. 2, pp. 135–151.
5. Sol Levine and Paul E. White. "Exchange as a Conceptual Framework for the Study of Interorganizational Relationships." *Administrative Science Quarterly*, March 1969. Vol. 5. pp. 583–601. James D. Thompson and Frederick L. Bates. "Technology, Organization, and Administration." *Administrative Science Quarterly*, December 1957. Vol. 2, No. 3. pp. 325–343. David Jacobs. "Dependency and Vulnerability: An Exchange Approach to the Control of Organizations." *Administrative Science Quarterly*, March 1974. Vol. 19, No. 1. pp. 45–59.

6. Robert B. Duncan. "Characteristics of Organizational Environment and Perceived Environmental Uncertainty." *Administrative Science Quarterly*, September 1972. Vol. 17, No. 3. pp. 313–327.

7. Karl E. Weick. *The Social Psychology of Organizing*. Reading, MA: Addison-Wesley Pub. Co., pp. 63–71.

8. Daniel Katz and Robert L. Kahn. *The Social Psychology of Organizations*. New York: John Wiley and Sons, Inc., 1966.

9. Alan D. Bauerschmidt. "The Calculus of Hospital Administration." *Hospital Administration*, Fall 1971. Vol. 16. pp. 50–68. Richard T. Viguers. "The Politics of Power in a Hospital." *The Modern Hospital*, May 1961. Vol. 96, No. 5. pp. 89–94.

10. Howard E. Aldrich. "Technology and Organizational Structure: A Reexamination of the Findings of the Aston Group." *Administrative Science Quarterly*, March 1972. Vol. 17, No. 1. pp. 26–43. Wolf V. Heydebrand. *Hospital Bureaucracy: A Comparative Study of Organizations*. New York: Dunellen, 1973.

11. Charles Perrow. *Organizational Analysis: A Sociological View*. Belmont, CA: Wadsworth Pub. Co., Inc., 1970.

12. Ibid.

13. Miriam M. Johnson and Harry W. Martin. "A Sociological Analysis of the Nurse Role." In James K. Skipper, Jr. and Robert C. Leonard (eds.). *Social Interaction and Patient Care*. Philadelphia: J.B. Lippincott Co., 1965. pp. 29–39.

14. Wilbert Ellis Moore. *Order and Change: Essays in Comparative Sociology*. New York: John Wiley and Sons, Inc., 1967, pp. 175–180.

15. D. S. Pugh, D. J. Hickson, C. R. Hinings, and C. Turner. "Dimensions of Organization Structure." *Administrative Science Quarterly*, June 1968. Vol. 13. pp. 65–105.

16. Richard H. Hall. "The Concept of Bureaucracy: An Empirical Assessment." *American Journal of Sociology*, July 1963. Vol. 69, No. 1. pp. 32–40.

17. John Child. "Organization Structure and Strategies of Control: A Replication of the Aston Study." *Administrative Science Quarterly*, June 1972. Vol. 17, No. 2. pp. 163–177.

18. James G. March and Herbert A. Simon. *Organizations*. New York: John Wiley and Sons, Inc., 1958. p. 160

19. David Mechanic. "Sources of Power of Lower Participants in Complex Organizations." *Administrative Science Quarterly*, December 1962. Vol. 7, No. 3. pp. 349–364.

20. James A. Knight, M.D. *Medical Student: Doctor in the Making*. New York: Appleton-Century Crofts, 1973. pp. 97–98.

21. Pugh et al. Ibid. Personal correspondence from Professor Pugh, June 19, 1973 in which he agrees that their first factor is similar to coordination by plans and procedures, Factor II is similar to hierarchical control by managers, and Factor III similar to self-peer control.

22. Jerald Hage and Michael Aiken. "Routine Technology, Social Structure, and Organizational Relationship." *Administrative Science Quarterly*, December 1969. Vol. 14, No. 3. pp. 366–376.

23. Richard H. Hall. "Some Organizational Considerations in the Profession-Organizational Relationship." *Administrative Science Quarterly*, December 1962. Vol. 7, No. 3. pp. 461–478.

24. Paul D. Montagna. "Professionalization and Bureaucratization in Large Professional Organizations." In Wolf V. Heydebrand. *Comparative Organizations: The Results of Empirical Research.* Englewood Cliffs, NJ: Prentice-Hall, Inc., 1973. pp. 534–542.
25. Thompson and Bates. Ibid.
26. David J. Hickson, D. S. Pugh, and Diana C. Pheysey. "Operations Technology and Organization Structure: An Empirical Reappraisal." *Administrative Science Quarterly,* September 1969. Vol. 14, No. 3. pp. 378–397.
27. Allen Newell, J. C. Shaw, and Herbert A. Simon. "Elements of a Theory of Human Problem Solving." *Psychology Review,* 1958. Vol. 65. No. 3. pp. 151–166.
28. Harold H. Kelley and John W. Thibaut. "Group Problem Solving." In Gardner Lindzey and Elliot Aronson (eds.). *Handbook of Social Psychology.* Reading, MA: Addison-Wesley Pub. Co. pp. 69–70.
29. Perrow. Op. cit.
30. Pugh (1968). Op. cit. Child. Op. cit.
31. Pugh (1968). Op. cit.
32. George Strauss and Leonard R. Sayles. *Personnel: The Human Problems of Management,* 3rd ed. Englewood Cliffs, NJ: Prentice-Hall, Inc., 1972. p. 324.
33. Aldrich. Op. cit.
34. Katz and Kahn. Op. cit.
35. Pugh (1968). Op. cit.
36. Joseph L. Fleiss. "Measuring Nominal Scale Agreement Among Many Raters." *Psychology Bulletin.* Vol. 76, No. 5. pp. 378–382.
37. Richard J. Light. "Measures of Response Agreement for Qualitative Data: Some Generalizations and Alternatives." *Psychology Bulletin.* Vol. 76, No. 5. pp. 365–377.
38. Henry Mintzberg. *The Nature of Managerial Work.* New York: Harper & Row, 1973.
39. Harold Koontz and Cyril O'Donnell. *Principles of Management: An Analysis of Managerial Functions.* New York: McGraw-Hill Book Co., Inc., 1955. pp. 22–28.
40. John R. Campbell, M. Dunnette, Ed Lawler, and Karl Weick. *Managerial Behavior, Performance, and Effectiveness.* New York: McGraw-Hill, 1970, pp. 74–81.
41. *Nursing Home Fact Book 1970-1.* Washington, D.C.: The American Nursing Home Association. p. 72.
42. John V. Therrell. "Top Management—In the Middle." *Medical Group Management,* July 1972. Vol. 19, No. 5. pp. 6–8.
43. Dorwin Cartwright. "Influence, Leadership, and Control." In James G. March (ed). *Handbook of Organizations.* Chicago: Rand McNally & Co., 1965. pp. 1–47.
44. Tom Burns and G. M. Stalker. *The Management of Innovation.* London: Tavistock Publications, 1961. p. 123. Bertram M. Gross. *The Managing of Organizations.* New York: The Free Press, 1964. p. 497.
45. C. J. Haberstroh. "Organization Design and Systems Analysis." In James G. March (ed.). *Handbook of Organizations.* Chicago: Rand McNally & Co., 1965. p. 1184.
46. Kenneth R. Andrews. "Toward Professionalism in Business Management." *Harvard Business Review,* March–April 1969. Vol. 47, No. 2, pp. 49–60.
47. C. Wright Mills. "The Chief Executives." In Barney G. Glaser (ed.). *Organizational Careers: A Sourcebook for Theory.* Chicago: Aldine Pub. Co., 1968. pp. 417–425.

48. Renato Tagiuri. "Value Orientations and the Relationship of Managers and Scientists." *Administrative Science Quarterly*, June 1965. Vol. 10, No. 1. pp. 39–51. Burns and Stalker. Op. cit. pp. 104–119. Robert Presthus. *The Organizational Society*. New York: Alfred A. Knopf, Inc., 1962. p. 438.
49. T. R. Sarbin and Vernon L. Allen. "Role Theory." In Gardner Lindzey and Eliot Aronson (eds.). *The Handbook of Social Psychology*, 2nd ed. Vol. 1. Reading, MA: Addison-Wesley Pub. Co., 1968. p. 555.

II

Managerial Actions to Implement Structural Changes

Introduction

Until fairly recently, the traditional view of the task of the manager has been one of structuring the work, of using the organization as a rational tool for achieving certain productive ends (Ullrich and Wieland 1980). The manager makes plans, designs organizational charts and institutes procedures so that the organization can produce widgets, make a profit, and so on. The task is one of articulating organizational means (usually structures, broadly conceived) so as to achieve the ends of the organization in the most rational way possible. More recently there has emerged another view of the organization as a social system and of the manager's role as one of working within that complex social system and taking into account human needs and their fulfillment. The manager cannot fully control and direct the organization because it is a living social organism in which unpredictable, interdependent groups and individuals strive to express themselves and to meet their own ends.

DESIGNING ORGANIZATIONS

In the traditional view of management organizational change takes place by first designing structural solutions to problems and then being concerned with implementation and acceptance. This traditional approach to change is introduced in the present section, while in Part IV we shall suggest that it is appropriate only for certain kinds of organizations, namely the highly structured bureaucratic organizations common when this traditional view of management evolved. A more recently developed approach to change—the psychological approach to be introduced in Part III—is more appropriate to another kind of organization, an organic organization. These distinctions regarding different modes of management and organizational change require the brief consideration of the nature of organizational design.

Current thinking about organizational design suggests that a contingency approach to structures is most appropriate. There is no single best structural design; this depends on the particulars of each organization. It especially depends on the kind of technology involved—whether individualized and nonroutine or routine (Perrow 1967; Scott 1972).

Individualized technology arises from variable, nonuniform inputs and from the lack of a transformation process based on a completely rational, cause-and-effect knowledge base. Such a technology requires a decentralized structure in which individual decisions can be made "on the shop floor," where the workers face the variable inputs and where they must use artistic and craftsmanlike judgment regarding the best course of action.

Routine technology, on the other hand, is feasible when inputs are uniform and when there is fully rational cause-and-effect knowledge. This kind of technology allows a rational assembly line to be set up and decisions to be made in a centralized, pyramidal structure. There will be few exceptions and the effects of the work operations are known and predictable, so a few managers at the top can lay out all the work and organize the workers in the most efficient arrangement for the organization as a whole.

Because of these differences in technology, the structural designs of the research laboratories and the manufacturing plants in the automotive industry are quite different. In the manufacturing plant, managers can establish rules and regulations, set up procedures and standards, and in general, create a highly formalized, hierarchical, and bureaucratic organization. This is a "mechanistic" organization (Burns and Stalker 1961). In the research laboratory, on the other hand, the structure is more informal and flexible, with considerable informal, horizontal communication, relatively few differences in status, relatively little use of authority based on hierarchical position, and a relatively low reliance on impersonal rules and regulations. This is an "organic" organization. This explains why the appropriate structure of the organization is dependent on the technology, and ultimately the environment, of the organization, since environmental conditions determine the inputs and the acceptance of the outputs, as they also determine the degree to which rational, cause-and-effect knowledge is available.

BETTER ORGANIZATIONAL DESIGNS FOR HOSPITALS

The hospital is a most interesting organization when viewed in terms of the contingency theory of organizational design, for it is partly based on a routine technology and partly on a nonroutine technology. The administrator concerned with laundry, dietetics, and most other departments is faced with a relatively routine technology, and consequently a centralized, hierarchical, and formal organizational structure is appropriate.

Doctors, however, work with a nonroutine technology. They deal with patients who vary considerably in their physical conditions; (if the physician has any bedside manner at all, he or she soon recognizes that each patient is unique). And they deal with a medical technology that is as much art as it is science. The medical organization, consequently, is decentralized, nonhierarchical, and informal.

This is all well and good if administrators and doctors stick to their own spheres, and never the two groups meet. Unfortunately, they do—on the ward floor, especially in the work of the nurses and others around the patient. One proposed solution for dealing with the interface between the administrator-directed departments and the medical staff is to form teams around each patient or group of similar patients, with both departmental participation and medical staff participation. In this design of the hospital as a matrix organization (Neuhauser 1972), the physicians ideally head temporary teams of nurses and other staff treating the patient. However, because this is such a temporary or constantly changing arrangement of personnel, it is likely that the functional units, nursing, social work, dietary, and physical therapy, provide most of the structure, and that there is poor coordination—even when the other staff are in the view of the physician in his or her great power (Charns 1976). Thus, while there are elements of a matrix organization, that is, lateral coordination by the physician, the hospital as a whole is still mostly organized (or disorganized) along traditional departmental lines.

To make the hospital more nearly a matrix organization requires an integrator to bring together the members of differentiated departments, so they can work as a team around the patient. Unfortunately, physicians often do not feel part of a team or responsible for integrating the team members' efforts (Charns 1976). Charns studied hospital staff to find a group which would be at the midpoint between the groups with the most different viewpoints and which would also be viewed by others as competent enough to influence the others. No group emerged as meeting these requirements.

Therefore, Charns advocates that integration instead be achieved by organizational practices such as continuity in staff (i.e., no rotation), use of physical space to locate team members close together, and increased use of devices for information exchange (scheduling procedures, improved medical records). Finally, he emphasizes that somehow "physicians must be drawn into the health care team." The section on psychological approaches to change will describe several projects which have apparently been successful in doing this (see especially Chapters 16 and 20). In this section, the implementation of service unit management (Chapters 11 and 12) is a step in the direction of more effective coordination on the ward floor, with the service unit manager performing various administrative coordinative functions and the head nurse performing various coordinative functions for patient care.

CHANGE IN DIFFERENT KINDS OF ORGANIZATIONS

The first reading in this section (Chapter 4) describes research by Hage and Aiken that suggests that different kinds of organizations have different propensities to change. The doctor's organic organization with its corps of highly trained professionals, informality, and lack of hierarchy tends to be quite creative. Doctors are continually striving to make care more individualized and appropriate to the particular patient. Administrators and their mechanistic organization, on the other hand, are not nearly so creative, they strive instead for greater efficiency which is achieved by stability and large production runs of a uniform product.

Hage and Aiken measured change in their organizations by the number of new programs added. The reader should be cautioned that this is not the same as change in the structure or technology of already functioning programs. To add a new program may be likened to an act of creativity—getting a new idea. But to take that idea and to change what already exists in the organization, to innovate, is another matter. As indicated in Chapter 4, this is very much a question of power, of the ability to change the way others think, so that they accept and commit themselves to new ways of behaving. Viewed in these terms, then, the administrator's organization may not be very creative in that there may not be new ideas all the time, but it can be quite innovative in that it has the internal power to implement the ideas that are generated. If superiors decide that new equipment for the laundry will be more efficient, it is likely that the organization will act on that decision. The same cannot be said of the medical staff in accepting a new drug en masse.[1]

We may speculate that the differences between the administrator's mechanistic organization and the doctor's organic organization imply two different processes of change. The relatively static and mechanistic organization of the administrator seems to entail a negative cybernetic feedback process. The organization is designed and controlled by those at the apex of the organization. Those in superior positions make changes to eliminate problems and to maintain appropriate functioning. Viewed by individuals and groups at lower organizational levels, there seems to be an external control system, with changes coming from outside to those at lower levels. Problems are communicated upward, and rectifying actions are passed downward. For this reason, we use the term "managerial action" to refer to change in the mechanistic organization typical of the administrator's domain.

The organic organization of the medical staff is less consciously focused on goals. Such a professional organization has been termed a "natural system" in contrast to the "rational system" of the mechanistic organization (Gouldner 1959). Individual physicians have goals, but it is less evident that the medical staff organization as a whole has a clear-cut set of goals.

Change in the organic system seems to be endemic but on a relatively low level. The heterogeneity and complexity of the highly trained staff are conducive to frequent exchanges and conflicts.[2] If an individual or a faction can "sell" an idea to enough of the others, if a critical mass can be convinced, then change occurs. In a sense, change is positive cybernetic feedback. Change arises out of a deviation among individual organizational members, a deviation that gains more and more committed adherents until the organization has more or less evolved into a new, changed state. The problem of change in this kind of organization seems to be one of diffusing the change, of eliciting enthusiasm and commitment among the interacting individuals in the organization. The psychology of the individual, and of interpersonal relationships, seems to be key.

The greater difficulty involved in gaining acceptance of a change in this kind of organization seems to rest in the presence of an internal control system guiding behavior. Along with their lengthy training in "facts," physicians learn what is "right" and "wrong." They learn standards of how to use their information. Most importantly, they learn that it is they, as individuals, who are to decide what is proper behavior. The controls come not from outside or from some higher level in the hierarchy, but from within the individuals. Thus, not managerial action, but a process of psychological change, a process of understanding the other in terms of psychological makeup, is the key to obtaining change in groups of highly trained professionals such as physicians. We shall return to the process of psychological change and understanding in Parts III and IV. In this section we focus on the manager, often an administrator, dealing with change in his or her sphere of the hospital organization.

THE PROCESS OF MANAGERIAL ACTION

Managers deal with changes every day they are on the job, because the organization is never the same from day to day or even from moment to moment. While he or she will have general goals or strategies, the manager usually reacts to events, attempting, for example, to maintain service despite absenteeism or supply shortages. The manager makes changes by dealing with these everyday problems, by ordering adjustments in staffing, a substitution in use of materials, or a temporary alteration in procedures.

When the same or similar problems recur, however, the manager no longer typically seeks temporary adjustments, he or she seeks a more major organizational alteration. As indicated above, such big changes often involve alteration in the structure or technology of the organization. Recurrent supply shortages may be due to a poor system for ordering supplies or for recording their use, or perhaps the procedures for using the supplies are inappropriate. For whatever reason, the manager must make a change in basic procedures rather than an ad hoc adjustment to get over a temporary difficulty.

The managerial process is typically the same, whether the manager is making temporary adjustments or major organizational changes. Academics have described this process entailing four to twelve or more steps. Most simply, the manager apprehends that there is a problem, gathers information and makes a decision about what to do (i.e., comes up with the solution), acts or implements the solution, and then controls or checks to see that the problem has been appropriately handled.

In actuality, the manager does not always act this rationally. Observational studies (for example, Mintzberg et al. 1976) show that managers may be presented with a solution and then look for a problem site to implement it, or because of time pressures, they may move directly from the problem to implementation without gathering information and assessing alternatives.

Nevertheless, the rational model for managerial problem solving is a useful normative model. That is, managers act as if they should be rational, as if they should work from problem assessment to decision, and to implementation and control. Chapter 4 presents such a model for managerial action in the case of major organizational change, a four-stage model developed by two sociologists: (1) determination of the need for change, (2) initiation of change, (3) implementation of change, and (4) routinization of change. This model makes organizational change sound mechanical, as if it were a matter of taking a thing and putting it on its proper shelf on the organizational structure. But organizations are people, as well as structures and technologies, so the chapter also describes a model devised by psychologists to help the manager understand how he or she must modify change actions to take into account psychological resistance.

MANAGERIAL ACTION FOR ADMINISTRATORS—AND DOCTORS

This section will also describe some actual managerial actions concerned with "big change," with the implementation of management controls for cost containment and the implementation of new structures to improve the quality and efficiency of patient care. In the second reading (Chapter 5) Robert Allison provides an excellent introduction to managerial actions in the area of hospital costs. He describes the evaluation of an experiment in eleven Michigan hospitals in which Blue Cross negotiated prospective reimbursements for hospital costs. As a result of the experiment, administrators in the eleven hospitals took action and improved various aspects of planning, budgeting, and cost control. After the onset of prospective reimbursement, for example, budgets were used more for control, rather than simply for prediction.

Allison also provides a model for understanding the variables that influence costs, and he shows how the pressures of prospective reimbursement have made administrators emphasize some of these variables in a different way.

However, the differences were not as great as they could have been. Some areas of potentially high cost-saving value were not emphasized, because administrators lacked power to act. For example, the number one potential cost-saving area—length of stay—was perceived as little subject to administrators' actions, but, rather, highly subject to physician control. The administrators in the experiment preferred to take action in areas where they themselves had power and had acted before (for example, changes in policies on plant maintenance or in-service education), even though these areas offered the least potential for cost savings.

The following reading (Chapter 6) briefly reviews the role of the physician in the hospital in relation to its management. Physicians have been reluctant to participate in management efforts, going their own ways and leaving administrators to do what little they can on the peripheral, nonmedical matters. A number of recent studies report, however, some involvement and some concern by physicians over better management of the hospital (including the imposition of control systems) with resulting benefits for both the quality and the efficiency of patient care.

ACHIEVING EFFECTIVE STRUCTURAL CHANGE

The next four readings (Chapters 7 to 10) describe aspects of an experiment in two community general hospitals undertaken by the Bureau of Hospital Administration at the University of Michigan. Members of the bureau helped devise and implement a variety of management controls for cost containment. The chapters here highlight the admission scheduling systems which were used to create a stable, high level of occupancy and, thereby, efficient utilization of facilities and personnel. In addition, such admission controls allow the creation of a system for preadmission diagnostic testing, which can in turn significantly shorten patient length of stay. Evaluation research (Griffith et al. 1973, 1976) in fact shows that a sample of 250 patients with diagnostic tests on day of admission had average savings of 0.7 day, or about 6 percent, in the hospital in which the admission scheduling program was successfully implemented.[3]

Chapters 7 and 8 describe the implementation of admissions scheduling systems in each of the two experimental hospitals, in one case a successful implementation, in the other, a failure. As expected, the role of the medical staff was central in determining the outcome.

Next, in Chapter 9, Munson and Hancock provide an excellent conceptualization of what must be done to implement a change in organizational structure or technology—in this case, the new hospital control systems devised by the outside management scientists. They describe the view of the typical management scientist (and of the typical manager, too): make the "right" decision, decide on the "right" changes, then worry about implementation in the organization. They contrast this view with that of the psychologist or social scientist: find out what organizational members want and are willing to do, study the organization as it is, and build up from there. In this view, people run organizations and their acceptance is necessary for whatever changes are proposed. The best new technical system is worthless if it cannot be implemented.

Of course, elements of both views are necessary for successful organizational change. For Munson and Hancock, these elements are: (1) a technically optimal method for reaching a given purpose, as well as (2) favorable attitudes by organizational members—at least key members or those who have power in the area of the proposed change, and (3) abililty of the participants in the change to take the required actions—for which training is usually required.

We can summarize Munson and Hancock by saying that for successful change, the first requirement is having the proper structural or technical change in mind, then more psychological matters come in to play a secondary role. Psychological changes are relevant to the degree that the implementation of the new structure is impeded without such changes.

PSYCHOLOGICAL ASPECTS OF IMPLEMENTING CHANGE

The fourth reading of the set (Chapter 10) provides a description of the hospital experiments by a psychologist member of the Michigan team. He recounts several factors which determined the success of the implementation of new controls in the experimental hospitals: continued exposure to the innovation and increasing familiarity by hospital personnel, their influence or participation in the implementation process, top management authority behind the innovations so as to overcome doubts and "testing" by resisters, (moderate) stress or tension which enhances motivation to change, and, finally, "chance," which is to say, psychologists can't ever expect to understand and predict everything about anything so complex as real human beings in real-life situations!

In general, Griffith and colleagues found that psychological changes came to be quite an important part of their program of structural changes to contain costs: "The installation of cost-reduction programs is a major organizational change that requires considerable human relations skills and change-process technology. Attitudes of all major participants in the institution must be changed, including those of the trustees and the medical staff" (Griffith et al. 1973, p. 138).

The great importance of organization-wide attitude change arises because of the great pressures toward the spending of money. There are pressures to order extra tests or increase staffing, so as to guard against shortcomings in patient care or even malpractice suits, pressures to spend because otherwise interpersonal conflict will result and organizational harmony will deteriorate, and pressures to spend because success is often measured by budget size or numbers of beds and staff. If attitudes are not changed systematically across the organization, Griffith and colleagues suggest, any savings achieved in one area are likely to succumb to the pressures to spend in other areas, by other staff.

FURTHER STRUCTURAL CHANGES

The next two readings (Chapters 11 and 12) describe the implementation of another structural change, service unit management (SUM), a complex reorganization of roles on the wards and the creation of a completely new role, the service unit manager. In the first reading Munson looks at the implementation process in a sample of fourteen hospitals, of which five succeeded and nine failed in introducing SUM. He finds a number of implementation stages common to the hospitals: introduction of the idea, preparation and training, unit shake down, expansion to other parts of the hospital, reorganization at the hospital level to deal with problems which have emerged, and adaptation to the overall environment of the rest of the hospital. Munson emphasizes the importance of aggressive leadership in the early stages, and also the importance of training for, and acceptance of, new roles.

In the next reading (Chapter 12), we review the work of a social psychologist who emphasizes psychological training and support and other organization factors which facilitate structural changes such as SUM. These findings are based on the intensive study of a group of eight hospitals as well as the nationwide survey of other hospitals introducing SUM. Changing structures in organization is more than a matter of redrawing boxes and lines on an organizational chart and then issuing assignments. Especially useful in the model presented here is the detailing of psychological problems at different levels in the organization—problems for the individual, for the relationships between individuals, among members of a unit, and between the unit and the rest of the organization.

The final reading in this section (Chapter 13) describes an experiment in "systems intervention," a way of helping managers solve major organizational problems which have ramifications throughout the organization. In this intervention technique, system flow diagrams are constructed for key top managers. These diagrams enable them to visualize the problem dynamics and interrelations among departments, and the likely effects of possible changes implemented in one or another department.

However, as one reviews what was actually done in the hospital described, it becomes apparent that the system diagrams may have served as a sort of cover for psychological change among the key managers. A psychologist might argue that the real work in the intervention was done by the discussion groups in which the key managers initially came together to discuss the systems diagrams, but very quickly moved to the interdepartmental and professional conflicts which were contributing to many of the problems. The discussions permitted the key managers to develop into a team which could then collaborate in solving hospital problems. Unfortunately, whether or not the psychological changes contributed more to the outcomes than did the systems diagrams per se cannot be assayed clearly in this single case study. But the study does provide a useful transition to the consideration of the psychological approach to change. In Part III (Chapters 14, 16, and 20) we shall describe team building as one of a number of organization development techniques.

REFERENCES

Abernathy, William J., and Prahalad, Coimbatore K. Technology and productivity in health organizations. In William J. Abernathy et al. (Eds.) *The management of health care.* Cambridge, Mass.: Ballinger, 1975. Pp. 189–203.
Burns, Tom, and Stalker, G. M. *The management of innovation.* London: Tavistock Publications, 1961.
Charns, Martin P. Breaking the tradition barrier: managing integration in health care facilities. *Health Care Management Review,* 1976, *1,* 4(Winter), 55–67.
Georgopoulos, Basil S., and Wieland, George F. *Nationwide study of coordination and patient care in voluntary hosptials.* Ann Arbor, Mich.: Institute for Social Research, 1964.
Gouldner, Alvin W. Organizational analysis. In Robert K. Merton et al. (Eds.) *Sociology today.* New York: Basic Books, 1959, Pp. 400–428.
Griffith, John R., Hancock, Walton M., and Munson, Fred C. Practical ways to contain hospital costs. *Harvard Business Review,* 1973, *51,* 6(November–December), 131–139.
Mintzberg, Henry, Rasinghani, Dury, and Theoret, Andre. The structure of "unstructured" decision processes. *Administrative Science Quarterly,* 1976, *21,* 246–275.
Neuhauser, Duncan. The hospital as a matrix organization. *Hospital Administration,* 1972, *16,* 4(Fall), 8–23.
Perrow, Charles A. A framework for the comparative analysis of organizations. *American Sociological Review,* 1967, *32,* 194–208.
Scott, W. Richard. Professionals in hospitals: technology and the organization of work. In Basil S. Georgopoulos (Ed.) *Organization research on health organizations.* Ann Arbor, Mich.: Institute for Social Research, 1972. Pp. 139–158.
Ullrich, Robert A., and Wieland, George F. *Organization theory and design,* rev. ed. Homewood, Ill.: Richard D. Irwin, 1980.

NOTES

1. Power is perhaps the most significant variable in organizational change, as in management generally, and the readings here will often point out its role. A general account of power in organizational theory is provided in Ullrich and Wieland (1980). Concerning the position of the doctors (their being relatively autonomous and free from the power of others to make changes), many observers have cited the increasing governmental pressures on doctors, pressures moving them toward greater dependence on the government and, consequently, providing the government with greater power for change. It will be of some interest to see whether physicians are able to coopt governmental pressures and maintain their autonomous position, much as the physicians did in Great Britain when the National Health Service was instituted. One might well speculate that the American Medical Association will not consider lightly giving up the great power that has stood American physicians in such good stead to date.

2. See Georgopoulos and Wieland (1964) for evidence that conflict *among* doctors is higher than conflict between any two groups in the hospital.

3. As part of their studies for cost containment, Griffith and colleagues also investigated the turn-around times for lab and x-ray reports. They found these relatively long—25 or more hours for routine reports. In addition, the reports often meshed poorly with the physicians' rounds, so that two or three days might elapse between the submission of a request for a test and the receipt of the results. As Griffith and colleagues indicate, "speed of reporting may eventually outweigh in importance the departmental load factor or measures of cost and efficiency."

    This point is very important. Since most hospital costs are somehow involved with the care of the patient by physicians and nurses, studies of the productivity or efficiency of particular parts of the hospital must always be reviewed for the effects of any savings on the medical and nursing costs of patient care. Take, for example, a study of the productivity of laboratory departments. Suppose the lab were able to increase productivity by accumulating tests of the same kind until a large batch could be analyzed (perhaps with labor-saving equipment). The lab might reduce its cost per test by 10 percent, but the increased turn-around time might require the patient to stay in the hospital another whole day, thus spending many more times the "savings" achieved in the lab. The moral is clear: the hospital is a system and savings in one area may mean cost in another, especially in the most costly areas of all, medical and nursing care.

    Abernathy and Prahalad (1975) make the important related point that economies of scale from mass production or "routine" technology may not yield in the hospital the ultimate savings that they have in other industries (usually manufacturing). They suggest that the technological facilities of the hospital and of patient care are young and still developing, and technological innovations should therefore be relatively small scale, flexible, and adaptable, or else they will become rapidly outdated and totally worthless in practice.

4 | Changing Organizational Structures

George F. Wieland
Robert A. Ullrich

ORGANIZATIONS THAT CHANGE

Hage and Aiken (1970) have been concerned with the rate at which organizations change themselves and the factors that foster or impede this rate of change. Why is it that some organizations are quick to adopt even untested ideas while others are slow to implement changes that have withstood the test of time? Although General Motors and Ford faced comparable circumstances during the 1920s, the former successfully developed a number of new products while the latter did not. Why do organizations with the same general objectives and comparable environments seem to differ in terms of the rate at which they change themselves? This is the question addressed by Hage and Aiken.

The focus of their study is *program change*, which they define as the addition of new services or products. Please bear in mind that these were the only kinds of changes studied and that, furthermore, the ultimate success or failure of these change efforts was not considered.

Hage and Aiken focus on seven organizational variables: (1) degree of complexity, (2) centralization, (3) formalization, (4) stratification, (5) production, (6) efficiency, and (7) job satisfaction. These particular aspects were selected because they were well studied in the literature and found to be related in one way or another to the rate of program change. Other aspects were considered but discarded when found to be more or less unimportant in determining the rate of change in organizations.

Adapted with revisions from Robert A. Ullrich and George F. Wieland, *Organization Theory and Design*, rev. ed. (Homewood, Ill.: Richard D. Irwin, Inc., 1980) Chapters 15 and 16. © 1980 Richard D. Irwin, Inc.

We shall take each of these variables in turn and examine evidence that suggests its relationship to the change process. Much of this evidence comes from Hage and Aiken's survey of sixteen welfare agencies which provided services in the areas of physical rehabilitation, mental rehabilitation, or psychiatry.

COMPLEXITY

Complexity refers to (1) the extent of knowledge and skill required of occupational roles and (2) their diversity. Organizations employing many different kinds of professionals are highly complex. One way to measure complexity is to determine the *number* of different occupations within an organization that require specialized knowledge and skills. An organization can be considered complex when it employs numerous kinds of knowledge and skills (occupations) and when these occupations require sophistication in their respective knowledge and skill areas. A general hospital is a complex organization. Typically, members of 50 different occupational groups will appear on the wards in the course of 24 hours. One will find a variety of nurses (having different amounts and kinds of training), dieticians, x-ray technologists, laboratory technologists, a variety of physicians of different specialties, occupational therapists, orthopedic therapists, medical social workers, psychiatric social workers, chaplains, ward clerks, housekeepers, janitors, engineers, various kinds of administrators, and others.

Organizations employing professionals of a single kind (or a few kinds) are less complex. An elementary school is of moderate complexity. Relatively few occupations are employed, and required levels of knowledge and skills within occupations are relatively modest. At the low end of the scale of complexity, one finds organizations such as automobile factories which employ a relatively homogeneous, unskilled, and unknowledgeable work force.

Hage and Aiken measured complexity in their sample of welfare agencies in terms of the number of occupational specialties employed, the length of professional training required by each specialty, and the extent of employees' involvement in professional societies and activities. It was found that the greater the complexity, the greater the rate of program change. The rationale for this relationship seems clear. In addition to their formal training, professionals engage in constant study to remain abreast of advances in their respective fields. Acquisition of new knowledge paves the way for change. Professionals may work themselves into new professions eventually. Alternatively, they may recognize the need for new kinds of professionals who can aid in the pursuit of their objectives. Social psychologists are results of the first kind of change, and media specialists who support faculty teaching are results of the latter. The professional's service ideal also contributes to the high rate of change in complex organizations. To be of service implies seeking the best ways to meet client needs. Obviously, improvements to existing service delivery practices frequently take the form of program changes.

CENTRALIZATION

Centralization is a measure of the distribution of power within the organization. According to Hage and Aiken, the fewer the occupations participating in decision making and the fewer the areas of decision making in which they are involved, the more centralized the organization.

Hage and Aiken find that the higher the organization's degree of centralization, the lower its rate of program change. An explanation of this finding is that a centralized organization, with power concentrated in the hands of a few individuals, tends toward the status quo because their power enables them to protect their own interests and to veto changes that are likely to threaten them. Michels' Iron Law of Oligarchy describes the situation well.

In a decentralized organization, where decision-making power is more widespread, a variety of different views will emerge from different occupational groups. This variety of opinion can lead to conflict, but also to successful resolution of conflict and to problem solving. In any event, decentralization appears to foster the initiation of new programs and techniques, which are proposed as solutions to various organizational problems. However, Hage and Aiken suggest that these organizations will be slow to implement the changes initiated. In a decentralized organization, it takes time for suggested changes in products and services to receive approval of all individuals party to the decision to implement them. A centralized organization may produce fewer new ideas, but once an idea is put forth its implementation is fairly straightforward. Lines of communication are clear and direct. The route to top management for ultimate approval or disapproval is traveled quickly. Nevertheless, in the long run, it is likely that the decentralized organization will experience more initiation of change and a greater number of actual program changes than the centralized organization. This, in fact, is what Hage and Aiken found in their study of welfare agencies.

FORMALIZATION

Formalization represents the extent to which jobs are governed by rules and specific guidelines. It may be recalled that this aspect of organization is typical of bureaucracies. Measures of formalization can be attempted in a number of ways. One may count the number of rules that apply to *jobs*, as these are found in formal job descriptions, rules manuals, or staff handbooks. In fact, the mere existence of such documents suggests a relatively high degree of formalization. Alternatively, one may count the number of rules and regulations that operate in the *organization* as a whole. These may be codified or unwritten as in the case of norms.

As one would expect, Hage and Aiken found that the greater the degree of formalization, the lower the rate of program change. Rules and norms discourage search for better ways of doing things. Furthermore, they rigidify the organization and promote homogeneity among its various units. Thus, implementation of change is made difficult, since even a minor change may have impact on extensive portions of the organization. Rules, regulations, job descriptions, and the like serve to stabilize an organization's behavior—to make it reliable and predictable. Obviously, they mitigate against change.

A study of the Teacher Corps, however, provides an example of how formalization (as well as centralization) can foster change (Corwin 1972). The aim of the Teacher Corps is to promote educational reforms in low-income schools through innovative teacher training programs. Corwin found that in the 42 schools studied, innovations (such as team teaching, introduction of black history, and mixed-age grouping) were associated with the organizational control exerted by the schools. Those with centralized decision-making procedures, stress on rules and procedures, and emphasis on pupil discipline were schools which innovated.

The contrast with the Hage and Aiken study is explained by the observation that implementation, not initiation of innovations, was studied in these organizations. While the universities and interns provided ideas, the administrators and their staff selected and implemented them. In this kind of situation, formalization and centralization foster change. In this situation teachers *had to change* the way they were teaching. Rather than "tacking on" a new program in addition to ongoing programs, a fairly simple matter for Hage and Aiken's professionals, top administration was responsible for selecting innovations and then seeing that they were implemented properly. A centralized administration with control of resources and the ability to formulate and enforce rules and regulations was able to enforce and also to *help* the process of innovation. (See also Gross, Giacquinta, and Bernstein [1971] for further evidence, and Wilson [1966], Zaltman et al. [1973] for a similar argument.) In sum, where emphasis is on implementation rather than initiation of innovations, centralization and formalization may be assets.

For each of the above—complexity, centralization, and formalization—Hage and Aiken found evidence (in both the research literature and their own study) of relationships with program change. Several further aspects of organizations discussed below, however, receive less support from the literature and the study, and they are to be viewed somewhat more tentatively as characteristics that influence an organization's propensity to change.

STRATIFICATION

Rewards are distributed fairly equally among members in some organizations and differentially in others. Stratification is a measure of this phenomenon. When some employees receive higher salaries, greater status, and more fringe benefits than others, their organization is said to be highly stratified. A second dimension of stratification concerns mobility between different parts of the organization. An organization is *not* considered highly stratified when employees are free to move vertically and horizontally among jobs, even when the rewards associated with these jobs differ markedly. Barriers to mobility (advancement), as well as heterogeneity in rewards, contribute to stratification.

According to Hage and Aiken, the greater the degree of stratification, the lower the rate of program change. Here again the Iron Law of Oligarchy seems to apply. Where rewards are distributed unequally, those receiving the largest share resist changes that threaten their advantage. Now, one might argue that differences in rewards will motivate individuals at lower levels of the organization to work their way up in the hierarchy, and that, consequently, they will seek improvements over the status quo to gain recognition that eventually will result in promotion. While this may occur, suggestions for change will be muted to the extent that they are perceived as criticisms of higher level employees. Thus, advocacy of change is undertaken reluctantly.

In general, high stratification discourages accurate upward communication. Lower level employees tend to tell their superiors what the latter want to hear. It has been argued that much of the distorted information in the Vietnam War was attributable to this phenomenon. Inflated body counts were reported because they were met with approbation by superiors. What evidence there is suggests that stratification blocks interaction and communication and, therefore, retards not only the initiation of change, but also its implementation.

PRODUCTION

As used by Hage and Aiken, production measures organizational emphasis on *volume* of output rather than *quality*. The number of units produced (or clients served) varies from one organization to another. Some automobile manufacturers engage in mass production of cars just as large state universities offer their services to a large number of students. These can be contrasted with manufacturers of limited production cars (e.g., Jensen and Jaguar) and small, private universities that employ low student-faculty ratios.

Hage and Aiken argue that the higher the volume of production, the lower the rate of program change. Their rationale is that emphasis on speed of production and volume, rather than on quality, leads management to resist interruptions of the productive process such as program changes are likely to entail. High-volume production permits the realization of economies of scale. Steady state efficiency becomes valued more than operating or strategic responsiveness (Ansoff and Brandenburg 1971). Success attained in operating the implied kind of technology will mitigate further against change. It is difficult to argue in favor of altering a system that produces satisfactory results.

Organizations with these characteristics can be contrasted with others emphasizing quality of production. The latter orientation will direct management's attention toward means for improving production standards or, at least, for preventing their deterioration. Research and development activities will be directed toward product (or service) improvement. These improvements often are found in the form of program changes.

EFFICIENCY

The sixth variable studied, efficiency, measures the relative cost of producing the organization's product or service. Some organizations are more concerned with costs than others; for example, research institutes generally are less concerned with operating efficiently than are the organizations that apply knowledge generated by the former.

A review of the literature provides some evidence that the greater the emphasis on efficiency, the lower the rate of program change. As Hage and Aiken suggest, new programs incur additional costs, some of which are unpredictable. Additional costs, especially those which are uncertain and, thus, uncontrollable, are unattractive to managers whose orientations are toward cost reduction and operating efficiencies. Of course, some innovations are sought as a means toward cost reduction. Necessity is the handmaiden of invention, as we say, and problems accompanied by high costs may lead to innovations directed toward their improvement. A close examination of such innovations, however, suggests that costs are *not* reduced in many cases. The application of computer technology to "paper work" problems is a common example of innovation that does not necessarily improve costs. Furthermore, cost-cutting innovations seem to be rarer than other kinds aimed at improving quality or providing hitherto unavailable services. In short, the efficiency-seeking organization is likely to play a "wait and see" game—to be a follower rather than an innovator in its industry.

JOB SATISFACTION

The final variable studied by Hage and Aiken is job satisfaction. Overall job satisfaction usually is assumed to be related to satisfaction with a variety of specific factors such as pay, fellow workers, supervision, working conditions, and the like.[1] One index of job satisfaction is the rate of employee turnover. Dissatisfied employees tend to leave their organizations in search of better jobs.

Hage and Aiken found a moderate relationship between job satisfaction and the rate of program change. The more satisfaction, the greater the rate of change. Apparently, satisfied employees become committed to their organizations. This commitment entails a desire to improve organizational effectiveness and a willingness to explore new ideas and try out the suggestions of others.

SYSTEMIC QUALITIES OF THE VARIABLES STUDIED

Hage and Aiken's most important point is that the seven variables and rate of program change seem interrelated. In static organizations the rate of program change is low and *all* of the seven variables seem to be configured to contribute to organizational stability. Organizations that do not change their programs frequently also seem typified by high degrees of (1) centralization, (2) formalization, (3) stratification, and (4) emphasis on high-volume production, and (5) efficiency and low degrees of (6) complexity and (7) job satisfaction.

In other words, these seven characteristics are *systemic qualities* of organizations. If one variable changes, the others tend to change as well in directions that are compatible with the change in the first. Hage and Aiken carry this analysis further. First, they argue that dynamic and static organizations arise in different kinds of environments. The dynamic organization arises in an unstable environment and the static organization in one that is stable. This analysis is useful since it enables us to anticipate changes in an organization based on our perceptions of changes in its environment. Second, Hage and Aiken suggest that changes in certain variables induce conforming changes in the remaining variables. A dynamic organization is most likely created by increases in its *complexity*. Alternatively, an organization can be rendered more stable by increasing its degree of *centralization*. These two observations provide us with levers, as it were, with which managers can attempt to move their organizations in desired directions.

Before examining the characteristics of static and dynamic organizations in greater detail, we are compelled to emphasize that neither kind is superior to the other. In general, it is appropriate to view the organization's degree of change propensity in terms of its adequacy in meeting environmental demands. Therefore, it is important to understand how both kinds of organization evolve, since it may be necessary for management to move the organization first in one direction and then in the other as its environment changes.

DYNAMIC ORGANIZATIONS

As the knowledge employed by an organization increases in quantity, complexity, and diversity, it becomes increasingly difficult for a few top managers to maintain a monopoly on power. As organizations become knowledge intensive, they make decisions on the basis of the combined inputs from experts and specialists. *Complexity* seems to require decentralization of power to make or influence decisions. Furthermore, experts and specialists seem to work best on a relatively informal basis. Gaining external control of professional activities is difficult, if not at times impossible. Generally, professionals require freedom sufficient to deal with problems that cannot be programmed in any simple fashion with rules, regulations, job descriptions, or plans. Knowledge-based organizations tend to rely on the quality of their professionals' training to control their behavior and ensure adequate job performance rather than on rules or programs. In consequence, the relative absence of rules and programs together with the associated distribution of decision-making power foster horizontal as well as vertical communication. Reliance on others for help in the coordination and execution of one's own tasks fosters teamwork and tends to diminish status differences among interrelated occupations. In other words, stratification is reduced.

As we saw earlier, highly trained employees may emphasize quality and service to the client as opposed to efficiency, "cutting corners," or cost reduction. Finally, highly trained employees (whose training is utilized in their occupations) seem to derive more satisfaction from their jobs than do employees possessing and using lesser skills. This may result from their power to demand or negotiate better, more satisfying conditions of work. In general, then, it seems that although each of the variables can affect the others, *complexity* is of paramount importance in determining the dynamic properties of the organizational system.

STATIC ORGANIZATIONS

Let us turn now to static organizations. The less complex an organization, the more it depends on unskilled employees who perform simple, specialized tasks. Similarly, these organizations do not depend on the knowledge and training of such employees to the extent indicated above. Such organizations tend to be highly *centralized*. Centralization (control from the top) implies that behavior in the rest of the organization is controlled via formalization, the use of job descriptions, rules manuals, evaluation systems, records, and the like. Also flowing from centralization is stratification—differences in rewards and low mobility in the organization.

The general policies of such organizations are likely to stress quantity of production and efficiency. As we indicated earlier, quantity is a less costly criterion of effectiveness than quality, which may require continual changes in the productive processes. Finally, external control, inequality of rewards, simple-minded jobs, and poor working conditions are likely to affect employee satisfaction adversely. In short, the qualities mentioned are likely to conform to one another in static organizations. Apparently, the critical factor among these is centralization, which seems to affect the others directly.

STABLE AND DYNAMIC ENVIRONMENTS

Hage and Aiken suggest that the environment becomes unstable (dynamic) as a result of increases in knowledge. Growth in knowledge can affect both the demand for products and services and the technologies used to produce them. As knowledge increases, new products become available and the demand for older products diminishes. When this happens, the organization must adapt accordingly, seeking innovations to replace services and products for which demand is waning and installing technologies capable of producing them.

Changes in technology sometimes require the addition of new occupations spawned by the technology itself; for example, consider the number of computer programmers and systems engineers employed today and recall that these occupations were not found in businesses, governmental agencies, or hospitals 30 years ago. Major organizational changes have resulted from the introduction of computer technology which, in turn, resulted from acquisition of knowledge in the information sciences. In summary, this suggests that environmental instability stems from increased knowledge which, in turn, requires organizations to become more complex. As we have suggested, increased complexity produces corresponding changes in other organizational qualities which allow the organization to become more change propensive.

This can be contrasted with a relatively stable environment in which organizations experience constant or steadily changing (predictable) demand for their products and services. Since knowledge develops slowly, technology changes gradually. Under these conditions, there is little need to launch new programs to produce new products or services, nor is there need to introduce new technologies and occupations. In a stable environment, organizations can pursue the modus operandi suggested by the rational school of thought. When goals are clear (e.g., market share in an unchanging market) and when means toward the achievement of these goals are stable (e.g., technology), the organization can centralize and structure itself to produce as efficiently as possible. From this follow the other characteristics of stable organizations, including low rates of program change.

Diversification

The environment can encourage or force diversification in a number of ways, and through diversification complexity is increased; for example, governments may force diversification through antitrust proceedings. Declining markets may encourage similar changes, although more subtly. For example, some colleges are seeking to diversify their services in the face of declining student populations.

The important point is that the addition of products and services requires employment of additional occupations which add to complexity. As we have noted, increases in complexity are likely to affect change propensity through the remaining variables. Diversification also seems to encourage decentralization. Problems of coordination increase as heterogeneous elements are added to the organization. The resulting overload of top management is ameliorated when decentralized profit centers are established. These centers are responsive to local circumstances and free top management's time for matters of strategic concern.

Similar to the effects of diversification are those of interorganizational programs. When organizations collaborate to produce a product or service, different occupational groups may be brought into contact. It follows that the creation of joint programs can increase organizational complexity.

Changing Existing Structures

So far we have emphasized organizational changes which primarily involved growth (either of new programs or in size), but much change focuses primarily on existing structure. Such change may alter the basic thrust of an existing structure, revise structural arrangements to improve efficiency, or perhaps install a computer to replace antiquated systems. These two different kinds of change, adding to the new and altering the old, may involve very different problems. Adding to structure primarily entails the problem of initiation. Once that is done, the implementation is often simply carrying forward and rubber-stamping the creative ideas of a well throught out process of initiation. In contrast, altering existing structure means a major problem of implementation. The old must be removed before there can be any new structures.

It is because of the differences in these two kinds of change that centralization, and perhaps other organizational characteristics, are likely to have a very different, and almost opposite, impact on change, depending on whether the initiation or the implementation stage is most involved. A centralized organization may not generate many new ideas, or initiate changes, but such an organization can bring considerable power to bear behind implementation. A centralized organization is thus very useful if change is the revision of already existing structure. The static organization may not be very change-oriented in terms of growth, as Hage and Aiken have shown, but when it comes to reorganizing and refining internal features for a more efficient output, then the static organization may come into its own. A review of some studies of such internal structural change will help explore the important factors involved, especially the role of power in facilitating change.

A MAJOR STRUCTURAL CHANGE

An account of a major structural alteration in a "giant" life insurance company has been presented by O'Connell (1968). The company engaged one of the world's largest management consulting firms for assistance with a problem in its hundreds of branch offices. Sales expenses were increasing, but insurance premium growth was lagging. Investigation by the consultants confirmed management's suspicion that problems were to be found primarily in the role of the senior sales agents. The existing role of the senior agent was primarily that of "supersalesman." This involved demonstration selling or putting business on the books for the regular agents. It was a "staff" or advisory relationship. It was proposed that this role be changed to emphasize supervisory behavior that would support increased selling by the regular agents.

The new behaviors were to be produced by means of structural changes. The special agents were inserted into line management, and they were given authority to plan and control the day-to-day work of the regular agents. Information flows were reorganized to facilitate this new role. The reward structure was also changed to make a supervisor and his or her agents more nearly a profit center, with rewards given on the basis of their productivity as a group. Even the physical arrangements were altered; instead of desks in a large general workroom with other agents, the new supervisors were given private offices and provided with a special conference room for meetings with subordinate agents.

The consultants acted to change the behavior of three pilot branches, with the senior managers of the firm looking on and learning. O'Connell emphasizes that the consultants used unilateral influence to institute structural changes. They altered the external forces or role demands on the senior agents, rather than collaborating with them to change their individual attitudes and cognitions directly. He contrasts the approach typically used by social scientists with the approach used here: "we might say the focus adopted by. . .social scientists tends to maximize human values within the constraints of economic values—in contrast to scientific management's. . .tendency to maximize economic values within the constraints of human values" (p. 6).

The consultants used a two-pronged plan. First, there was an "information and exhortation" phase of four days of orientation for the superiors of the new first-line supervisors, and two days for the new supervisors themselves. Detailed 100-page guides were distributed for these orientations. These explained the changes in the positions and why they were being made, e.g., "this relationship (between branch manager and first-line supervisor) should be on a first name basis if the discussion is to be full and frank" (p. 71). There were filmstrips and slide presentations, an enthusiastic presentation by a senior manager, and discussion and answering of questions—all used to sell the new role. What could not be done in a short time, was to help the agents learn the behavioral skills for their new role. Skill training was to be on the job. This second component of the consultants' plan was to be "supervised learning by doing."

The structural change program, as evaluated by O'Connell, yielded "relative success." In the branches sampled, there was an ostensible modest improvement in performance in terms of new premiums, fewer lapsed policies, and lower costs. Unfortunately, the simple before-and-after research design without control or comparison groups does not provide much confidence about the source of whatever improvements occurred. Furthermore, O'Connell attributes the lack of greater improvement to a failure in achieving the requisite behavioral outcomes. Some of the new supervisors continued to be "supersalesmen," rather than supervisors. In addition, they often spent two times as much time doing in-office paperwork than was proposed in the guides.

Other problems were instigated by the decision to install the new structure full-blown in each branch, but allowing installation in the entire company to take three years. This meant that rumors were rife and that "unofficial" preparatory steps sometimes interfered with the ultimate, planned installation. Furthermore, the new regional managers (one level above the branches) had to spend most of their two initial years working on installation at lower, branch levels rather than perfecting their own new roles. O'Connell argues that a formal behavioral training program designed for the different managers, and properly articulated with the change effort, might have alleviated these problems.

ROLE OF CONSULTANTS IN STRUCTURAL CHANGE

The direction of influence in the change was almost completely unilateral on the part of the consultants. Outside of top management, there was little participation by clients. The consultants used their expertise and their rational arguments (and probably their prestige) to convince their sponsor within the company (the senior vice-president of sales management who called them in). They then worked with the authority of top management to engineer or implement the changes.

This approach to change was taken because there were time pressures, and there was "a sense of urgency arising from a worsening competitive position." Furthermore, "this was a goal-oriented project." There were specific problems, and "the sponsor expected an expert who would say what to do and how." Top management officials had neither the time nor the resources to deal with the problem themselves. The consultants' focus on the structural and technical systems rather than on the social system (e.g., "interpersonal competence") also arose because of the magnitude of the problem. There were several hundred branch offices, and the consultant could hardly focus on the specific social system or interpersonal problems of each branch.

In assessing the role of the management consultants in this study, O'Connell suggests that their unique contribution is in implementation. Many managers get creative ideas, he suggests, but creativity is only the conception of an idea. It is innovation, or the implementation of the idea, that brings birth: "knowing what to do is less important than knowing how to do it" (p. 61).

O'Connell suggests that the operating manager often emphasizes maintenance of his system—keeping things running, rather than innovating. Of course, in the long run innovation is required, and the manager must therefore perform a balancing act between maintenance and innovation. Many times, however, the plethora of operating information available to the manager encourages an emphasis on corrective actions, on creating negative feedback to maintain the system. In a sense, there is a failure of success. Innovation is left either to the staff specialist (internal consultant) or to the outside consultant. In other words, the management consultant (or sometimes a new top manager) must be called in to break the negative feedback cycle and to implement some new ideas that are very different from current management thinking.

DESTRUCTION AS PART OF ORGANIZATIONAL CHANGE

What is lacking in O'Connell's description of structural change is an account of the politics of change—the use of power to "win" the change either for the dominant coalition or for some other contender for power. A recent description (Biggart 1977) of the reorganization of the U.S. Post Office Department into the U.S. Postal Service (USPS) provides just such a picture. According to Biggart, successful reorganization required a number of actions to consolidate the new structure and prevent chaos and backsliding under pressures by publishers, unions, and constituents. The new U.S. Postal Service had to destroy the old organizational ideology and also destroy the former power alliances and leadership.

To destroy the old ideology, a number of tactics were used. The 200-year-old name of the organization was changed, the old logos and colors were removed and new ones selected, and symbolic birthday parties were even held at each post office in the U.S. An internal communications effort was also launched to preach the new ideology. The house organ advocated aggressive selling of stamps, for example, and former policies, such as nit-picking inspections, were denigrated. The staff of the post office training school was increased to handle a heavy load of retraining for supervisors and on-site training and management games were carried out at major post offices.

While all this was going on, plans were made to eliminate senior staff who either would not, or could not change with the organization. Just before the changeover, a one-time bonus of six months' pay was offered to staff members who would leave immediately, and about one-third of the 6,000 senior regional and headquarters staff accepted. Furthermore, Biggart says, "in order to assure a steady supply of leaders loyal to the USPS the organization had to dismantle the former management recruitment system" (p. 422). Lower ranks were made eligible for earlier advancement, competition for positions outside one's own post office was allowed, and outsiders with MBAs were recruited for the first time.

The Postal Service also moved on the external front to protect its changes. When postal unions complained to Congress about job cutbacks, the head of the post office issued an order that all communications between the post office and Congress go through his office. The post office also cut its external dependencies: rather than get money interest-free from the Treasury Department, it issued bonds on the open market. Similarly, a new personnel system was instituted, one which was not compatible with that administered by the Civil Service Commission elsewhere in government.

In conclusion, then, organizational change is affected by the fact that the dominant coalition must protect organizational changes, must maintain its hegemony, and must further its ends (including the organizational change) against those either within or without the organization who would subvert the changes for their own ends. Organization change requires destruction as well as construction. Without destruction, competing elements may prevent the implementation of the new.

THE CHANGE PROCESS

It is useful to take an overall look at the process of successful planned change in organizations. Greiner (1967) provides just such a look in his review of the apparent differences in a sample of eleven successful and seven unsuccessful change programs. He found that successful programs seemed to consist of identifiable sequences of steps undertaken in the following order.

PROBLEM RECOGNITION

Successful change programs were found in organizations whose top management was under considerable pressure to change. Furthermore, pressures emanated both from the environment and from within the organization. In contrast, unsuccessful change programs were launched in response to pressures originating either internally or externally *but not both.*

Furthermore, it should be emphasized that these pressures were quite serious from top management's point of view. Typical sources of external pressure were stockholder discontent, decreasing sales volumes, and breakthroughs by competitors. Internal pressures emanated from strikes, low worker productivity, rising costs, and interdepartmental conflict. Greiner emphasizes the probable significance of the simultaneous existence of internal and environmental pressures. Pressure from one source or the other, by itself, can be rationalized as temporary or even inconsequential, as is likely to happen, for instance, when low employee morale is accompanied by high profits. Such rationalization is less likely when poor morale and declining profits are experienced together. If Greiner's observations are valid, one is led to question whether an outside consultant alone will be able to develop a need for change.

SEARCH FOR SOLUTIONS

The second stage observed in successful change programs involves top management's search for solutions. Presumably, success at this stage precludes the next stage. However, problem-solving activities do not arise automatically in response to problems. Even under severe pressure, management may rationalize its problems by blaming them on the union, government, or other entities over which they lack control.

ARRIVAL OF A CHANGE AGENT

Failing to react successfully to pressures, management will seek out (or have thrust upon them) the services of an outsider, known for his or her ability to improve organizational functioning. Sometimes organizations in dire straits find their top management replaced by a "man of the hour." More frequently, existing management employs a consultant. The newcomer's position is advantageous. Having no vested interests in the organization or historical loyalties to one manager or another, he or she can provide a relatively objective appraisal of the organization. Furthermore, the consultant's reputation (or "aura") as a change agent will provide leverage to influence top management's behavior.

COMMITMENT OF TOP MANAGEMENT

The fourth stage involves the newcomer's attempts to commit top management to one change strategy or another. Dealing with top management appears to be critical to success, since changes are most likely to come about if the organization's power structure is behind them. In successful change programs, the newcomer encourages top management to examine past practices and current problems. He or she encourages the power structure to suspend temporarily its preconceptions and accustomed ways of viewing problems. In this vein, management is led to original perceptions of the causes of organizational behavior.

COLLABORATION

Successful change efforts tend to involve the head of the organization and the immediate subordinates in extensive reexaminations of past practices and current problems. After having secured the collaboration and support of top management, fact-finding and problem-solving discussions are begun in lower levels of the organization. Top-management support is important at this stage, since it enables subordinates to view their own efforts as legitimate, having the backing of important people in the organization. Greiner suggests that subordinates have evidence that top management is willing to change, since they are involved in the diagnosis and change efforts. They have evidence that important problems are being acknowledged and faced up to and furthermore that ideas from lower levels are being valued by upper levels.

CREATIVITY

At some point, management may become convinced that its problems, as they have been redefined, defy solution using available techniques. Here, the change agent's function is to provide new ideas and methods for developing solutions. Management generally is involved in learning and practicing new forms of behavior that permit creative problem solving. As unique solutions are generated, top management's commitment increases. Greiner notes that none of the less successful change programs reached this particular stage of development. The seeds of failure, sown in previous stages, grow into severe resistance to change prior to this. As this occurs, top management usually gives up or regroups for another effort.

REALITY TESTING

Solutions developed in the previous stage are tested on a pilot basis to determine their efficacy. This must be done before attempts are made to broaden the scope of change to larger problems and the entire organization. Difficulties are nearly inevitable in the pilot run. Rather than presenting problems, they serve as opportunities to modify solutions and enhance their effectiveness.

DIFFUSION

Following pilot testing, adequate solutions are introduced on a larger scale. With each successful implementation, management support grows and the change is gradually absorbed into the organization's way of life.

This is a bird's-eye view of the change process, but from the manager's perspective things are not at all so clear. Here, it seems, to undertake change means to confront a continual series of dilemmas.

DILEMMAS IN THE PROCESS OF CHANGE

The change process may be viewed (Hage and Aiken 1970) as comprising four different stages: (1) determining the need for change, (2) initiation, (3) implementation, and (4) routinization.[2] During the first stage, the organization becomes aware of problems that suggest the inadequacy of the status quo. Perhaps goals are not being met as adequately as in prior periods, or as projected by forecasts. In any event perception of a gap between desired and actual performance initiates the process of organizational change.

An external consultant might think of this as the diagnostic phase of the process. However, from management's point of view, this term is not exactly appropriate. Most organizations have ongoing surveillance and monitoring procedures as well as programs for gathering information in nonroutine situations. Identification of gaps between actual and intended performance is a routine activity. When interpreted according to the theories, constructs, or paradigms employed by management, these gaps suggest both the sources of problems and tentative remedies for them.

An interesting question at this stage concerns the extent of consensus about the need to change. Need for change is indicated by the perception of gaps between intended and actual performance, as we have said. But it can also be said that organizations typically pursue a number of goals which occasionally are in conflict. Goals and shorter run objectives constitute statements of intended performance. Depending on the goals most salient to managers and the accuracy with which performance toward them can be measured, conflicts may arise due to different perceptions of the need for change. The processes by which these perceptions are communicated to top management as well as the negotiation and compromise strategies that lead to consensus should interest us here. Unfortunately, these aspects of the change process have received little attention from behavioral scientists, perhaps because they occur so early in the change process that they precede the scientists' interventions. A modified rational theory of perception of the need for organizational change is found in March and Simon (1958) and, more recently, in Downs (1967). The interested student may wish to pursue these theories for a view of how the first stage of the change process would look if managers behaved "rationally."

One dilemma facing management during the early part of the change process is whether to engage in a large-scale or modest change effort. Modest changes are relatively simple to make and bear proportionate risks. Large-scale changes are more difficult to bring about, more costly, and riskier, although more likely to remedy serious problems. One way to analyze the magnitude of a change effort is in terms of its depth of intervention (Downs 1967). Relatively shallow structural changes modify a limited portion of the organization; for instance, a university may create a new associate dean's position in its school of business in response to administrative overload. A deeper change affects the organization's rules for decision making. At this level, the university in our example may alter the formula by which funds are allocated to its various schools. Still deeper are changes in the organization's structural arrangements for making and enforcing rules. This depth of change would be observed in a university that granted students a vote in decisions to tenure faculty members. Finally, the deepest level of change modifies the purposes of the organization, and would be found in a university that divested its traditional goals to become a training center.

Different managers and consultants have different predilections for shallow and deep changes. Some will prefer to operate at shallow levels while others will be attracted to more dramatic efforts. Similarly, different individuals will entertain different theories of organizational behavior and change. These will give rise to contrasting opinions of the ends and means of change efforts. Please bear in mind that these differences are based on attitudes and predilections as well as on objective scientific experience. Thus, a series of dilemmas can arise. We shall introduce some of these dilemmas below.

INITIATION OF CHANGE

The initiation stage of the change process arises when it is decided that change is necessary and when one alternative solution is perceived to be more desirable than competing alternatives. At this stage, management must decide *who* is to conduct the remainder of the change process. Should the organization employ external consultants or rely on the talents of its own employees?

Using insiders is preferable if management wishes to avoid major disruptions. However, because of existing obligations, loyalties, preconceptions, vested interests, and the like, insiders may find themselves unable to bring about major changes. The opposite is true of outsiders, of course, who can bring new ideas and directions for change to the organization, but who are likely to create conflict and resistance in the process.

A second dilemma concerns the source of financial support for the change effort. Use of existing resources will curtail other planned or ongoing activities. Thus, reallocation of a fixed budget is likely to engender conflict or at best a lack of whole-hearted cooperation from segments adversely affected. Going outside the organization for financial support will create dependency on the source of funding. The various arrangements described by Thompson (1967) are relevant here, namely, cooptation and cooperation. The form of dependency experienced will depend on the nature of the arrangement; for example, a bank loan will be accompanied by the bank's insistence on safeguards such as limitations on the organization's activities, the right to certain kinds of surveillance, and the right to specific reports.

The need to identify the starting point for a change program gives rise to another series of dilemmas. An organization contemplating changes in its branch offices has a choice of targets for its initial change attempts. Should the parent organization begin the change program in units that are weak or powerful? Should it begin with independent units or those that are linked with other units? Should integrated, cohesive units be selected, or should the program begin with personnel who are not so closely knit?

A stronger effort is required to change powerful, integrated, or cohesive units than to achieve the same initial results with those that are relatively weak, independent, or fragmented. However, the long-run effectiveness of the change program may be enhanced by starting with units having the former characteristics. Powerful and cohesive units may serve as models for others. The latter may follow the lead of the former to the extent that changes will be emulated. Interrelated units must remain compatible. A change in one unit will create pressures in the others to change accordingly. Where this is the case, change tends to be diffused throughout the organization more readily.

The degree of risk inherent in the intended change is an important factor in the decision to select a particular starting point. If the change is modest and experience suggests that attendant risks are slight, it is probably well to begin with the more difficult units. When the change program is envisaged to be difficult or to portend substantial risks, it is appropriate to begin with a pilot project in a unit separate from the others and weak enough to offer minimal resistance to change. Having demonstrated the effectiveness of change in the pilot unit, management can turn its efforts to more difficult areas of the organization.

IMPLEMENTATION OF CHANGE

Top management tends to operate on its own, without involving others, throughout the first two stages of the change process. In the implementation stage, lower level personnel must become involved as well. Awareness of a need for change and exploration of alternative courses of action tend to disrupt (unfreeze) top management's habitual ways of thinking and acting. We shall examine the phenomenon of "unfreezing" habitual behavior in Chapter 14. At this point, it is important to note that lower level participants must be "unfrozen" as well.

Habits, rules, structures, and procedures contribute to organizational stability. The more stable the organization, the more readily its steady state activities can be predicted and controlled. This situation can be described as one of equilibrium. Hage and Aiken note that the implementation of change increases organizational disequilibrium. At this point, more of the staff have become "unfrozen." In the utopian world of the rational school of thought, this is the point at which a plan for change is implemented, behavior refrozen, and equilibrium reestablished. In actual practice, we find this stage to be a prolonged period of "muddling through."

Management cannot make complete plans for change. For one thing, they lack a science of organizational change. For another, they lack vital, detailed information residing at lower levels of the organization. Furthermore, intended changes may be resisted by various personnel. When organizational objectives and the self-interest of participants conflict, employees appear perverse, unpredictable, and stubborn. The behavioral sciences are inexact. We cannot predict all responses to change accurately. As these and other shortcomings compound the situation, mistakes are made. Thus, the change process must proceed gradually, using feedback to correct mistakes and accommodate unforeseen contingencies. The organization must be unfrozen for the initiation of change and *remain* unfrozen for the duration of the change.

Hage and Aiken note that conflict is prone to arise during the implementation stage. Units undergoing change or newly created by change frequently demand additional resources, authority, and changes in rules. However, these demands can affect other units adversely. Resources may be taken directly (or indirectly) from the budgets of other units. Changed rules may impede their functioning. Newly acquired authority may encroach on established "turfs." If top management does not accede to legitimate demands of this sort, the change effort may die on the vine. If it does accede, it may disrupt the organization and possibly limit its effectiveness.

A related dilemma concerns the extent to which change programs should be made participative. Should all parties affected be allowed to participate, as human relations practitioners suggest? An expected result of such participation is increased commitment to the process. Another expected outcome is that participants will express their desires and change the program to suit their own ends, possibly hindering or curtailing those of top management. Cooperation is bought at the price of alterations to the change program envisaged. Alternatively, the integrity of the change effort may be maintained at the cost of resistance to change and conflict.

Top management may decide to make structural changes unilaterally, expecting that, in the long run, interpersonal conflicts and adverse attitudes will die out—that eventually behavior will conform to new structural arrangements. Alternatively, behavioral scientists may be brought into the organization to alter behavior prior to making structural changes. Changing people is costly, risky, and occasionally subject to question on ethical grounds. However, appropriate changes may foster intended structural modifications.

Another dilemma arises in attempting to decide whether to use a highly structured or unstructured change effort. On the one hand, management can plan changes in considerable detail beforehand and then proceed to implement its plan systematically. On the other hand, it may be decided that planning is infeasible, or too costly. In this event, change will be implemented and coordinated by feedback. The advantage of planning is that it provides a degree of security when it can be done effectively. Contingencies are foreseen, costs projected, and pitfalls, perhaps, avoided. Management can determine its progress by comparing actual to planned results at any point in time. Anxieties of those responsible for implementation may be reduced to the extent that the direction of the effort is foreseen. The existence of a plan, similar to the existence of rules, may reduce potential for interpersonal conflict.

However, flexibility is lost in the process. In relatively deep change efforts containing risk and uncertainty, mistakes in the initial planning effort are difficult to correct. The mere existence of a detailed plan may cause those charged with its implementation to become relatively insensitive to feedback. Accomplishment will be measured in terms of executing the plan rather than in terms of the achievement of objectives which may entail modifying what has been planned.

ROUTINIZATION OF CHANGE

A problem arising in both the implementation and routinization stages concerns identifying the point at which changes will be consolidated. One strategy is to prolong the unfrozen state and to work numerous changes simultaneously—to move from one change to the next without attempting to freeze behavior. The alternative strategy is to consolidate each change as it is accomplished. An advantage of the latter approach is that management can devote its attention to other portions of the organization without worrying about backsliding in previously changed units. This outcome may be offset by the very attributes that make it seem advantageous. Interdependent units must remain compatible despite changes undergone. We may find that a change in unit 2 requires modification of unit 1. If unit 1 was previously changed and refrozen, it must be unfrozen, changed, and refrozen once again if resistance to change is to be overcome. At the extreme, the situation becomes expensive, frustrating, and baroque.

This may be contrasted with the strategy of leaving change efforts unfrozen temporarily. As change proceeds in one unit, interdependencies will affect other, unfrozen units influencing them to change appropriately and reinforcing them for these responses. In fact, the situation can be mutually reinforcing. Changes made in the second unit reinforce and stabilize those made in the first. The problem with this approach is that it disperses the attentions of management across numerous units. Although the total change effort may be substantial, the effort directed to any one unit may be meager.

The timing of efforts to consolidate changes is contingent upon the degree to which changes have been completed. Ideally, consolidation occurs after the gap between intended and actual performance is eliminated. In reality, it may be impossible to measure this gap precisely. Alternatively, the gap may have shrunk as a result of organizational change, but not completely. In this case, the question arises whether major or minor effort is required to complete the process. Continued major effort is costly and time consuming. Oftentimes, the costs of change are salient while the benefits are not. Time and money spent, conflict and anxiety suffered, and inefficiency and confusion endured are readily identified with attempts to change organizations. Benefits, such as improved morale, are intangible. Improvements such as organizational growth and survival are remote in time from changes intended to cause them. In short, when costs are more apparent than benefits, change efforts may be terminated prematurely.

RESISTANCE TO CHANGE

As the manager contemplates and initiates change in the organization, one theme is likely to emerge time and again—resistance to the change process. These reactions have been emphasized in the psychological literature, perhaps overly so (Gross et al. 1971), but resistance to change is a major problem that can develop at any point in the change process. As Gross indicates, there is little research on the actual process of change or overcoming associated resistance to change. For this reason, we are forced to rely primarily on the day-to-day experience of change agents, who work with management to bring about organizational change.

The organization members' responses to change depend on their perceptions of the proposed change and, of course, on the effects they think the change will have on their needs and aspirations (Mann and Neff 1961). If they experience ambiguity, individuals may engage in search behavior which may appear as resistance from the perspective of those initiating change. Also related to search behavior are the individuals' perceptions of their ability to control the situation and their general trust in those in charge of proposed changes (see Figure 4–1). Ambiguity may not lead to resistance if individuals are permitted a degree of control over their destiny, as is the case when they are encouraged to participate in the change process. Participation in the planning phases of change, of course, provides not only the opportunity for control, but also clarity about the nature of the intended change. Trust also affects the degree to which the individual views prospective changes positively. Mann and Neff suggest that information, participation, and the organizational culture determine the individual's perception of a proposed change by operating through the mediating variables of ambiguity, control, and trust. Participation is useful in overcoming resistance to change because of its potential to increase the accuracy of perceptions and extent of control, and to reduce ambiguity. However, trust may or may not increase, depending on what is observed in the act of participation. The individual's perception of participation as a facade, used to increase manipulation, or as an opportunity openly granted, with openly stated risks and trade-offs, is likely to affect trust.

This is basically a rational model in which individuals respond to change situations by considering the implications and acting in their self-interests. Ambiguities and anxieties enter into the model by coloring perceptions. It is assumed that individuals react either positively or negatively, depending on how the change is presented. Sometimes, however, we can expect to find individuals with basic predispositions toward change—who view either change or the status quo as an end in itself (Barnes 1967).

If the individual perceives change to be compatible with his or her personal goals, and management concurs in this estimate, there are few problems. However, if the individual's perception is inaccurate (e.g., if he or she sees change as compatible when it is not), management will need to clarify the situation even though the individual's resistance may increase as a result. If management were to deliberately mislead employees, the longer-range effects on trust and acceptance of future changes (even those clearly within the individual's interest) would be costly.

When management experiences resistance from individuals who perceive changes to be incompatible with their goals, even when management's view is to the contrary, increased communication is also advised, although the

Figure 4-1

A Model for Understanding an Individual's Response to Change

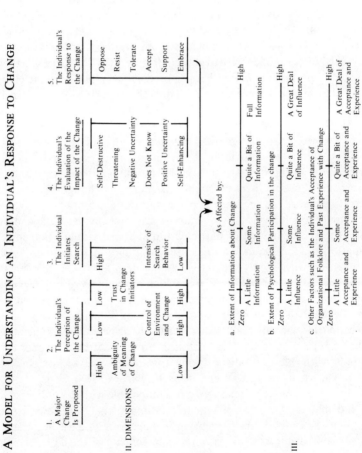

Source: Mann and Neff (1961, p. 69).

climate of trust may be such that perceptions of negative implications of change cannot be altered. Mann and Neff suggest that management emphasize its *actions* when these are compatible with individual goals, and that the proposed change be differentiated from other, past changes.

When individuals see change as incompatible with their goals and management concurs in this view, then, Mann and Neff suggest, management must review the objectives of the change and either alter them or proceed with the original change program (assuming that the wherewithal to overcome resistance is available, and that the various costs of change do not outweigh its benefits).

Sometimes, management is uncertain about the effects of a proposed change. Here the offer of employee participation may be in order. When employees are involved in decisions concerning change, its implications for both management and employees become clearer.

In general, then, Mann and Neff suggest that the management of change can be improved by giving those affected more information and allowing them to participate in the change process. While these are useful suggestions, we shall explore change phenomena in greater depth, developing more detailed, specific approaches to organizational change.

REFERENCES

Ansoff, H. Igor, and Brandenburg, Richard G. A language for organization design, Parts I and II. *Management Science,* 1971, *17,* B705–B731.

Barnes, Louis B. Organizational change and field experimental methods. In V. H. Vroom (Ed.), *Methods of organizational research.* Pittsburgh: University of Pittsburgh Press, 1967.

Biggart, Nicole Woolsey. The creative-destructive process of organization change: the case of the post office. *Administrative Science Quarterly,* 1977, *22,* 410–426.

Corwin, Ronald G. Strategies for organizational innovation: an empirical comparison. *American Sociological Review,* 1972, *37,* 441–54.

Downs, Anthony, *Inside bureaucracy.* Boston: Little, Brown, 1967.

Greiner, Larry E. Patterns of organizational change. *Harvard Business Review,* 1964, *42,* 3 (May–June), 119–30.

Gross, Neal, Giacquinta, Joseph B., and Bernstein, Marilyn. *Implementing organizational innovations: a sociological analysis of planned educational change:* New York: Basic Books, 1971.

Hage, Jerald, and Aiken, Michael. *Social change in complex organizations.* New York: Random House, 1970.

March, James G., and Simon, Herbert A. *Organizations.* New York: Wiley, 1958.

Mann, Floyd C., and Neff, Franklin W. *Managing major change in organizations.* Ann Arbor, Mich.: Foundation for Research on Human Behavior, 1961.

O'Connell, Jeremiah J. *Managing organizational innovation.* Homewood, Ill.: Richard D. Irwin, 1968.

Thompson, James D. *Organizations in action.* New York: McGraw-Hill, 1967.

Wanous, John P., and Lawler, Edward E., III. Measurement and meaning of job satisfaction. *Journal of Applied Psychology.* 1972, *56*, 95–105.

Wilson, James Q. Innovation in organization: notes toward a theory. In J. D. Thompson (Ed.) *Approaches to organizational design.* Pittsburgh: University of Pittsburgh Press, 1966. 193–218.

Zaltman, Gerald, Duncan, Robert, and Holbek, Jonny. *Innovations and organizations.* New York: Wiley, 1973.

NOTES

1. The nature of this relationship, though, is anything but clear. See, for example, Wanous and Lawler (1972).
2. Hage and Aiken term the first stage "evaluation." We have changed their terminology since we use the term in a different sense elsewhere.

5 | Administrative Responses to Prospective Reimbursement

Robert F. Allison

With both major political parties advocating increased federal participation in financing the cost of hospital care, policy makers are investigating alternative methods of controlling hospital costs. Since, historically, changes in hospital costs have corresponded roughly with changes in methods of reimbursement by third parties, attention is currently directed at controlling costs by varying the form of payment. That is, if guaranteeing retroactive payment of full costs itself contributes to increases in costs, will reversing that process by determining in advance what a hospital will receive at the end of its fiscal period moderate cost increases during the period? In such experiments, the interest has been primarily in establishing *whether* costs have been influenced by reimbursement.

As could be expected, administrative officials of hospitals have a different interest and perspective in this matter. While interested in whether prospective reimbursement [PR] influences costs, hospital officials are equally concerned with *how* this occurs. To the skeptical, "hard-headed businessman" official, it is important to know what action hospital administrators took in such experiments to affect costs, if such experiments are to have any value to other hospitals.

This article describes one of the few, if not the only, PR experiment which investigated how hospital officials made cost-influencing changes in response

This research is supported by Contract SSA–PMB–74–344 from the Office of Research and Statistics, Social Security Administration.

Reprinted from *Topics in Health Care Financing*, Vol. 3, No. 2, "Administrative Responses to Prospective Reimbursement," by Robert F. Allison, by permission of Aspen Systems Corporation, © 1976.

to PR. Although this article relies primarily on the Blue Cross of Michigan experiment, the discussion will not be confined to Michigan, and the emphasis will be on information of value to all hospitals. Given the centrality of the Michigan experiment to the discussion, a brief description of its origin and nature is appropriate.

DESCRIPTION OF THE MICHIGAN EXPERIMENT

With the passage of Medicare and Medicaid legislation in the mid-1960s and the resulting dramatic increases in hospital costs, interest shifted to control of costs. After a series of Blue Cross rate increases of 16 percent to 19 percent, the state Insurance Commissioner of Michigan in 1970 "strongly encouraged" Blue Cross of Michigan [BCM] to institute PR as a cost control measure. After a delay for the Economic Stabilization Program, BCM began in July 1973 a pilot experiment in eleven community hospitals which had volunteered to be included.

Because some readers might wish to know how these hospitals compare with their own institutions, key descriptive characteristics of the experimental hosptials are presented in Table 5-1.

DATA FORM PACKAGE

In the Michigan experiment, each hospital completes a package of data forms and submits them to BCM prior to negotiations. The hospital thus provides detailed reports of its last completed fiscal year, the year to date, estimates of the remainder of the current year, and a budget for the

TABLE 5-1
EXPERIMENTAL HOSPITAL CHARACTERISTICS
(Averages for all 11 hospitals)
1973

Beds [Range: 34 to 400]	159
Admissions	6254
Length of Stay	7.3
Days Covered by Blue Cross	38.3%
Per Diem Cost	$97
Occupancy	81
Scope of Services*	26

*Count of number of services shown in AHA Annual Guide Issues 1973. No university teaching hospitals are in the experiment.

prospective year. BCM reviews these data and meets informally with hospital personnel to resolve nonsubstantive, clerical questions. Although they are chronically behind schedule, formal negotiations are supposed to occur about three months prior to the beginning of the prospective year. In negotiations, several high-level representatives of BCM meet with the administrator, controller, and sometimes other hospital representatives such as the chairman of the board, key officials, and possibly the hospital's external auditor.

Actual negotiations center on the forms completed earlier by the hospital. BCM assumes hospital costs increase primarily because of three factors: inflation, utilization, and productivity. Since BCM feels the hospital can most affect productivity, attention in negotiations is directed at significant changes in departmental administration. When differences of opinion occur, BCM is at a disadvantage to the hospital because of the hospital's "insider" knowledge and the absence of generally accepted productivity standards. Typically, negotiations conclude in a series of offers and counteroffers, separated by caucuses of the negotiating teams. Since this experiment was voluntary, should a hospital have refused to agree to BCM's final offer, the alternative was withdrawal from the experiment. (This never occurred.)

DETERMINING TOTAL EXPENSES

Throughout the negotiations, total hospital expenses for each hospital are determined in advance. Actual hospital expenses in excess of this contractually fixed amount must be met in full by the hospital. If a hospital is able to keep expenses below that figure, it can retain all savings. Thus, a hospital has both an incentive to avoid losses and a possibility of earning a surplus. The participating hospital receives weekly cash payments from BCM equal to 1/52nd of Blue Cross's share of the total budget. Since all other hospitals receive biweekly checks that vary in amount depending on utilization, this feature of PR contributed greatly in encouraging hospitals to enter the experiment.

Other features of the experiment reduce its potential to provide an incentive to control costs. First, only 38 percent of the average hospital's costs are covered by the contract. Second, many contracts contain provisions for retrospective payment of costs that are unpredictable or uncontrollable, i.e., malpractice insurance premiums or utilization of new services or units. Third, the physicians in these hospitals are neither at risk nor directly involved in this experiment. Since physicians exert primary control over utilization (one of the major determinants of hospital costs), their exclusion diminishes the effectiveness of a PR plan.

Considering both factors that enhance and factors that diminish the constraining power of this experiment, it seems reasonable to conclude that the Michigan experiment provides only a moderate incentive for hospitals to contain costs. Indeed, this conclusion is consistent with interview responses in which officials in these hospitals indicated that their primary reasons for entering the experiment were not to earn a surplus or to contain costs but to receive the regular weekly checks and to gain expertise in a system they predicted would soon be mandatory for all hospitals. Regardless of the theoretical potential of this PR plan to provide incentive or these respondents' reasons for entering the experiment, the plan has, in practice, motivated officials to behave differently once in the plan. Changes that occurred in these hospitals are examined next.

Structural Changes

PR and Decision Making

A natural expectation one could hold toward this plan is that it would increase the already high level of "bureaucracy" within hospitals; so, several aspects of hospital operations generally thought to constitute bureaucratization were measured. First, changes in formalization were considered. Formalization is defined as the extent to which standard methods of performance exist, the degree to which they are written, and the extent to which efforts are made to ensure that they are followed in actual practice. Results indicate only an insignificant increase in formalization. Since the increase that did occur was only slightly greater than that of control hospitals, it is clear that PR was not responsible for significant changes in this factor.

It might also be expected that hospitals would employ more personnel specializing in accounting and finance to contend with the added work load associated with PR. Apparently, these hospitals are adding such specialists over time at a rate similar to that occurring in control hospitals. Therefore, one can conclude that thus far PR has not created the need for additional financial specialists.

One might also reason that PR would enhance the power of the central administration over lower level supervisors and vis à vis the board and medical staff. Our results to date indicate administrators do not perceive their power in relation to these other groups as having increased. Although they do perceive minor shifts have occurred in their power over individual cost-influencing variables [CIVs], increases have been offset by decreases. Since this is similar to the situation in controls, one can conclude PR has not materially affected the level at which final decisions are made.

Related to the question of the level at which decisions are made is the broader question of the effect of PR on the decision-making structure. Our data indicate the medical staff is the last major decision-making body affected by PR, and the least affected. However, in year two of the experiment physicians were being affected—primarily by being denied new equipment they had failed to include in the budget. One should not conclude, however, that this will reduce costs. The effect is more likely to be the inclusion of such capital purchases in the next budget, not denial of the request. Although the governing boards of these hospitals were virtually unaffected by PR in the first year of the experiment, at least one-half were affected by the end of the second year. Administrators indicated the effects were beneficial (i.e., increasing the board's interest, involvement, and information pertaining to planning, budgeting, and cost control). Clearly this is an "educational effect" of the PR plan.

The first and most affected by PR are the department heads. In year one about 50 percent of the administrators indicated their relations with department heads had been affected. By the end of year two, this figure had increased to over 60 percent. Looking horizontally at the hospital, across functional departments, PR most affects personnel associated with the controller and business office. Looking vertically at the hospital, PR most affects the highest administrative and supervisory levels. Administrators seem to agree that PR is primarily and narrowly a financial program, the success of which depends heavily on the expertise and commitment of department heads.

EDUCATION AND IMPROVED PRACTICE

In addition to regularized cash flow, the single greatest benefit of this PR plan is its educational effect. The administrative and clerical requirements of participation in any PR plan force improvements in planning, budgeting, and cost control procedures in all but the most well-run hospitals. Such improvements are front-loaded, one-time gains occurring early in the hospital's experience with PR. This is one of the main reasons for the success of PR in Indiana. Being in *any* PR plan over 15 years will improve hospital budgeting practices and cost performance. PR improved existing practices rather than caused hospitals to do entirely new things. Most hospitals have always forecasted, planned, budgeted, and monitored performance. PR, in the study hospitals, caused them to do these things better. Also, poor financial planning was unrelated to hospital size. Respondents were asked what type of hospital could best survive under PR—the anticipated response being large hospitals. They seemed to agree that success within PR is primarily a matter of financial expertise, regardless of hospital size. Observation confirmed their opinions.

EXPENSE AND REVENUE

It is not too much of an exaggeration to say that under retrospective reimbursement, expenses determine revenues. That is, when all budget requests of the various departments of the hospital are totaled that figure determines what changes will be necessary in the charge structure to generate sufficient revenues to pay expenses. Interviewers asked specifically what they did at that point in budgeting when they found projected expenses exceeded projected revenues: did they reduce budgeted expenses or increase charges? The typical response in both PR hospitals and control hospitals was, as one respondent phrased it, "Put projected expenses and revenues together, then adjust charges accordingly." Only a monopolist can ignore the market in setting budget totals. Our data indicate PR did not materially affect this aspect of budgeting. PR improved utilization and cost estimates, but budget totals were the last, rather than the first, step in budgeting. To paraphrase one respondent, "if the budget components are justified, the budget total will be justified." Of course, in other forms of PR a hospital would begin budgeting knowing the budget total constraining all the components. This is at least one difference between a voluntary PR plan in which budgets are negotiated and other, more rigorous PR plans.

A surprising number of experimental and control hospital officials are, in effect, "cash managers." To them, the real goal is to ensure adequate cash flow rather than recovery of full cost and generation of a surplus. Although it is impossible to document, it seems that a slowdown in Medicaid payment to all Michigan hospitals in recent months had more effect on cost containment than PR. If cash determines costs, restrictions on the timing of payments to hospitals might have as great an impact on hospital costs as restrictions in the size of payments.

COST PREDICTION

In hospitals operated by cash managers, the budget is used more for prediction than control. Of course, the avowed purpose of a budget is to constrain actual expenditures. Prospective reimbursement did affect actual expenditures, and the effect seemed to exceed the actual constraint provided by the budget. For example, even though only 37 percent of a hospital's costs might be constrained by the PR contract, officials would act *as if* the entire budget were similarly constrained. Some of this incentive could be due to Medicaid policies unique to Michigan; therefore, these findings should not be overgeneralized. Nevertheless, using budgets to constrain costs, a practice the sophisticated reader simply assumes, is a new experience in some hospitals. One administrator of a control hospital boasted that his actual expenditures were never more than one-half of one percent different from budgeted expenditures; he called his method "variable budgeting." However, "variable" to him meant revising his budget upward each month on the basis of expenditures department heads remembered during the year that they had not reported during the budget preparation! Letting actual costs determine the budget, rather than the reverse, might seem strange to the reader; but it is not so uncommon in hospitals. It seems fair to conclude that PR, perhaps any PR, causes hospital officials to use budgets not only to predict costs but also to control them.

COST CONTAINMENT

The data underlying the analysis of the actions taken in PR hospitals to control costs are shown in Table 5–2. Cost-influencing variables (CIVs), a term coined by William L. Dowling,[1] are shown in the first column of the table. These are believed to be among the major determinants of total hospital costs. Each of these CIVs is, in turn, influenced by specific actions of the hospital. For example, to affect efficiency, the hospital might conduct special studies to determine the procedures and type of personnel appropriate for a given task. A lengthy list of actions that affect the 10 CIVs was constructed for this study. For each action the administrator indicated: (a) whether they had already done it ["previous emphasis" column in Table 5–2]; (b) whether they were either just beginning to perform that action or increasing/decreasing their past emphasis on that action; and, (c) how much they thought that particular action affected total hospital costs in the long run ["cost-saving potential"]. The responses for two years of the experiment are averaged and shown in rank order in Table 5–2.

TABLE 5–2
COST-INFLUENCING ACTIONS

CIV	Current Emphasis	Previous Emphasis	Cost-Saving Potential	Administrator's Power
Investments	1	1	10	1
Quality	2	2	3	7
Admissions	3	9	2	6
Scope of Services	4	10	7.5	8
Teaching	5	4	5	4
Length of Stay	6	6	1	5
Case Mix	7	8	9	10
Efficiency	8	5	6	3
Intensity	9	7	4	9
Input Prices	10	3	7.5	2

What a hospital is currently doing about cost containment depends on a number of factors, the three most important of which are presented here: previous emphasis, potential for saving costs, and the power to do it. The "administrator's power" refers to the administrator's perception of his/her ability to influence an action *relative* to the medical staff's influence over this action. For example, these administrators felt they had maximum power over the medical staff to control investments in capital and human resources and minimal power to control the types of patients admitted (case mix). The choice of this research design was partly in response to two hyptheses often expressed by academics and practicing managers: some complain that the administrator's failure to take an action that will significantly reduce costs is not due to a lack of will or knowledge but to the fact that the medical staff controls such action; others maintain administrators ignore taking actions that will save money and focus on actions having a low payoff because those are the actions that they have the expertise and power to perform. Available data do not permit a rigorous test of these hypotheses, but perhaps the analysis will provide some fresh insights on the topic.

Examples of actions to control the hospital's investment in human and capital resources are changes in policies regarding plant maintenance, inservice and professional education, etc. Even though these types of actions were emphasized in the past and offered the least potential for cost savings, they are the ones currently being given the most emphasis relative to other actions administrators might take. Administrators also perceive that they had more power to control this CIV than any other. A possible explanation is that administrators are, like the rest of us, creatures of habit and inclined to take the course of least political resistance. These findings might suggest that such expenditures are among the first to be cut or deferred when resources are mildly constrained by PR.

QUALITY CONTROL

In the broadest sense, it is hard to conceive of an action that does not somehow affect "quality." It is also difficult to think of a single action affecting quality that does not simultaneously affect another of the CIVs. As used in this experiment, quality is not a separate CIV but a unit of measure for the other CIVs. Because only physicians may practice medicine, hospitals can only indirectly affect quality—by taking actions affecting the other CIVs. Respondents were asked for their definition of quality, and they defined it primarily in terms of the scope of services offered by the hospital and the type and number of nursing personnel providing bedside nursing care. That is, they see "quality" as a combination of two other CIVs: scope of services and efficiency. The reader should keep these qualifying remarks in mind when interpreting the comments to follow concerning this CIV.

Although actions related to quality received much attention in the past, hospitals continue to give this CIV emphasis. On the surface quality appears to offer the classic example of the CIV having great cost-saving potential, yet being relatively uncontrollable by administration. There are two possible explanations why such actions were stressed despite the fact that administrators perceived the medical staff to have more power than they to control it. First, the types of actions involved are those currently being mandated by government programs and regulations (utilization review). Second, if public statements can be accepted, quality is a central value shared by physicians and administrators; therefore, the administration can act in this area without conflicting with the medical staff.

OTHER POLICY AREAS

Compared with other CIVs, admissions received less past emphasis yet offered more potential for saving costs than all but one other CIV. Programs such as outpatient screening and surgery and preadmission certification are examples of actions affecting this CIV. Despite the physician's relative dominance in this policy area, the survey hospitals gave it third highest priority among the ten CIVs. The reason for this seems to be similar to that for quality: government intervention.

Actions related to scope of services have been given the least emphasis in the past, yet they are fourth in current emphasis. This is a policy area in which the cost savings and administrator's power are both perceived to be low. Actions related to this CIV are decisions to add, expand, or contract services or units and to monitor utilization of existing services. A plausible explanation for past inattention to this policy area is the absence of certificate of need legislation. Under PR major changes in services approved by state officials and utilization must be monitored if costs are to be kept within the budget.

Teaching is a CIV in which most of the factors influencing current actions seem fairly consistent. The item includes actions pertaining to both in-service and occupational-type educational programs. It was given moderate emphasis both in the past and currently, has moderate potential for cost savings, and is a policy area where the power of the administration and the medical staff is fairly balanced. In other words, the emphasis on this CIV is about what would be expected.

Length of stay is a CIV offering a good example of the conflict between economic and political determinants of decisions. Despite the fact administrators feel this CIV offers the highest potential for cost savings, only moderate emphasis was and is being given to this policy area. Apparently the lack of emphasis is related to the administrator's perceived inability to take such actions. It is also possible some administrators might not be familiar with policies and programs affecting length of stay (i.e., home care programs, seven-day workweeks. or decreases in turnaround times in lab and x-ray).

The best example of the influence of the dual hierarchy within hospitals is offered by case mix. Administrators feel least able to affect case mix; yet if any CIV is germane to the practice of medicine in hospitals, it is this. Indirectly, hospitals affect case mix through changes in the scope and quality of services offered. More directly, case mix is affected by such actions as policies affecting the composition of the medical staff. It is a CIV that was and is relatively ignored. The administrators surveyed seem to feel relatively powerless to affect this CIV and that the low potential for cost savings is not worth the effort. If administrators were to perceive a large payoff in controlling this policy area, it would clearly invite conflict with the medical staff.

The reader may be surprised to see the low priority given to actions associated with efficiency. This exists despite official perception of this policy area as being highly controllable by administration. Actions typical of those affecting efficiency are merit programs, work studies, use of part-time employees, and admissions scheduling. There has been only moderate emphasis in the past on such actions; they are given even less current emphasis. Apparently the reason for this is the administrator's lack of appreciation for the cost-saving potential in this policy area. Considering the emphasis most college hospital administration programs place on tools to increase efficiency, it is hard to understand the relatively low priority given it by practitioners.

Another explanation for the lack of attention to efficiency is the lack of standards. Hospital officials simply might not recognize that they have efficiency-related problems! As discussed earlier, Blue Cross negotiators gave much emphasis to productivity changes yet were hampered in their efforts by lack of productivity standards. As a bargaining concession, two hospitals in the PR experiment agreed to permit productivity studies by outside consultants paid by Blue Cross. In the absence of such standards, Blue Cross tried in negotiations to disallow budgeted decreases in productivity. In summary, though PR might have stabilized or frozen productivity at historical levels, no data exist to indicate PR improved it. (These conclusions could change as more definitive data are analyzed in the near future.)

"Intensity" refers to the types of diagnostic and therapeutic procedures performed on patients. As the case mix, it is a physician-controlled CIV that was and is given little emphasis. However, unlike case mix, administrators perceive that changes in intensity have relatively more payoff in terms of cost savings. The most logical explanation for this lack of emphasis seems to be the same as that for length of stay, i.e., lack of administrative power vis à vis the medical staff.

Actions related to controlling the prices paid for inputs received the least attention of all the CIVs. Since administrators perceive very high control over this policy area, the most obvious explanation is the past high levels of emphasis on this CIV (third out of ten). Either for this reason or from the belief that factors beyond hospital control determine prices and wages, administrators perceived controlling this CIV had a low potential for saving costs.

IMPLICATIONS OF THE MICHIGAN EXPERIMENT

Certain lessons from the Michigan experiment seem obvious. A voluntary PR experiment of the negotiated budget type is not feasible for two reasons: it is administratively too burdensome on both Blue Cross and hospitals to be feasible on a statewide basis in any but the smallest states, and the voluntary aspect reduces the negotiating leverage of Blue Cross to the point that "negotiations" with hospitals become exercises in cooperative problem solving. However, one can conclude that procedural requirements of even a voluntary PR plan will improve budgeting practices in all but the most well-run hospitals. Finally, the experiment has increased the cost consciousness and expertise in cost control of Blue Cross officials in Michigan. Given that, historically, Blue Cross officials have been oriented more to serving hospitals than controlling them, this is a major benefit of any PR plan. Beyond these three obvious lessons are three more fundamental lessons from the Michigan experiment.

PR's INCENTIVE NOT ENOUGH

First, experience with these hospitals had led one to certain conclusions about the *incentive* value of PR. A major assumption of the Michigan experiment was that the state could control hospital costs through Blue Cross. It appears that such control of only 41 percent of hospital costs provides an inadequate incentive to hospitals. Blue Cross simply cannot do the job alone. To be effective, PR must include Medicare and Medicaid revenues. If this had been done in Michigan, approximately 75 percent of all hospital costs would have been covered by PR. In addition, it is debatable whether any form of cost control is workable since there is much to recommend the view that cost-based reimbursement by Blue Cross, Medicare, and Medicaid is the reason costs are now out of control.

PERCEIVING CIVs ACCURATELY

Second, it appears cost control depends greatly on the *perception* of factors causing costs. Figure 5-1 presents an understanding of how the major CIVs relate to costs.

Any action taken to control costs is based on some assumption of how that action affects a CIV, which in turn affects costs. Usually these assumptions are implicit rather than explicit. For example, the administrator who devotes most of his time to selection, training, methods improvement, and supervision implicitly assumes efficiency is the major determinant of costs. The administrator who tries to control costs by improving the composition and performance of the medical staff implicitly believes that CIVs related to utilization are the largest determinants of costs (i.e., admissions, case mix, intensity, length of stay). Everyone has such a set of mental assumptions, or a "model."

As shown in Figure 5-1, the length of stay and the types of services received (intensity) are the immediate determinants of cost per case. They require a certain type and quantity of resources (productivity), which must be purchased at certain unit prices. However, cost per case is not fully controllable by manipulation of only these four CIVs because each is, in turn, influenced by other CIVs. For example, although various "markets" might largely determine input prices, location largely determines the markets relevant to the hospital. The hospital located in midtown Manhattan certainly experiences input price problems different from those of the upstate New York hospital. Similarly, intensity is largely determined by the type of patient admitted (case mix, patient condition). However, the type of patient admitted depends largely on the scope of services available in that hospital and the specialties represented within that hospital's medical staff.

It can be seen that, ultimately, cost per case depends on characteristics of the service area population and the size and specialty composition of the medical staff. The major factors of cost per case are those in the middle row of boxes in the figure, and CIVs to the left are factors influencing those on the right.[2]

NEED FOR ADMINISTRATOR POWER

Every administrator realizes the relationship between the medical staff and hospital *revenues*. The current boom in construction of medical office buildings adjacent to hospitals is evidence of this understanding.[3] However, not every administrator sees a comparable relation of the medical staff to *costs*. One rarely meets the administrator who has attempted to control costs by limiting the size or specialty composition of the medical staff. Where

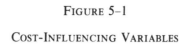

FIGURE 5–1

COST-INFLUENCING VARIABLES

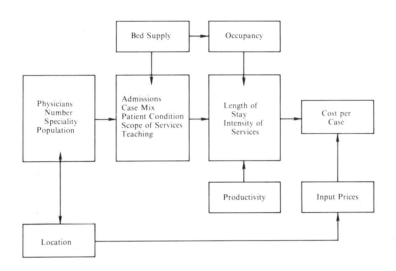

actions are taken to control length of stay or case mix, they are usually taken to meet government regulations or to control quality rather than cost. With the exception of the investment CIV, the CIVs currently being emphasized in actions taken by administrators within the PR experiment are roughly consistent with the model shown in Figure 5–1 (see Table 5–2).

It seems clear that administrators now know more about controlling costs than they are able to implement because of a real or perceived lack of *power* to do so. Controlling costs in the short run depends primarily on the variability and controllability of costs. In the short run, variable costs are, by definition, the ones that can be controlled. By these estimates, only 30 percent of all hospital costs are variable in the short run. Also, as has been discussed at length above, certain hospital costs are seen as being controlled more by the physicians than administration. In Table 5–3 are listed hospital administrators' perceptions of the influence of the medical staff over the CIVs. Scores for administrators of both the experimental and control hospitals for two years of the experiment were combined and averaged in Table 5–1, since the scores were virtually identical for both groups and for both years.

It is clear from Table 5–3 that these administrators have judgmental perception concerning the CIVs that are inherently linked to the practice of medicine. The first five CIVS *are* the major aspects of the practice of medicine in hospitals; and the sixth CIV, quality, is merely another aspect of these five.

TABLE 5-3
PHYSICIAN CONTROL OF CIVs AS
PERCEIVED BY THE ADMINISTRATOR

1. Case Mix	3.65
2. Admissions	3.50
3. Scope of Services	3.45
4. Intensity	3.35
5. Length of Stay	3.25
6. Quality	3.05
7. Teaching	2.65
8. Efficiency	2.30
9. Amenities	2.30
10. Input Prices	2.25
11. Investments in Resources	1.65

Notes: N = 33. Scoring key: 4 = very great influence, 3 = much influence, 2 = some influence, 1 = little influence.

The last five CIVs are part of the administrative half of the so-called dual hierarchy in hospitals. Given the perceived power of physicians to control certain hospital costs, what part of controllable costs are most controllable by administration? To help answer this question, Table 5-4 was constructed using national averages for short-term, voluntary hospitals in the United States for the interval 1962-66.

Although the method, and to some extent the data, in Table 5-4 are partially supported by prior studies, for the most part the analysis is a judgment of the author.[4] It is doubtful that such data have never before been presented despite the importance of this issue to health administration. Administrators probably feel the matter is so obvious it needs no documentation; academics avoid it because of lack of data and the untenable number of assumptions underlying the analysis. Regardless, the basic thrust of the data is unassailable: those with the formal authority to control hospital costs do not have enough power to control them. The estimate in Table 5-4 is that, at most, administrators control less than 25 percent of total hospital costs in the short run. When asked, most administrators and academics will provide much lower estimates.

For PR to be effective, these three conclusions from our research should be given recognition in the plan's design. First, the plan should include Blue Cross, Medicare, and Medicaid revenues to the hospital. Second, the information gap concerning five of the CIVs should be closed. The five CIVs related to quality of medical practice are not now seen primarily as *cost*-influencing variables, but as *quality*-influencing variables. That is, adminis-

TABLE 5-4
CONTROLLABILITY OF EXPENSES:
PERCENT OF TOTAL OPERATING EXPENSES

Administratively Controlled Departments	Total	Fixed	Variable
Administration and General	.12	.06	.06
Laundry and Linen	.03	.015	.015
Dietary	.09	.045	.045
Housekeeping	.04	.02	.02
Plant Operations	.04	.02	.02
Maintenance	.02	.01	.01
General Nursing	.22	.176	.044
Medical Records	.01	.005	.005
Pharmacy	.04	.02	.02
Education	.01	.005	.005
	.62	.376	.244
Physician-Controlled Departments			
Medical and Surgical Supplies	.05	.04	.01
Operating Room	.04	.032	.008
Delivery Room	.02	.016	.004
Anesthesiology	.02	.016	.004
Radiology	.05	.04	.01
Laboratory	.06	.048	.012
Physical Therapy	.01	.008	.002
Emergency Room	.01	.008	.002
	.27	.216	.054
Subtotals	.89	.592	.298
Depreciation, Interest, Other	.11	.11	
TOTALS	1.00	.702	.298

trative officials are focusing on the five administratively controlled variables having the least impact on cost and letting the medical staff continue to control the five variables having the most impact on costs. Third, for this to occur, administrative officials will need more than education; they will need more power. Certainly an onerous PR plan imposed by the state would increase management's negotiating power with the medical staff; PR *was* well received in these eleven Michigan hospitals, and it brought about the beneficial changes described in this article. It is too soon to know if PR slowed the growth of costs; but it is evident that had the experiment incorporated the three recommended changes, its impact on both actions and costs would have increased considerably.

NOTES

1. Dowling, W. L. "Prospective Reimbursement of Hospitals." *Inquiry* 11:3(September 1974) p. 163–180.
2. Lave, Lave, and Silverman. "A Proposal for Incentive Reimbursement for Hospitals." *Medical Care* 11:2 (March–April 1973) p. 79–90. Lave. "The Extent of Role Differentiation Among Hospitals." *Health Services Research* 6:1 (Spring 1971) p. 15–38. Shuman, Wolfe, and Hardwick. "Predictive Hospital Reimbursement Evaluation Model." *Inquiry* 9:1 (March 1972) p. 17–33. Shuman and Wolfe. "The Use of Case Mix and Case Complexity in Prospective Hospital Reimbursement." [Unpublished manuscript from the University of Pittsburgh] 1974.
3. Toland. "A Hospital Should Own and Operate Its On-Site Medical Office Buildings." *Hospitals* 50:14 (July 16, 1976) p. 80–84.
4. Bauer. *Containing Costs of Health Services Through Incentive Reimbursement* (Boston: Harvard Center for Community Health and Medical Care, Cases in Health Services Series No. 4 December 1973) p. 154–55. Davis and Foster. *Community Hospitals: Inflation in the Pre-Medicare Period.* (Washington, D.C.: D.H.E.W., Social Security Adm, Office of Research and Statistics, Research Report No. 41, 1972, Table 32. Also: *Six-Month National Comparison for Period Ending December 31, 1973*, Hospital Administrative Services, A. H. A., Chicago, Illinois). Houser. "Cost Variation With Volume in a Short-Term, Non-Federal General Hospital" [Unpublished Ph.D. dissertation from the University of Wisconsin] 1971. Davis. "Community Hospital Expenses and Revenues: Pre-Medicare Inflation." D.H.E.W. Pub. No. [SSA] 73-117000, Reprinted from *Social Security Bulletin* (Oct. 1972) p. 10–11.

6 | Physician Participation in Hospital Management

George F. Wieland

It is useful to consider the recent history of hospitals and their physicians. As Perrow (1965) indicates, earlier in this century influence in the hospital lay primarily with the trustees since their financial contributions were so important. Then, with the development of medical practice, influence shifted to the physicians who could bring patients into the hospitals. More recently, the growth in the specialization and complexity of medicine has made for much more complex organizations which need specially trained administrators to coordinate them.

ADMINISTRATIVE CONTROL OF DOCTORS

Predictions of the increasing influence and authority of the administrator began almost as soon as it was recognized that the hospital was a very anomalous organization with "two lines of authority" (Smith 1955). The other line is composed of physicians, who are not employees of the organization. A number of recent developments in the hospital's external environment may indeed provide the administrator with more leverage over the physicians: complex reimbursement schemes (such as prospective reimbursement, described in Chapter 5), utilization review regulations, a more demanding public, and even legal decisions which may make the hospital responsible in malpractice suits brought by patients against the independent physician. These external pressures would seem to give the hospital managers an opportunity to integrate the nonmedical and medical spheres of the hospital rather more closely.[1]

Despite these emerging factors of recent years, the medical staff is quite free from managerial controls and from integration with the nonmedical side of hospitals. Physicians seem to achieve this freedom by virtue of their complete authority in the realm of patient care. They are trained to expect to be individually responsible for the patient. They are the ones who have the most expertise, and who can claim that matters of life and death provide emergency powers. This enables the physician to exert a "professional dominance" over the other health care professions (Freidson 1970). In addition, the training of the physician in autonomous, individualistic decision making is reinforced subsequently by the profession's emphasis on personal achievement and on improving one's own performance (see Weisbord, Chapter 15). Any diminution of autonomy thus is a direct threat to the physician's status, and a threat to his or her basic identity.

A final factor which probably contributes to the freedom of the physician from managerial controls is the general lack of any role definition. The physician is responsible for the patient, and this allows any behavior—or the evasion of any behavior. Even when the physician takes on a multiplicity of roles, such as teaching, research, and clinical reponsibilities, as in the university medical center, he or she can use these role possibilities creatively, in carving out an idiosyncratic combination (Bucher and Stelling 1969), which can give even greater freedom by allowing one to manipulate (or evade) responsibilities in one role by using the leverage of the other role.

The almost absolute power of the physician in the domain of patient care—power to act, but also power not to act or to resist—helps explain a report by Kaluzny and Veney (1972) entitled "Who Influences Decisions in the Hospital? Not Even the Administrator Really Knows." A survey of 49 hospitals in New York State showed that administrators felt that the physicians had "considerable" influence over factors such as "adoption and implementation of new hospital-wide programs and services," "allocation of total hospital income," and "development of formal affiliation with other organizations." The physicians, however, felt that physician influence in these areas was "none." The discrepancy must lie to some degree in the individualistic behavior of physicians. Although physicians seldom initiate hospital-wide policy (yielding physician reports of little influence), their independence can make for considerable negative or blocking influence (yielding administrator reports of high physician influence). An individual physician, for example, can block administrator-initiated cost-saving procedures in the area of patient care and can block a relationship with another institution by behavior such as refusing to refer patients.

PHYSICIAN PARTICIPATION IN MANAGEMENT

A manager's response to physician independence would seem to lie in the creation of structures which help to integrate the medical staff into the management of the organization. Neuhauser (1971) provides a vivid picture of how much patient care can be improved if physicians play a more influential role in running the organization and, especially, in structuring their own activities. Studying 30 Chicago-area hospitals, Neuhauser measured physician participation in terms of the percentage of medical membership on the board of trustees and also in terms of the frequency of meetings of the joint conference committee (in which the chiefs of the medical staff meet with the executive officers of the board). Such physician participation is positively associated with the quality of medical care as measured by outside expert evaluators, by the accreditation evaluation, and by the severity-adjusted death rate.

Neuhauser found physician participation to be correlated with a rating (by the chief or president of the medical staff) of the influence of the physicians in the hospital. This provides some insight into how participation could operate to improve care. Both participation and influence are positively correlated with the autopsy rate and with an index measuring the presence and frequency of various reports (on incomplete medical records, percent normal tissue removed, consultation rates, postoperative deaths, anesthesia deaths, etc.). These factors are all-important because they help make the medical care process more visible and thus more amenable to control and improvement (see also Becker and Neuhauser 1975; Shortell et al. 1976). As Freidson and Rhea (1963) indicate, the visibility of medical performance is usually very low and only the most gross cases of incompetent performance are likely to become known to other colleagues and thereby amenable to sanction (see also Millman 1977). Thus, Neuhauser has documented the great importance of medical staff participation and its improvement of the "visibility of consequences."

In addition, Neuhauser found medical staff participation and influence to be positively associated with the imposition of certain procedural constraints on the practice of medicine. These constraints dictated the extent to which certain admission tests (e.g., chest x-ray, urinalysis, blood count) were required for all patients and the extent to which limitations were placed on the activities (e.g., surgical, obstetrical) each physician could perform in the hospital. Neuhauser suggests that these constraints were imposed by the medical staff itself, not by the administration or board of trustees (since physicians will benefit financially from the tests and from the monopolies on surgical or obstetrical activities). These self-imposed constraints apparently help to structure the care process; they give the medical staff more influence over their own activities in providing good patient care. Neuhauser found these procedural constraints to be positively associated with the quality of care as measured by the three different indicators (see also Flood and Scott 1978).

Procedural constraints *imposed by the hospital*, on the other hand, were found to be negatively associated with the quality of care. Hospital imposition of a formulary (a limited range of drugs stocked in the pharmacy), or a policy of suspending admitting privileges for those having too many incomplete medical records, has a negative effect, according to Neuhauser, because these are inflexible bureaucratic constraints which hinder the complex process of medical care. (The particular constraints here serve only to benefit the pharmacy or medical records department, respectively.)

SOME BENEFITS OF PHYSICIAN PARTICIPATION

Using regression equations, Neuhauser shows that if the average autopsy rate were raised from the observed rate of 41 percent to 60 percent and if medical staff participation were increased modestly from no medical membership on the board to (very roughly) 10 percent membership, the severity-adjusted death rate in these 30 hospitals would decline from 3.87 to 1.96 deaths per 100 admissions. This is, of course, a post-hoc analysis that requires cross-validation and there is no assurance of causal direction. Nevertheless, taken with the research of other investigators, there would seem to be some evidence that physicians' participation in hospital management is important for improved patient care.

Support for the view that physician participation is important comes from a study by Roemer and Friedman (1971), finding that highly structured medical staffs accompanied higher-quality hospital performance. They measured structure in ten California hospitals primarily in terms of the numbers of physicians who worked for (i.e., had a contract with) the hospital, the extent of departmentalization, and the number and the diligence of control committees. Not only were severity-adjusted death rates lower in hospitals with highly structured medical staffs, but the total expenditures per patient day were also lower.

Participation of the medical staff is likely to have an additional effect, the increased visibility and the structuring of appropriate medical care activities. Participation should give the medical staff some exposure and insight into the views of other staff. This increased awareness of the problems of others and their perspectives is likely to foster improved coordination and eventually improved patient care (see Chapter 1).

Participation can be of potential use in a variety of areas. The hospital manager, in addition to encouraging medical staff participation in matters such as budgeting, clarifying goals, and planning resource management (see Weisbord, Chapter 15), should also consider medical staff participation in some very specific matters. It is probably not wise for the manager to commission an operations research study of operating room schedules and present the results to the medical staff for implementation. Participation would be better. The manager might instead ask a medical staff committee to study the matter with appropriate staff support (see, for example, Chapters 22 and 23). Success for management interventions with the medical staff may depend very much on how the intervention is conducted (Kovner 1972).

PARTICIPATION—OR POWER

Of course, participation is no panacea. Many times the manager is likely to need a more power-oriented, negotiating strategy, convincing physicians to institute some procedures or constraints by offering inducements such as office space in the hospital in exchange for support by a key physician. Unfortunately, many organization behavior and management texts relegate power and conflict to a negligible role, but the great relative autonomy of physicians (and other professionals, too) together with the interdependence of the patient care process inevitably make the hospital an arena for power struggles and conflict. As Weisbord (Chapter 15) indicates, managers will often need to "engineer consent," and to play a "political game," not the "managerial game of implementing decisions."

In this connection, the manager is wise to consider that tensions among medical staff members are often higher than between medical staff members and other groups (Georgopoulos and Mann 1962; Georgopoulos and Wieland 1964). The manager may wish to seek to build coalitions with particular subgroups in the medical staff, as well as with members of the board of trustees and other influential groups (see, for example, Metsch and Levey 1974).

REFERENCES

Becker, Selwyn, and Neuhauser, Duncan. *The efficient organization.* New York: Elsevier, 1975.
Bucher, Rue, and Stelling, Joan. Characteristics of professional organizations. *Journal of Health and Human Behavior*, 1969, *10*, 3–15.
Flood, Ann Barry, and Scott, W. Richard. Professional power and professional

effectiveness: the power of the surgical staff and the quality of surgical care in hospitals. *Journal of Health and Social Behavior*, 1978, *19*, 240–254.

Freidson, Eliot. *Professional dominance: the social structure of medical care*. New York: Atherton Press, 1970.

Freidson, Eliot, and Rhea, Buford. Processes of control in a company of equals. *Social Problems*, 1963, *2*, 2, 119–131.

Georgopoulos, Basil S., and Mann, Floyd C. *The community general hospital*. New York: Macmillan, 1962.

Georgopoulos, Basil S., and Wieland, George F. *Nationwide study of coordination and patient care in voluntary hospitals*. Ann Arbor, Mich.: Institute for Social Research, 1964.

Kaluzny, Arnold, and Veney, James. Who influences decisions in the hospital? Not even the administrator really knows. *Modern Hospitals*, 1972, *119*, 6(December), 52–53.

Kovner, Anthony R. The hospital administrator and organizational effectiveness. In Basil S. Georgopoulos (Ed.) *Organization research on health institutions*. Ann Arbor, Mich.: Institute for Social Research, 1972.

Metsch, Jonathan M., and Levey, Samuel. Organizational analysis: theory or anecdotes. *Association of University Programs in Health Administration Program Notes*, 1974, No. 57 (February), 6–17.

Millman, Marcia. *Life in the backrooms of medicine*. New York: William Morrow, 1977.

Neuhauser, Duncan. *The relationship between administrative activities and hospital performance*. Chicago: Center for Health Administration, University of Chicago, 1971.

Perrow, Charles. Hospitals: Technology, structure, and goals. In James G. March (ed.) *Handbook of organizations*. Chicago: Rand McNally, 1965. Pp. 910–71.

Roemer, Milton I., and Friedman, Jay W. *Doctors in hospitals: Medical staff organization and hospital performance*. Baltimore: Johns Hopkins Press, 1971.

Shortell, Stephen M., Becker, Selwyn W., and Neuhauser, Duncan. The effects of management practices on hospital efficiency and quality of care. In Stephen M. Shortell and Montague Brown (Eds.) *Organizational research in hospitals*. Chicago: Blue Cross Association, 1976. Pp. 90–107.

Smith, Harvey L. Two lines of authority one too many. *Modern Hospital*, 1955, *84*, (March), 59–64.

Weisbord, Marvin R. Why organization development hasn't worked (so far) in medical centers. *Health Care Management Review*, 1976, *1*, 2 (Spring), 17–28.

NOTE

1. That this integration is no foregone conclusion is shown by the results of the government nationalization of the health care system in Britain. The physicians were able to negotiate a very favorable arrangement in 1948, allowing them a very influential position relatively free of managerial controls till this day.

7 | The Failure of Admission Scheduling at Able Hospital

Kurt R. Student

THE SETTING

Able Memorial Hospital is a 287 bed, voluntary hospital, one of three in a city of 70,000. Its medical staff is composed entirely of allopathic physicians, most of whom also maintain active privileges at the 201 bed Martin Hospital. The community is also served by a forty-four bed osteopathic hospital, but there is little interchange between the allopathic and osteopathic physicians.

The community rate of utilization is 957 per thousand population which is below the average for the state of 1,223 per thousand; this was not due to a shortage of beds. In 1969, the average census in Able was eighty-three percent; in Martin the average census was seventy-one percent. A study in late 1969 estimated that thirty adult medical-surgical beds were in excess of current requirements of the community. There were possibilities for reducing the bed needs in obstetrics. At the same time, there were shortages of psychiatric beds and shortages of long-term care beds at the basic nursing care level.

In a series of six meetings between October 1969 and March 1970, project personnel from The University of Michigan Bureau of Hospital Administration and the Able administrator confirmed the willingness of the administrator to have his hospital participate in the demonstration, and identified the scheduling of patient admissions as the first major project.

These initial discussions supported a prior conviction of the University

Reprinted from *Cost Control in Hospitals*, John R. Griffith, Walton M. Hancock, and Fred C. Munson, eds., "The Failure of Admission Scheduling at Able Hospital," by Kurt R. Student, by permission of the Health Administration Press, Ann Arbor, Mich., 1976.

team that a service area planning study should be undertaken. During this initial period a presentation to all hospital department heads and supervisors was made by the administrator and the Bureau team. Funding, which also was approved during this period, was followed by a publicity release in the community paper. Based primarily on the opinion of the administrator, no formal discussion was deemed necessary with either the board of trustees or the medical staff. Some previous research by others from the University had involved collecting data from Able's medical staff. In the opinion of the medical staff, these data were not properly fed back and, as a result, the staff was somewhat reluctant to participate in another research program.

THE ADMISSION SCHEDULING MODEL

The original suggestion to work on admission scheduling came from the Bureau team. It was chosen on the basis of evidence of wide variation in daily census at the hospital. The initial thrust of the project was to control census by forecasting emergency admissions and discharges and controlling the scheduling of elective and urgent admissions. The initial quantifiable savings were expected to come from reduction in nursing staff. Intangible benefits were seen by the University as reducing the probability of serious overload upon nursing personnel and in providing firm future dates for elective admission to both the physicians and patients. It was envisioned that a second round of savings might come from the further refinement of nurse staffing needs once census had been stabilized and from the use of admission and discharge forecasts in work scheduling, and planning manpower needs in social service, dietary, housekeeping, and pharmacy. The project was begun in January 1970.

A doctoral candidate in industrial engineering was assigned the task of review of the existing literature, and the construction of a practical scheduling system. With guidance from two senior members of the Bureau team, he worked for the next two months to devise a theoretical model, analyze the historical variation in census, and establish the goals of a new scheduling system.

The initial work by the Bureau team established a number of postulates which appeared desirable in an admission scheduling model. The admissions office performs three principal functions, the *scheduling* of patients for admission, the *assignment* to specific beds or units, and the completion of certain legal, financial, and clerical tasks associated with the patient's physical *admission* into the hospital. While many admitting offices have a variety of other tasks, these three are central. An ideal admission system would develop appropriate measures of performance of each of these three tasks and also give the admitting officer mechanical aids to complete the necessary work and make the necessary decisions. It was clear that the most cost-effective area for study was in the scheduling portion of the activities. The average occupancy on the four medical-surgical floors during 1965 was 82.6 percent, and average weekly occupancy ranged from 52.4 percent to 95.3 percent. Except for obvious seasonal fluctuations, the variation did not appear to be predictable.[2]

It was clear to the Bureau team that the goal of the admitting office should be to handle the scheduling decisions in a manner which optimally used the resources of the hospital without interfering with the medical needs of the patient. This desired goal statement was different from the actual goal of the Able admitting office, "to keep the hospital full." The actual goal meant that any patient would be scheduled immediately as long as a bed was available and not reserved for possible future emergency. The desired goal under the proposed system was optimal use of beds and other resources. Patients could be deferred for three reasons: the lack of a bed; the lack of nursing staff; and the lack of necessary ancillary services (principally on weekends).

Implementing this scheme would require an assessment of overall demand, forecasts of likely admissions and discharges, and an analysis which changed these data to a daily guideline for the number of elective patients to be admitted. Guidelines for several days into the future would be given the admitting officer each day. Whenever the guideline was reached for a given day, elective patients would be deferred to a later day. Thus, the proposed guide would inevitably introduce short delays for some patients, but would, at the same time, eliminate the "feast or famine" characteristic of occupancy and of nursing workload.

It soon appeared that the critical technical problem was the forecast of occupancy, and the critical policy question was the trade-off between dampening occupancy swings and delaying elective patients. If the forecast of discharges could be made accurately, not only in terms of the number of patients to be discharged but also the identification of patients to be discharged, then the next process of the admitting office, assigning patients, could be facilitated by such information. This led the study group to conclude that estimates provided by physicians with revisions as the individual patient's stay progressed would be most likely to yield the necessary accuracy.

Presenting the Model to Able Staff

This formulation of the admitting office problem (in expanded detail) was reviewed in April 1970 with a key group consisting of the hospital's administrator, director of nursing, controller (and supervisor of the admitting office), and the chief admitting officer. On their acceptance, more intensive work was begun with them in weekly meetings aimed at establishing the specific procedures to be used, developing the necessary information to measure potential achievement, and establishing the desired occupancy levels. From April first through June of 1970, meetings were held weekly with most of the members of this group. The administrator attended occasionally; the controller and the admitting officer were the most frequent participants.

These meetings were generally well received. The controller and the admitting officer were clearly interested in the project from the outset. They and the Bureau team contributed substantial amounts of work on their own between the meetings. The director of nursing was cooperative, as were members of her department, although their role was not large at this point in the project. A number of important findings and outcomes came from the discussion at these meetings and the analysis of relevant data. These were: 1) *There was at the time essentially no constraint on the admitting decision by the admitting office.* Except in periods of extreme crowding called "emergency conditions" which occurred about ten days a year, any patient was accepted and usually admitted the same day as the request. 2) *There was substantial variation in daily census and in nursing hours per patient day.* Variation was caused by both day-of-the-week and seasonal cycles in demand and also by random factors. 3) *The opportunities to improve control of the occupancy level differed in the various parts of the hospital.* Obstetrics, pediatrics, intensive and coronary care were felt to have almost entirely emergency admissions; orthopedics and psychiatry were specialized floors with different occupancy patterns. Eliminating these six units left four nursing units of varying size serving essentially the adult medical-surgical population. 4) *Data were developed which showed high variation in census and in nursing hours per patient day in these four floors.* These data, a portion of which are shown in Figure 7–1, were used to explain the goals of the project to both other members of the hospital staff and the medical staff. The justification was explained in terms of the opportunity to eliminate peak periods of census by deferring some elective admissions to the future. As a result, other periods when the census was low and nursing capabilities were underutilized would be reduced as well. 5) *Studies of the demand for beds in the hospital's service area confirmed that there were more adult medical-surgical beds available in the area than were necessary to meet present or near future forecasts of demand.* This finding verified the impression that the administrator and others in the community had had for some time. 6) *There was considerable uncertainty about the exact bed count on the four floors of interest.* The admitting officer treated the private rooms as available for two-person occupancy whenever necessary to follow her practice of accepting any patient for whom a request was made. The "ideal" capacity of these floors was 133. This could be increased when necessary to 144. The result of this policy, of course, was to

FIGURE 7-1

COMPARISON OF ACTUAL NURSING HOURS AND HOURS NEEDED FOR UNIFORM HOURS PER
PATIENT DAY, FIFTY WEEKS, ABLE HOSPITAL

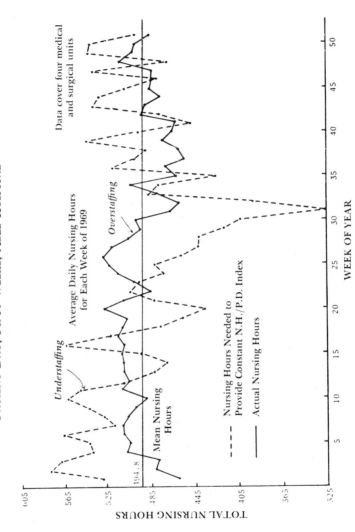

heighten the possibility for variation in census and for overtaxing the available nursing supply. The guideline for establishing an emergency condition was not precise but was approximately a census of 140. The remaining capacity was felt necessary to handle true emergencies which might occur. 7) *Although the hospital had clear policies for defining emergency, urgent, and elective patients, the fact that this classification was only applied in peak occupancy periods resulted in a lack of accurate data on distribution of emergencies.* A special data collection effort was necessary by the admitting office to gain this distribution which was critical in the design of the scheduling model. 8) *Elective surgical patients were accepted by the operating room, not by the admitting office.* The admitting office was notified of these bookings with varying lead times before the patient's arrival and processed them in the usual manner. The operating room functioned well below its physical capacity but was also staffed below maximum levels. When the "emergency" condition existed, it was necessary to cancel prior surgical commitments for some elective patients. 9) *There was no advance notification of discharge given to the admitting office.* In emergency conditions, the admitting office sought out additional information on discharges. At other times the admitting office was notified after the patient had left the building by a discharge slip left at the admitting office by a ward aide who escorted the patient to the door.

After considerable discussion, the appropriate manual and telephone systems for coordinating scheduled admissions between the admitting office and the operating room were arranged and it was agreed that the system of obtaining discharge estimates from physicians on the nursing floors and delivering the information to the admitting office was feasible. It was also agreed that the admitting office could obtain estimates of the approximate length of stay of patients from physicians at the time the admission request was made. It was determined that the hospital computer, an NCR Century 100, could be used to implement the model of a desired occupancy level and provide the admitting office with guidelines on the number of admissions for each of the next eight future days. The program could be fit into the accounts receivable routine of the computer and could use the in-house computerized accounts receivable file as a data base. By June 1970, the hospital management and the Bureau team were convinced of realistic opportunities for smoothing occupancy on these four units. The next steps were to gain the support of the medical staff for an experiment in scheduling elective patients and to begin development of the necessary computer programs and new procedures for implementing a scheduling model.

The key role of the physicians in the admitting scheduling system had been recognized in general, but only in April and May of 1970 did the specific changes required of them in their hospital practice begin to take shape.

Specifically, physicians needed: to accept delays in their elective admissions when the desired occupancy level was reached; and to provide estimates of when their patients would be discharged. They obviously would need explanation of why they should do these things. Strategy was discussed by the Bureau team with the hospital administrator. He favored a discussion with the key leaders of the medical staff rather than a formal presentation by the Bureau team to the executive committee of the staff. He held a luncheon meeting for six doctors representing the medical and surgical services and pathology, and containing the chief of staff as well as several present or former elected officers. This group heard the presentation and were cautiously favorable. They, rather than the Bureau team, made the presentation to the staff executive committee, which agreed to support the project on a trial basis. In September (1970), the matter was presented by the chief of staff as an informational report from the executive committee to a quarterly meeting of the full staff. The project director made a presentation of the goals and methods and identified the two key elements of interest to the staff. There were questions and some misgivings about the discharge estimates: (1) the doctors did not always know, and some were reluctant to guess, when the patients could be discharged, and (2) some doctors worried that their estimates would somehow be used against them by the utilization review committee, or even by Blue Shield. They were not completely reassured by promises of confidentiality. (Blue Shield had no access to the estimates, nor any legitimate reason to request them.) The discussion was brief, however, and the chief of staff and chairman of the meeting moved on to other items without a formal vote, reemphasizing the trial nature of the proposal.

COMPUTER PROBLEMS

Acceptance by the medical staff left only the technical problem of producing the printout which would provide the basis for requesting physician discharge estimates, and the policy issue of determining current occupancy levels. The data processing requirements were in principle easily interrelated with an existing inpatient billing routine which was part of the software package of a recently purchased small computer, adding about ten minutes to a four-hour daily run updating patient ledgers. Unfortunately, an employee hired to install the computer packages proved to be unfamiliar with both the language and with the hospital billing systems. By October, the hospital was falling behind in inpatient billings, and some three months behind in outpatient billings. Such delays caused the controller and the administrator to feel a natural concern for the hospital's cash position, and the admission scheduling system was given little attention. In November, the

Bureau team finally proposed that their personnel assist in catching up in the billing, simply to provide computer time to debug the scheduling subroutine and to provide a current data base for the scheduling system. One member of the Bureau team spent much of his Christmas vacation helping to work down the backlog, learning the computer language, and debugging the scheduling subroutine. By then, two months had passed since the nurses had been informed that they would shortly be receiving training on when to request discharge estimates from physicians, and three months since physicians had been told of the impending experiment. In December the planned training of the nursing staff was again postponed, while the Bureau team learned a great deal more than they ever had wanted to know about the internal storage, disc capacity, unidimensional arrays, and other interesting features of the hospital computer and its software. The project director pressed the administrator to seek a data processing manager skilled in the equipment. He was hired in December and spent most of January familiarizing himself with the packaged routines. In the meantime, the Bureau team completed the debugging. In February 1971, nearly six months later than the September 1970 estimate, the first pilot runs of census data were produced.

IMPLEMENTATION

The continuing expectation that the computer problem could be solved "soon" had led to a decision to start securing an expected length of stay estimate at the time a patient was scheduled for admission before the system was ready to utilize the estimates in setting the number of admissions required to stabilize occupancy. This procedure had some unexpected problems because the admitting request was often made by the doctor's secretary who did not know the estimated length of stay. Also, a clear explanation of why the unused estimate was being requested proved difficult for the admitting staff. The intended use of estimates, to accurately predict bed supply so that elective admissions could be scheduled (delayed) to stabilize occupancy, required considerable physician interest in stable occupancy in order to be effective. During early 1971, the admitting officer indicated she was experiencing considerable pressure. The design and preparation for introducing the system had caused tension with the nursing department, but by now the controller was anxious to see the system get started and appeared unsympathetic to reports of additional problems from nursing, the physicians, or their secretaries. All of these problems were traceable to the Bureau team, but only rarely did the admitting officer show irritation with them. Like the controller, she had become an active proponent of the system.

When all elements of the admitting scheduling system were finally started at the end of February 1971, two members of the Bureau team were on hand full time to help the hospital personnel keep things running as smoothly as possible. One team member was based in the admitting office to assist in using the scheduling allowances and other admitting oriented tasks. The second team member circulated among the four nursing units in the system, to deal with questions and problems in collecting discharge estimates from the individual patients' physicians. Much of the time on the nursing units was spent attempting to persuade nursing unit personnel both that the system would actually work and that when it did there would be significant advantages to them and the hospital. The understanding of the physicians was a key element to their accepting and participating in the system, but achieving that understanding in individual physicians was a time-consuming, difficult, and often frustrating assignment. These difficulties prompted the Bureau team to supplement individual contacts with a more formal communication effort:

> In answer to specific questions which had been raised by members of the medical staff, a four minute slide-tape presentation was assembled in the latter part of May. This presentation, in addition to addressing specific questions, again reviewed the value of accurate discharge estimates and the need for the acceptance of some non-emergent delays in admissions. A small projector and screen which could be easily operated were placed in one corner of the physician's library daily and many observed the presentation.[3]

One must remember that a key feature of the admitting scheduling system was that it explicitly connected one aspect of medical need (admission on request) with one aspect of efficiency (stable occupancy) in a trade-off relation. An increase in stability could be achieved by lowering the desired occupancy level, but only at the cost of increasing the probability that a requested admission would be deferred. The key policy decision was setting the desired occupancy level, agreed upon by the administrator in December 1970, at 135 (ninety-five percent occupancy, ten percent probability of a delayed admission).

Late April and early May was a period of unusually high admission requests, and it was apparent that the admission scheduling system was not working as well as hoped. The census of the whole hospital, including the four units controlled by the scheduling system, was lower in the last week of May than it had been for several years. Further, the total patient days of care rendered since January were down and, except for the three-week spurt, had been down consistently during the five-month period. Patient days are a critical factor in the revenue of a hospital, and the Able administrator and the controller were quite sensitive to any possible loss of inpatient revenue. At the same time, some members of the medical staff were becoming more vocal in their complaints.

PHYSICIAN DISCONTENT WITH ADMISSION SCHEDULING

The effort to constrain the occupancy level which occurred in the early part of May resulted in deferring the admission of about thirteen elective patients. A number of doctors involved announced that they would take those patients to Martin Hospital, and at least nine of the thirteen patients were admitted to Martin. The doctors also were annoyed at the requests for advance notification of discharge; this annoyance was experienced most directly by the head nurses, staff nurses, and ward secretaries responsible for securing estimates from the doctors. The original director of nursing had been replaced several months before for reasons highlighted perhaps by the Bureau team activities, but not directly connected with them. Rather difficult problems of communication between the former director and other members of the administrative group had been experienced before the study team arrived. The new director was more supportive of the admitting scheduling system, and with some encouragement from a team member, she began to visit the four units several times a week to talk with nurses and encourage them to continue asking for estimates. But the problem was acute for some nursing unit staff who were not comfortable requesting the doctors to provide estimates and who became very upset when doctors attacked them for doing so. A study team member also would visit the units regularly and would regularly find one or two nurses ready to abandon the requests because of treatment received from physicians when requesting discharge estimates. In spite of this, some head nurses appeared to honestly support the system, and tried to make it work.

Exaggeration and rumor generation occurred in late May. Some doctors cited instances of thirteen-day delays for elective patients, eight-day delays for urgent patients, and the routine delay of elective patients even when there were "empty beds all over the house." These statements were inaccurate in substance, but fairly represented physician annoyance with the system. Patients were actually deferred because of scheduling model constraints for less than two weeks in early May. After that time demand had slacked off and the admission scheduling limits were not reached. No emergency patient was ever deferred; no urgent patient was ever deferred longer than three days. On June 2, the administrator and project director met and agreed to review the general situation with both the hospital and Bureau groups and also to meet with the full medical staff at their quarterly meeting in the evening of June 8. There was substantial question as to whether the system could be made to work.

At the meeting of the medical staff, the administrator encouraged wide-ranging discussion which touched upon the relationship of Able and Martin

Hospitals and the doctors' obligation to assist in the control of the cost of hospital and medical care. The project director reviewed the goals of the admitting project and asked for continued support of both the discharge forecasts and the short delay of elective admissions. The discussion was animated. In addition to reiteration of several of the rumor statements, it revealed several aspects of the impact of the system as seen by the physicians. One physician cited a case of a middle-aged man with alcoholism and a bleeding ulcer whom he thought might exacerbate his ulcer to the point of an acute hemorrhage by drinking if he could not be admitted to the hospital immediately. The doctor was annoyed because he had to reclassify the patient as emergency when in his mind the patient's condition at the moment was only urgent. His definition of emergency clearly was limited to those conditions which were immediately and directly life threatening although the staff's formal definition, and the one assumed by the Bureau team, was much more lenient. Another doctor remarked that if he had to wait to admit elective patients he forgot some of the details of the workup he completed in his office, and thus was forced to repeat parts of the history and physical when the patient was admitted two or three days later. This remark drew some nodding heads. Another doctor added that since physicians were in short supply the community owed it to the doctors to meet their needs. The physicians were not more enthusiastic when it was pointed out that reducing the variation in nursing census would reduce the costs of hospital care for the people of the community. The implication was quite clear that the system should optimize physician convenience and whatever extra cost was involved should be paid.

Other comments were directed to the forecasts of discharge requested at several different points during the patient's stay. The doctors felt that repeated requests three days, two days, and one day prior to expected discharge were unnecessary. Some commented that they were frequently asked for a discharge estimate before they had a chance to work the patient up and others noted that they were at one point being pressed for discharge dates on patients awaiting transfer to nursing homes when they in fact had no control over discharge dates. (This had been corrected several weeks before the meeting.) Another level of concern was indicated by the remark: "Blue Shield might get hold of these estimates and not pay our fees if we do not discharge the patient on the estimated day." This appeared to be a serious concern to at least a few physicians. Several doctors indicated or implied that they were deliberately giving long forecasts because of this possible danger, a fact which was obvious by comparing their patients' estimated and actual discharge dates. The restatement that these estimates were not even given to the hospital's own utilization review committee did not noticeably reassure these doctors. The team director again asked for cooperation on an experimental basis and the meeting closed without action by the medical staff.

RECONSIDERATION OF THE SYSTEM

Very shortly after this meeting the nursing department noticed a new wave of complaints, with some doctors promising to eliminate the system and routinely refusing to supply discharge estimates. These remarks and actions were sometimes made in a manner highly upsetting to the nursing staff and ward secretaries. On June 16 the operations group, consisting of the administrator, controller, associate administrator, director of nursing, admitting officer, supervisor of ward secretaries, operating room supervisor, and assistant administrator, met with three members of the Bureau team. The administrator had requested the meeting to consider whether or not the system should be continued. Both nurses reported very serious concern with the attitude of the physicians. The director also noted that the response rate to the discharge requests was falling despite constant reminders by ward secretaries and nurses. The operating room supervisor reported some additional problems with the scheduling of surgery which appeared to be independent of the admission scheduling system. The admitting officer reported little problem, either in getting the initial discharge estimates or in managing the system from her point of view. The supervisor of ward secretaries reported that his people were increasingly reluctant to ask for estimates. Discussion moved to the competitive position of Able and Martin Hospitals. There was extensive discussion of the rumor that Martin Hospital was quite full of patients and of the problem of low occupancy which had plagued Able for most of the year.

In the course of the discussion it became clear that the general census loss had been from floors not involved in the scheduling system and that there was a lack of data on exactly what the impact of the scheduling system had been. The administrator again indicated that it might be better to discontinue the system and requested members of his staff to comment. The controller and admitting officer were strongly in support of continuing the system with modification for thirty days, with further discussion at that time. The administrator agreed to this, and decided to meet with the administrator of Martin Hospital to permit verification of rumors about their census and of the transfer of patients whose admission had been delayed. It was also agreed that the nursing staff might themselves supply estimates when they were reasonably sure of the accuracy. Finally it was agreed that the administrator, director of nursing, and team director would meet with the head nurses, ward secretaries, and ward managers of the four floors involved to attempt to counter the rumors and to communicate both management's understanding of the burdens being placed on these people and the decision to continue the system for an additional thirty days.

The meeting with the Martin Hospital administrator occurred on June 22.

She confirmed that the hospital had renovated and improved inpatient accommodations and added a chemotherapy service. Martin Hospital had also installed new dictating equipment in the past year. This equipment could be reached by ordinary telephone and used to update medical records. She also noted that Martin did not check specifically for history and physical within seventy-two hours of admission, but relied instead on postdischarge review by the appropriate medical committees on the quality of care as a whole. This policy, she noted, was much more popular with the doctors, and she believed that they recognized the other advantages to the use of Martin Hospital.

She agreed to release data on census and to trace the patients who allegedly changed from Able to Martin admissions and also agreed to provide data for a study of the potential cost reduction of sharing services between the two hospitals. She declined to participate in any admission coordination procedures.

The meeting with members of the Able nursing staff was held late in the same day. One of the hospital's most senior head nurses said that the doctors on her floor were now supplying discharge estimates and that she felt their attitude would improve as time went on. Another senior head nurse noted that it was difficult to supply a reasonable estimate for some kinds of patients (particularly the aged, chronically ill). A ward secretary pointed out that estimates were being requested on the day of surgery when the patient, the doctor, and the medical record were all off the nursing unit. This made compliance very difficult. Several versions of what appeared to be the same rumors as encountered among the medical staff were brought out.

It became clear that there were two concerns among the people present. One belief was that the hospital was taking a series of actions which invaded the prerogatives of the physician, such as forcing him to defer emergency admissions; the second was that the system appeared to be resulting in a reduction of work available for nurses. One nurse commented that the hospital was turning patients away, but at the same time the opportunities for part-time work for nurses had decreased. The administrator noted the potential advantages of the scheduling system, and that the nursing department would avoid being overworked as it has been during peak census periods in the past. The team director stressed the new option of the nursing department to use their judgment in requesting estimates from the physicians, and in the case of registered nurses to supply estimates on their own when appropriate.

The early summer of 1971 saw the admitting scheduling system in place and operating, but by no means stabilized as a part of Able Hospital's standard procedures. The controller was a strong supporter because the analysis preceding the innovation had clarified for him the possibility of budgeting quarterly adjustments in nurse staffing, with a potential savings estimated at $40,000 per year. The simple good sense of the system appealed to the admitting officer, and the increase in significance which it gave to her own role made it attractive to her. The pressures she experienced had come fully three months before the problems of securing estimates had hit the nursing floors, and in a sense were investments she had already made in the system. Floor personnel, notably nurses, saw few benefits, some level of irritation if it continued, and some degree of job insecurity and usurping of doctors' prerogatives if it were successful. Only a minority felt it made sense and were truly willing to support the system. The administrator had a vivid memory of the emotions generated in the medical staff during the two weeks when the system seriously constrained admissions. He also recognized that the cost savings of the system were proportional to the number of delayed admissions. Among physicians there was now a vocal minority that opposed the system in principle, a minority which would probably increase in size if admission delays were experienced again.

Analysis of Martin data by the Bureau team showed no evidence of a significant shift of patients to that hospital. Martin had had two near-capacity weeks with the adult medical-surgical service in May and June, but like Able, its occupancy was subject to wide and unpredictable swings. It was not true that it had been "crammed to the gills" after the Able scheduling system had been installed. Analysis of the revised and less demanding discharge estimate system showed that accuracy had not declined, and that the response rate was somewhat better. The data were reviewed with the administrator and his key personnel, and again there was consensus that continuance of the system required that the desired occupancy be set at a level which generated very few patient delays. In fact only three patients were delayed during the last half of 1971.

FAILURE

By midsummer of 1971 it became somewhat easier for the Bureau team to assess the implications of a continuing desired occupancy level that generated very few delayed admissions. Among these implications were a rather low return on the bad will and emotional strain that the repeated requests for discharge estimates were producing. An August meeting with the medical staff's executive committee had confirmed that the executive committee did not think it appropriate for them to help make the discharge estimate system work, but that further revisions in it might reduce the irritations it caused. The executive committee determined that the medical staff should be polled on the continuation of the system at its September meeting. The result was enough continuing criticism that the initial request for a discharge estimate was dropped, and only a single estimate, to be provided voluntarily by the doctor twenty-four hours before discharge was retained. The last collection of data to estimate the accuracy of estimates had been done in July, and there seemed little reason to collect further data.

At this point the system was functioning at a level scarcely different from the original admissions procedures. A minimal control of overcrowding was in effect which would eliminate the highest five percent of daily census values. Even assuming that the nursing department could adjust staffing uniformly, this would result in insignificant savings, little different than the added cost of maintaining the system. The reason for retaining the system was because the costs of reinstalling it were great and it was hoped that attitudes might change over time.

Instead, the opposite happened. An article appeared in *Medical World News*, January 7, 1972. This brief and rather inaccurate article confused Able Hospital with other programs in other institutions, even to the point of placing the Able administrator in the wrong hospital. At least one member of the medical staff was highly offended, apparently because the article failed to give sufficient recognition to the amount of work and support the Able doctors had given the project. He also served as a hospital trustee, and in this role he urged that the program be discontinued. The medical executive committee recommended discontinuance, and the admitting scheduling system was dropped in February 1972.

NOTES

1. [Chapters 7 and 8] record detailed histories of the implementation process as the Bureau team observed and experienced it. The reports were written by members of the research staff, and therefore are not impartial. The authors were conscious of this problem, and three steps were taken to overcome it. A member of the project team who had no responsibility for achieving results within the hospital guided the preparation and in two cases wrote the reports; multiple reviews of draft reports were made by members of the research team not directly responsible for the innovation; and a guideline for writing emphasized reporting sequences of events, rather than plausible explanations for them. In many cases daily notes, working memos, and similar documents by team members were the principal sources of information. The guidelines for report preparation also emphasized the protection of persons, and incidents which might have added color but would have embarrassed hospital personnel are not recorded.
2. Galen P. Briggs, Jr., "Inpatient Admissions Scheduling: An Application to a Nursing Service," Doctoral dissertation, The University of Michigan, 1971.
3. *Ibid.*, pp. 62–63.

8 | The Success of
Admission
Scheduling at
Baker Hospital

Kurt R. Student

THE SETTING

Baker Hospital is a modern 290 bed facility which serves a number of industrial communities on the outskirts of a major urban area. Baker is one of four general community hospitals controlled by a hospital authority. Baker has neither internship nor residency programs. Some of the medical staff are active at other hospitals located in nearby communities. Some are specialists, but most are general practitioners. A small number are osteopaths. Baker has neither an associate administrator nor an assistant administrator; all department heads report directly to the administrator. (See organization chart, Figure 8-1.) One reason for this is that some functions such as planning, public relations, purchasing, and some accounting are centralized in the office of the hospital authority to whose executive director the Baker administrator reports. Such an organizational structure requires the administrator to be involved in all major interdepartmental decisions because the organization is linked together only in the top management position.

Admission scheduling was introduced in Baker in early 1972, after several other activities initiated by the University of Michigan Bureau of Hospital Administration team were underway. There were significant differences between the admission scheduling system designed for Baker and the one implemented at Able. The Able system was designed to stabilize occupancy at

Reprinted from *Cost Control in Hospitals*, John R. Griffith, Walton M. Hancock, and Fred C. Munson, eds., "The Success of Admission Scheduling at Baker Hospital," by Kurt R. Student, by permission of the Health Administration Press, Ann Arbor, Mich., 1976.

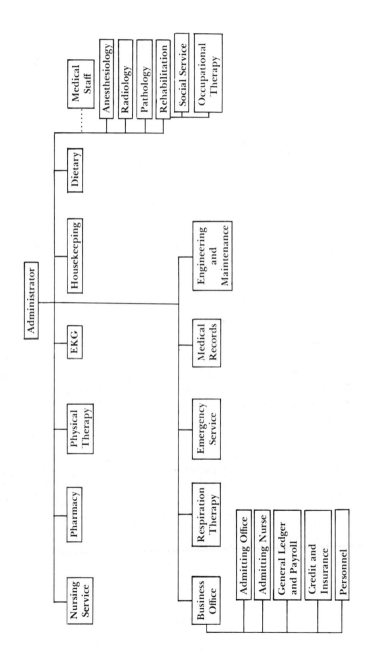

FIGURE 8-1

BAKER HOSPITAL ORGANIZATION, 1972

a level below the bed capacity of the hospital. At Baker, the occupancy and the demand for beds in the three medical and surgical units covered were already stable at relatively high levels, and a Bureau planning study indicated demand would increase. The threefold objective of the Baker admission scheduling system was: (1) to reduce cancellations and transfers under the conditions of high and stable census levels; (2) to control the mix of medical and surgical patients in the hospital; and (3) to schedule a significant number of medical admissions so that preadmission testing could be performed.

Prior to the scheduling system development, physicians scheduled surgical admissions with the Baker operating room supervisor and the admitting office held beds open for these surgical patients until about 3:00 P.M. Any beds not assigned to surgical patients by that time were then filled, if possible, by medical patients. Four or five admitting office clerks telephoned patients on the medical waiting list and requested that the patients come in for immediate hospitalization. Frequently, these prospective patients could not arrange for their hospitalization on such short notice, and beds remained unfilled. For that reason the occupancy level was somewhat lower than the demand for services would indicate, and the variation and inconvenience were borne mainly by the medical service. The initial settings of the medical and surgical admission allowances for Baker were based on the hospital's historical data so that there would be no change in the balance between medical and surgical admissions.

In 1970, the Bureau team conducted a long-range planning study which indicated that the demand for inpatient beds at Baker was high and that this demand would increase. By July 1970, community demand required that Baker operate at an approximate occupancy level of ninety percent, while the planning study determined that the expected twenty percent increase in Baker's service area population over ten years would decrease Baker's share of admissions from its service area unless inpatient beds were added or the occupancy level was increased. Since there were no immediate plans to increase the number of Baker's inpatient beds, there was pressure to increase the hospital's occupancy level to offset as much as possible Baker's decreased potential to serve its growing service population. This desire to maintain high occupancy without increases in admission cancellations and organizational stress was a primary factor in the decision by the Baker administration and the Bureau to design and implement an admission scheduling system for the hospital.

THE ADMITTING NURSE ROLE

In February 1971, the Baker administrator had established the position of admitting nurse within the admitting office. His motivation for doing so was primarily the success he had experienced with such a position in his former hospital. Initially, her purpose was to expedite the admissions process for scheduled surgical patients, so that they could receive the necessary tests and exams on the day of admission (in anticipation of surgery the following day). Although there were certain routine presurgical tests, the admitting nurse normally contacted the admitting physician to obtain specific orders for each patient. Since surgery was performed essentially on a Monday through Friday schedule, the admitting nurse position was staffed five days a week. Because of the strong nursing orientation of the admitting nurse function, the position was initially established so that she was administratively responsible to the director of nursing. However, she performed her job geographically and functionally within the admitting office (which is a component of the hospital's business office). A number of conflicts arose. The situation was resolved within a few months by making the admitting nurse directly responsible to the business office manager, while retaining professional liaison with the director of nursing.

Preparatory activities for the implementation of the admission scheduling system began in November 1971. The Bureau staff analyzed PAS data on patient discharges in order to establish a basis for the historical discharge estimating system used to establish "flag dates." The analysis indicated that patients' age and service categories were the best explainers of length of stay; the attending physician was the third best explainer.

THE EARLY TESTING TRIAL

One of the early efforts was to determine the feasibility of sending medical patients to the laboratory and to radiology for diagnostic testing early in the morning of their day of admission prior to going to the nursing floor. The test results could be made available to the attending physician on his visit the day after admission instead of two days after admission, thereby possibly reducing the length of stay of adult medical patients. The experimental results indicated that patients had to be at the hospital by 9:00 A.M., that fifteen minutes of laboratory time was needed for the usual blood sampling, and that seventy-five percent of the adult medical patients required radiological tests, usually chest x-rays or flat plates. Two conclusions were reached as a result of this trial: (1) early testing was feasible and should be presented to the hospital for consideration, and (2) successful implementation of early testing, as well as of the admission scheduling system, would require much greater coordination between the admitting nurse, the admitting office, the laboratory, radiology, housekeeping, and the nursing unit personnel.

IMPROVING COORDINATION

In late January 1972, the Bureau team discussed the lack of coordination evidenced in the early testing trial and the coordination which would be required for implementing an innovation as encompassing as the admission scheduling system. The Bureau favored an internal steering committee to plan a series of meetings which would establish the required interdepartmental coordination at Baker. On February 2 a conference was held with the administrator. The Bureau staff explained that during the early testing experiment, patients had appeared on the nursing floors without any knowledge by nursing personnel as to what was occurring. The nursing department had been notified, but communication to head nurses and staff nurses was failing. The need and value of several coordinating meetings was clear, and the first meeting was scheduled for February 17.

The chief of the internal medicine department, a prominent surgeon representing the surgical department, the chiefs of radiology and pathology, the administrator, the business office manager, the director of nursing, and four members of the Bureau team attended the first meeting. The Bureau team reviewed the admission scheduling proposal and stressed the meeting's importance for its success. The early testing trial was reviewed to illustrate the need for coordinated cooperation. A particular effort was made to seek comments and support from members of the medical staff.

The internist was particularly enthusiastic about implementing early testing. He stated he had long favored better screening of medical admissions, and he realized that scheduling diagnostic tests in a medically preferred sequence would have great potential for reducing patient length of stay. The surgeon was also enthusiastic about the proposal. The radiologist and the pathologist made no comment about the admission scheduling system and were concerned only in their departments' involvement in early testing activities. The acceptance of the Bureau's proposal by the internist and the surgeon made quite clear to the others attending that they believed the medical staff would want to implement the innovations quickly. When the Bureau's staff explained that the requests for discharge estimates were based on analyses of Baker's PAS patient discharge data, both the internist and the surgeon indicated they wanted to use these analyses for medical staff utilization review purposes. However, the Bureau cautioned that releasing the data for this purpose might be viewed as threatening by some of the medical staff and might result in their reluctance to provide estimates and to cooperate in implementing the system. It was agreed, with some reluctance by the surgeon, that the discharge estimates would be used solely for admission scheduling purposes. The meeting ended with agreement that the admitting nurse would meet with the chief of medicine and doctors from pathology and radiology to establish the preferred diagnostic test sequences. The Bureau agreed to assist her in compiling these lists and arranging their distribution. It was also agreed that the admitting nurse should attend the next task force meeting.

The second meeting held on March 9 included those attending the first meeting, the admitting nurse, and the housekeeping department manager. Prior to the meeting, agreement had been reached on the role of the admitting nurse for administering the early testing sequences, and at this meeting it was decided to implement early testing concurrently. Agreement was also reached to start up the admission scheduling system on April 10. The director of nursing voiced some reservation about getting the physicians to cooperate with nursing personnel in securing the discharge estimates; she stated that some members of the medical staff were well-known for their lack of cooperation with nursing. The chief of medicine replied that he would personally "straighten out the troublemakers;" the surgeon also agreed to help secure medical staff cooperation. This outspoken support by two influential members of Baker's medical staff set the stage for initiating the implementation activities. Although the director of nursing voiced some lack of conviction and lingering reservations about the nursing department's role in securing discharge estimates, there was a strong desire from the doctors to begin implementation as soon as possible. The medical staff executive committee met on April 6 and approved the beginning of the admitting scheduling system.

Admitting Office Reorganization

In January, Baker's admitting office was found to require extensive reorganization in order to raise its effectiveness to the level required by the admission scheduling system. The Baker office received intensive attention from the Bureau staff during February, March, and April. It should be remembered that the office had been given expanded responsibilities only a year and a half earlier. Well developed traditions and even written protocols were missing. Communications within and from the office were incomplete. Both the employees and first line supervision seemed unclear as to their full responsibilities.

The general admitting procedures and the specific admitting clerk tasks were studied in detail for all three shifts. As a result, the procedures were categorized into three activities: direct patient admission activities: patient transfer activities; and census activities. A detailed work flow was made for each of these activities, and three major problem areas were identified: there was a lack of job definition on the afternoon and midnight shifts; there was too great an overlap in responsibility between shifts for the performance of many of the activities; and there was need for greater communication from the admitting clerks to the admitting office supervisor and the business office manager. On March 1, the Bureau recommended strengthening supervision of the second shift as well as a number of changes in office procedures and work flow. The admitting office's second shift was deemed particularly crucial to the admission scheduling system because second shift personnel were to input Baker's data. Because the second shift admitting clerks were less experienced than the first shift clerks, the admitting office's second shift received particular attention from the Bureau's implementation team. An experienced second shift supervisor was hired, and several clerks were trained to operate the terminal. The adoption of these changes proceeded slowly and required the extensive involvement of Bureau personnel.

Start-up occurred April 10, 1972. Four broad and interrelated problem areas developed almost immediately and consumed major efforts of the Bureau team for the next two months. These problem areas were the discharge estimating system; the communications between nursing, admissions, lab, and x-ray; surgeons' dissatisfaction with allowances; and resistance from the operating room supervisor. These problems were simultaneous and interconnected but are described separately below for clarity.

The Discharge Estimating System

The Bureau team was familiar with the resistance which physicians had to making discharge estimates for their patients, and considerably modified the system which had been used in Able. A study of historical data indicated that patient age, diagnosis and admitting physician were the best predictors of length of stay; they were used to determine a probable discharge date for each admitted patient. Three or two days before this date each patient's record would be flagged, and the physician would be asked to estimate a discharge date for the patient on this "flag day." Such a system relies on a computer for three functions: to identify the flag day for each patient (for about twenty percent of the patients each day); to provide printout for discharge estimate requests and to process the estimates obtained from the physicians; and to provide the scheduling guidelines for the admitting supervisor's use. A computer terminal was installed to support the dynamic system, and the data collection and the processing system were begun in April.

Initially, the computer output was not used for scheduling decisions. It was understood that discharge estimates would be difficult to obtain and the initial results would not be sufficiently accurate to provide a stable system. Beds available through discharge were calculated manually, based on the average number of expected discharges for each day of the week. The intention was to change over to the dynamic system once it proved stable.

The provision of patient discharge estimates soon proved troublesome. On April 21 a meeting was held with the head nurses and ward clerks to review the discharge estimate situation. Two of the clerks attending were quite negative; one stated that she believed the system would not work and that she would not participate in securing estimates. The percentages of requested estimates actually supplied were forty-seven, forty-nine, and sixty-one percent, respectively, for the medical, medical-surgical, and surgical units. The head nurse on the surgical unit was more receptive when the physicians visited the unit. She was more interested in making an effort to ask each physician personally for the required discharge estimates, and she also felt that estimates were easier to obtain on her unit.

During the middle of May, the overall discharge estimate response rate on the three nursing units declined, and varied from ten percent to forty percent, indicating an apparent lack of interest on the part of both nursing personnel and physicians. During a period in July, the overall physician response rate was twenty-two percent with an accuracy rate of thirty-four percent.[1] Since previous research indicates that if physicians are asked to provide an estimate of discharge one day prior to a predicted discharge based on historical data for the patient's service classification, the accuracy rate can be from eighty-five to ninety-five percent correct,[2] an accuracy rate of thirty-four percent suggested an apparent unwillingness on the part of Baker's medical staff to cooperate with implementing this aspect of the admission scheduling system.

The Bureau was dealing with two problems simultaneously, the problem of improving the physician response and accuracy rate, and the problem of making the manually based scheduling system work. There was a shortage of resources to handle both problems thoroughly and an inevitable tendency to concentrate on the scheduling system, which was producing real decisions, and therefore had to work if the hospital was going to admit patients. It was argued that heavy emphasis on getting the physicians to do better on estimating would cause further antagonism. Moreover, there was no readily available mechanism to reach individual physicians in order to get them to do better. The manual system of estimating available beds was adequate, and after several months of indecision, the effort to secure physicians' estimates was terminated.

COORDINATION AND COMMUNICATION

Shortly after the start-up of the admission scheduling system, it became clear to the implementation team that greater coordination was needed both within the nursing department and between nursing and the other departments involved in the system. Unwittingly, problems were being created simply because one department lacked knowledge of the impact of its actions on the other departments. One example of such problems involved the assignment of a specific bed to a specific patient prior to or at the time of admission. Traditionally, it had been the responsibility of nursing unit personnel to assign surgical patients to beds based on the list of patients scheduled for surgery the following day. With the need for bed control in the admitting office in order to make the scheduling system work well, the Bureau team tried to have the bed assignment function switched to admitting office personnel. However, because of the feeling among nursing personnel that the admitting clerks would not be able to make "good" assignments based on both the personal and medical considerations of the patient, they resisted giving up their control.

The computer-printed nurses' reports used to collect discharge estimates for individual patients from their physicians created other problems. The reports were produced on the computer terminal in the admitting office, and were distributed to the nursing units early each morning. Nursing unit personnel attempted to obtain the discharge estimates from the physicians, and filled in certain information on the reports. Since this information was to be input data for the next day's reports, both the format and content were crucial. In fairness, it should be noted that the entire situation was aggravated by a number of technical problems in producing accurate and timely reports. Corrections were not always completed and computed in the system.

Such problems appeared to be attributable to a lack of organizational coordination, and the Bureau proposed that a communication meeting be held with nursing supervisors and head nurses, the admitting officer, and the admitting nurse. After continued urging by the Bureau an initial "gripe session" was held on May 16. This meeting had an immediate cathartic effect.

As these meetings continued to be held, they became an increasingly important part of Baker's operating structure. When the meetings began to deal with more important interdepartmental matters, decisions had to be delayed because, in the absence of an associate or assistant administrator, only the administrator, himself, could deal with these new issues coming before the communication meetings. In January 1973 the meetings were rescheduled so that the administrator could attend all the meetings personally.

CHANGING THE SURGICAL ADMISSION ALLOWANCES

The Bureau's system of medical and surgical admission allowances helped to increase the number of medical admissions in May 1972, and there was also a small increase in the number of surgical admissions. However, during the period 1969–1971, forty additional physicians had been granted hospital privileges at Baker, and a considerable number of these physicians were given surgical privileges. Consequently, the number of procedures per physician had been decreasing for reasons independent of the Bureau's activities. For whatever reason, implementation of admission allowances became the immediate focus. This brought the Bureau into direct conflict with a powerful group within the hospital—the surgical department of the medical staff.

On May 22 a surgeon known for his volatile temper became angered because he observed a number of empty beds in the surgical nursing unit. This occurred because the operating room supervisor, who scheduled surgical admissions, had not implemented the Bureau's surgical admission allowances. The surgeon demanded that one of the nurses present write a note verifying that there were ten empty beds, and then met with two of his colleagues, one of whom was a former chief of the medical staff. These three then went to the administrator and voiced a vigorous complaint. At the next regular surgical department meeting, a surgeons' ad hoc committee was formed to review the surgical admission allowances. This committee was appointed on the spot by the chief of surgery, and consisted of the three surgeons who were most vocal in their complaints, plus the administrator at his request. Shortly thereafter, the administrator told the Bureau's project principal that he was under pressure. Some of the surgeons were apparently talking to board members and the executive director of the hospital authority. The project principal, the administrator, and the executive director met promptly. After a thorough discussion, the executive director authorized further work with the system. He noted that the overall impact was helpful to the patients and to the doctors and that the slight slack in the summer months would give time to settle disputes and smooth the system's operations.

On June 7 two of the Bureau's investigators met with the surgeon's committee in order to resolve the conflict. The surgeons objected to the Bureau's basing the allowances for medical and surgical admissions upon historical data which did not reflect Baker's increased occupancy level, and they claimed the allowances favored the medical department of the medical staff. The allowances actually gave the surgeons a slightly higher fraction of total hospital admissions than they had held historically. However, the surgeons requested a redefinition of equity between medical and surgical admissions. According to the surgeons on the ad hoc committee, equity was equal waiting times for medical and surgical patients. Because the surgical length of stay is about thirty-six percent shorter than the medical, 7.2 days compared to 11.2 days, this would allow the surgeons to admit proportionally more patients.

At the surgeons' request, the Bureau readjusted the allowances by basing them on an arranged balance in the length of the waiting times for medical and surgical admissions. At the same time, the administrator was able to transfer six pediatric beds to the adult medical-surgical unit. (This decision had resulted from other studies.) As a result of these negotiations, the surgical admission allowance was increased by eight per week; the medical admissions allowance was decreased by two per week. The Bureau anticipated pediatric scheduling problems due to the bed reduction, and preliminary pediatric admission allowances were determined. However, the pediatric system was not implemented because both the Baker administrator and the Bureau wanted to concentrate on the adult medical and surgical units. In addition to changing the allowances, it was agreed that the business office manager would periodically review the length of the waiting lines and make admission allowance adjustments in order to maintain equity in the length of the admission waiting times. Shortly thereafter, on June 21, the new allowances were implemented. The surgical department was satisfied; the revised allowances were accepted without further resistance. Curiously, the change did not arouse resistance from the internal medicine department.

THE OR SUPERVISOR AND THE SURGICAL ALLOWANCES

Prior to the Bureau's intervention, the Baker operating room supervisor had the responsibility of controlling surgical admissions by virtue of her surgery scheduling function. When most admission control was transferred to the admissions office, she kept this power. Moreover, the hospital had an admissions process in which surgical patients received preference. Surgical patients were scheduled first; medical patients were then called to fill whatever open beds remained. As a result of her crucial role, the operating room supervisor established close relationships with the surgeons. She viewed the Bureau's activities as a reduction in her role and in her power vis-à-vis the surgeons. She alone kept records of surgical admissions and surgery schedules. When the Bureau's representatives asked to see these data to establish the admission allowances, she claimed the data were not available. Her lack of cooperation continued; as already noted, she did not implement the initial allowances correctly. On some days she would exceed the allowances, on other days she would schedule fewer surgeries than the allowances. This practice continued after the revised allowances were agreed to on June 21. However by this time, the Bureau had arranged for the admitting office to keep records of surgical admissions. These deviations from the revised allowances were brought to the administrator's attention, and he wrote a sharply worded memo to the operating room supervisor, ordering her to implement the surgical allowances. A copy of the memo was sent to the chief of the surgical department; another copy was posted in the physicians' staff room. The memo had its intended effect and the surgical allowances were implemented properly. Shortly thereafter, the operating room supervisor became a regular participant in the communication meetings. She became an important and cooperative member of this group; on several occasions she praised the Bureau's system and stated that the Bureau had improved the operation of the hospital.

With the change of heart of the OR supervisor, the initial installation problems subsided. Three of the four—communication, the supervisor, and the allowances—were solved by specific adjustments. The fourth, discharge estimating, had been deferred.

TERMINATION OF THE DISCHARGE ESTIMATING SYSTEM

The discharge estimate response rates and the accuracy of estimates remained at unsatisfactory levels through early September. On September 7, the executive committee of the medical staff formed an ad hoc committee of doctors who were interested in meeting with the administrator and representatives from the Bureau to discuss the discharge estimate situation. Significantly, only three doctors attended the meeting on September 20. At a subsequent surgical department meeting, the chief of the surgical department also discussed this matter with his colleagues. These two meetings produced no change; the surgeons ignored any suggestion for altering or improving the system to facilitate getting better estimates. As a result, it was decided to discontinue the discharge estimating system; this was done on October 26. Shortly, thereafter, the computer terminal was removed from the admitting office. The "dynamic" system had never reached operational level, because of the estimating performance.

The success of the allowance-based system indicated that precise discharge estimates were not necessary to maintain high occupancy and low cancellations. The occupancy level of the three units involved was maintained at an average occupancy level of ninety-six percent during April to September 1972. A simple system, not requiring daily computation was found to be feasible, and with this system no computer terminal was required.

MAINTAINING THE ADMISSION SCHEDULING SYSTEM

During an eight-week period beginning in December the Bureau team left the administration of the admission system completely in the hands of Baker's personnel. This was done to determine whether they had developed the internal capabilities to administer the system without outside intervention. Prior to December the Bureau had developed a system for holiday scheduling which would minimize the expected drop in admissions during the coming holiday season. However, the Bureau learned that the holiday scheduling system had not been well implemented, and by the beginning of 1973 Baker reported increasingly serious problems administering the system. A marked increase in the number of cancellations of surgery drew ire from the physicians while nursing complained of extra workloads as a result of an increase in the number of transfers.

By mid-January the Bureau team decided to begin a series of analyses to identify problems which had arisen during the period when the hospital was solely responsible for maintaining the system. Before withdrawing from active involvement with the system, the Bureau and the hospital had agreed upon the data base required to administer the system. It was arranged for the admitting office to keep weekly graphs which plotted the following data: the predicted census and the actual census for the three units in the system; the number of emergency admissions before 1:00 P.M., the number after 1:00 P.M., and the total number of emergency admissions to the units; the total weekly cancellations; the total weekly transfers; weekly totals of the actual and allotted number of surgical patients; weekly totals of the actual and allotted number of medical patients; weekly totals of the actual and allotted numbers of both surgical and medical patients; the number of days in the future medical and surgical patients were being scheduled, and the delay (in days) for both medical and surgical admissions. Periodic adjustments to the system, as well as its daily administration, were to be based on these records. When the Bureau team asked to see these data in order to begin their analysis, they learned that the data had been collected but not regularly summarized. Without the summarized data, the system could not be administered properly. Basing the system on the above sixteen data points added administrative as well as data collection problems and was in fact a somewhat cumbersome system. Yet the data requirements were clear, and it had appeared that these requirements were well understood by hospital personnel when the Bureau stopped direct assistance in December.

At near full occupancy, the system is highly sensitive to small changes in the number of additional admissions. Usually, the hospital overreacted to immediate conditions. When occupancy was lower than expected, too many patients were called in, and several days later cancellations had to be made. The Bureau underrated the time required and overrated the organizational resources available at Baker to administer the system. It was also learned that a system so sensitive requires considerable administrative experience.

Further study identified several other factors which contributed to the problems. The most important of these was a large and unexpected increase in the number of emergency admissions. The emergency admission allowance in the initial admission scheduling system was based on historical data which indicated an average of six emergency admissions per day, about three of which occurred after 1:00 P.M. However by the spring of 1973, the emergency admission rate had risen to an average of eleven per day. This near doubling of the number of emergencies was responsible for much of the increase in cancellations and transfers.

A health records analyst was hired in November 1972 and was asked to study the increase in emergency admissions. He learned that three physicians accounted for approximately half of the hospital's emergency admissions. The admissions of the three doctors were studied and given to the executive committtee of the medical staff for review and possible action. The three physicians were brought before the executive committee in order to defend their practices. Two of the three did not receive specific sanctions. The third was suspended for the month of April and placed on probation for the remainder of 1973.

The January analysis also identified two secondary factors which suggested that refinements in the system would bring the admissions process under greater control. The initial allowances for the three nursing units did not include a provision for transfers from the hospital's intensive care units (ICU/CCU) to units in the system. This factor would not be important with lower occupancy levels, but when occupancy approaches 100 percent, transfers into and out of the units in the system became critical. At near capacity, the system would not have been able to absorb what equaled two admissions per day without very serious problems had it not been for an offsetting factor which had also not been included in the initial allowances. It was learned that some patients coming within the surgical allowances who were admitted for clean gynecological surgeries were placed instead on the obstetrical unit. These admissions did not completely offset additions due to transfers from the intensive care unit, but they did help to reduce the number of potential cancellations.

The various implementation problems were not minor, and it was by no means possible to say as of May 1973 that the system was stable and permanently a part of the admission process at Baker. It was reasonable to assess the introduction as successful, both in economic and organizational terms. The role of the admitting nurse had been expanded, and this increased the effectiveness of the admitting process. The admitting office was reorganized, strengthened, and made more efficient. The communication group created an important new organizational mechanism for improved problem solving and decision making as well as for better interdepartmental communication. The admission allowances enabled the hospital to provide firm future admission dates, an important benefit to both patients and physicians. The Bureau's activities resulted in strengthening the hospital's supervisory staff, not only by employing a more experienced second shift admitting office supervisor and a health records analyst, but by increasing the skill and competence of those who came in contact with the system. Finally, the overall system allowed the hospital to operate at near full occupancy without the organizational stress that existed prior to the introduction of the system. By May 1973 the situation was viewed as favorable for future work. Among the encouraging signs were the decisions to look at emergency admissions and approach physicians who were responsible for excessive emergency admissions, and to look at the admitting office's practice to determine if they were following the revised procedures. An alternative to either would have been to blame the system. The shared willingness to look for other explanations of difficulty suggested that key actors in the system had begun to acknowledge an investment in the innovation, and that it was on the road to acceptance, if not there yet.

NOTES

1. Response Rate = Number of responses ÷ Number of times asked.
   Accuracy Rate = Number of patients accurately estimated ÷ Number of patients with estimates provided.
2. G. H. Robinson, L. E. Davis, and G. C. Johnson. "The Physician as an Estimator of Hospital Stay." *Human Factors*, 8, 1966, pp. 201–208.

9 | Implementation of Hospital Control Systems[1]

Fred C. Munson
Walton M. Hancock

Organizational requirements for the successful introduction of control systems are outlined here. It is easy to state a requirement, more difficult to know how to meet it. Therefore we will also outline the mechanisms we found useful in implementing our control systems in the study hospitals.

Successful organization change usually happens only when a good idea is well implemented. These normative criteria, excellence of idea and application, often cause attention to focus on one or the other of two distinct bodies of knowledge. Assuring the merit of the innovation requires technical experts in whatever discipline or profession is relevant; assuring the success of the implementation process requires the use of behavioral experts in the unique, dynamic, and richly complex sociotechnical system in which the innovation will be introduced.

From the technical and behavioral orientations come separate streams of scholars (industrial engineers versus organization psychologists), scholarly literature (*Operations Research* versus *Human Relations*), and indeed conceptions of purpose. The behavioral group defines success within a homeostatic model, the technical group in an optimization model. Thus a fertile ground for conflict is provided. Behavioral specialists ridicule the management scientist who designs a cost-saving innovation that is never accepted; technical specialists ridicule the change agent who labors mightily for participation in the design of a system that a beginning student in plant

Reprinted from *Cost Control in Hospitals*, John R. Griffith, Walton M. Hancock, and Fred C. Munson, eds., "Implementation of Hospital Control Systems," by Fred C. Munson and Walton M. Hancock, by permission of the Health Administration Press, Ann Arbor, Mich., 1976.

layout could improve. Although the title of our chapter suggests the behavioral point of view as a starting point, our purpose is to consider the necessary interfacing between the two approaches.

Implementation is a process, a set of events which occur in sequence. The underlying framework is one of unfreezing, moving, and refreezing the task behavior of individuals, and our purpose is to operationalize certain concepts when this framework is applied to the introduction of control systems.[2]

In changing control systems, many persons may be involved. Figure 9-1 shows the major linkages in the admitting process for adult, nonemergency, surgical patients. The content and order of communications is not shown. For other admissions, minor differences would appear, and for the associated discharge process, a separate diagram with additional boxes would be needed.

A change in the admitting/discharge process would not only involve persons linked in these networks, but one or more persons in central administration, the same in nursing administration, the medical staff (as an organization) and its executive committee, plus the external group if the source of the innovation is outside the hospital. The importance of mere numbers arises from the complex nature of the change process. To unfreeze, move, and refreeze the conception of task in a large number of individuals is not a trivial problem.

We are satisfied that success in implementing a change in a control system has three basic requirements:

• The innovation be well devised in a technical sense, so that it clearly achieves the objective that gave rise to it.

• The attitude of critical actors be favorable, or at least neutral, toward the innovation.

• Those who must perform new tasks learn to perform the required actions correctly.

We understand each of these to be necessary and, taken together, sufficient conditions for the successful implementation of change. Excluded here is an important precondition for change, that goals of powerful members be consistent with the purposes of the innovation. We specify this as a precondition because the basis of power for such members often arises outside of the organization, and is therefore likely to be impervious to internal modifications of structure. We cannot ask the change process to do well on something it cannot affect. Therefore we treat goal congruence among powerful members as a precondition, rather than as a variable within the control of the innovators. The balance of this chapter will spell out the significance of the three criteria and will identify a process of negotiating and renegotiating the substance of the innovation. The final paragraphs will discuss some typical problems of handling the negotiating process.

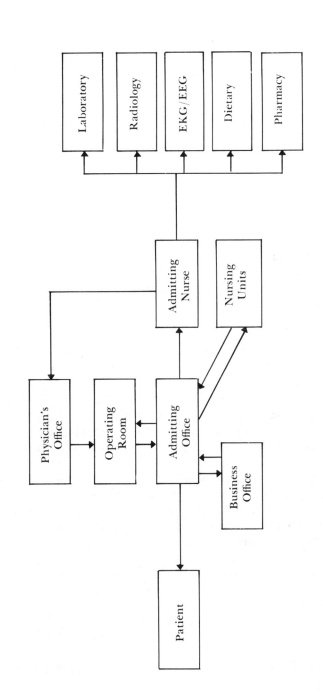

FIGURE 9–1

ADMITTING PROCESS FOR ADULT, NONEMERGENCY, SURGICAL CASES

The Innovation Be Well Devised
in a Technical Sense

Technical requirements for an innovation require an explicit statement of the objective, so that the technical requirements can be continuously reviewed against it. Examples of objectives that exist in the hospital field are as follows:

a. To minimize the cost of community health care.

b. To minimize the cost of operating a hospital where the quality of care is maintained at stated levels.

c. To provide a radiology service that will minimize the total cost of care per patient.

d. To provide a radiology service at minimum cost with respect to the radiology department's budget.

Each of the above objectives is sufficiently different that the technical requirements of designing an innovation would be affected. For example, **objective a** would require a detailed examination of duplicating services between hospital facilities within a community; **objective b** would not contain such a requirement. **Objective c** and **objective d** are different because **objective d** would require an examination of the use of resources used to meet a predicted demand where the radiology department would be considered a separate entity. **Objective c** would require that not only the operation of the department itself be examined, but the interaction of the department with the physicians and nurses be examined regarding the timeliness of the information. It is quite conceivable that the implementation of **objective d** would result in a nonoptimum solution with regard to **objective c**.

Once an objective is stated, the role of the technical expert in the innovation process is to provide an explicit statement of the best method with respect to contemporary technology. The technical requirements must be stated without consideration of the local environment under which the innovation might occur. The reason for the emphasis on a technical solution independent of local conditions is that the technical expert's initial function is to provide the most complete solution possible to accomplish the objective. The explicit statement of the solution then forms a basis for evaluating the cost of the compromises that may have to be made during any particular implementation of the system. Knowing this cost, in terms of what is being considered versus what is technically possible, decision makers will be in a better position to evaluate whether or not the compromise should be made. Once we permit the technical expert to take into account local conditions, it is very difficult to evaluate whether or not his recommended solution is consistent with contemporary technology.

As an example of the role of the technical expert, let us consider **objective b**—that we desire to minimize the cost of operating a hospital with quality levels maintained. This, in terms of operation research methodologies, is an optimization problem with quality constraints. If there is sufficient legitimate demand (demand that excludes unnecessary admissions or excessive lengths of stay), one of the ways to minimize the cost is to maximize throughput. The correct technical solution to this problem should contain the following elements:

• An analysis of the demand placed upon the hospital with respect to the patient inflows for the day of the week, between weeks, and between seasons. Specific applications would include separate analyses for inpatient and outpatient services, medical, surgical, psychiatric, or other subclasses of patients within the hospital.

• Any constraints imposed by the physical structure should be examined. Where actual physical constraints exist, then patient waiting lines will also exist. The significance of the constraints in many cases can be measured by the length and rate of turnover of the waiting line. Characteristic of typical constraints are the number of beds or the number of operating rooms.

• The operating procedures which affect the allocation of resources should be examined. For example, since the admissions department in many hospitals commits the resources of the hospital to the patient upon admission for a period of time in the future, the role of admissions, the interaction of admissions and the service departments and the knowledge of the state of use of resources at any given time have to be determined. A minimum cost solution requires that the resources available are sufficient to meet all quality needs, but not in excess.

Sufficient resources must be available at the time the service is needed for it to be rendered. Resources here clearly include personnel, and the training and qualifications of people necessary to give the service have to be examined.

In brief, a technically feasible model to minimize the cost of operating a hospital requires that we allocate resources as a function of the input demand, subject to the constraints that all of the resources will be consumed and that no physical or quality constraints are violated. For example, in Able Hospital the analysis of demand indicated that the hospital physical facility would not be fully utilized over a ten-year horizon. In addition, there were wide variations in the census in the hospital which reflected an admissions policy of admitting patients immediately. A result of these procedures was that personnel and other resources were established to meet all possible levels of demand. The adoption of **objective b** indicated that the admission of some patients should be delayed in order to stabilize demand so that the labor resources of the hospital could be reduced to a level consistent with the steady state need for these resources. In Baker Hospital, analysis indicated that demand was equal to or greater than the physical facilities (beds) of the hospital. Yet, the hospital was operating at approximately eighty-five percent census. There were empty beds in the hospital even though the demand was available to fill the beds. Since there was a physical constraint as well as other constraints imposed by the operating procedures of the hospital, the variations in demand were quite low. The accomplishment of the objective required improving the hospital operating procedures and then determining the size of the nursing staff and service staff so that when the beds were all full the quality constraint would not be violated. In the two facilities the objective was the same, but the technical requirements differed depending upon the relationship between demand and whether or not the demand was constrained by a physical or nonphysical constraint.

A technically optimal solution must also be a complete solution. Developing parts of an innovation is easily rationalized as "allowing full participation" but leads to wasted effort and ill will. A proposed change in radiology scheduling should not only include technically correct solutions for the radiology department, but also for the interfacing of these changes with nursing units, the outpatient department, and other hospital units which form the environment of the radiology department. We have found it quite common to dispose of such a connective as "a minor detail," only to discover upon investigation it is neither minor in the technical difficulty of solving it, nor in the consequences to the success of the innovation. It is not necessary or desirable to have the organizationally best solution, a point which will be developed in the following section. It is both possible and necessary to identify obvious connectives of a new procedure with other hospital systems, and to determine the technically correct method of information, patient, or other flows between the systems.

To summarize, if an innovation is well devised in a technical sense, it will be referenced to an explicit statement of objectives, will be the soundest technically available solution, will be complete in covering observed connections with other parts of the system, but will not contain the compromises and adjustments necessary to make it the organizationally best solution. This is the initial requirement for successful change, but only one of three requirements.

THE ATTITUDE OF CRITICAL ACTORS BE FAVORABLE

The problem of securing favorable attitudes from system members is important only for those system members with a relevant basis of power. It is nice to have favorable attitudes in everybody, but it is necessary to have them only in those whose support determines the success or failure of an innovation. Our understanding of the relevant literature suggests that many supporters of participation claim too much, seeking to prove that participants with little power have much power in determining productivity.[3] We will consider later the practical problem of defining who counts, after we have discussed the mechanism of attitude change.

Resistance to change rarely arises from mindless opposition to everything new. It is usually a reasonable response to avoiding one or more of three problems. Change may cause a member to lose status, influence, or valued relations, in short, to lose something of value.[4] The "may" (the uncertainty) is as much a part of the problem as what will be lost. Second, a specific change may simply not fit within the complex social and technical networks that bind any organization together.[5]

Finally, a change requires a person to raise "why am I here?" type questions, to rethink relations between means and ends, and therefore to consider whether some hitherto unexpressed purposes are in fact legitimate.[6] A reasonable approach to overcoming resistance to change will deal with these causes.

The most direct method is to involve the system members in the change, fully engaging them in the development of the innovation. Only by this involvement can a system member learn enough about the innovation to decide how much it will add or detract from the balance of benefits he receives under the status quo. If the member suffers a clear loss, he rationally must either oppose the change or seek modifications in it. In our experience the individual gain or loss is less often a basis for resisting change than a well based conviction that it will not work. Drucker is correct in suggesting that General Motors executives (or hospital head nurses) will find many compromises with the technically correct solution, but one must recognize that these people are true experts in defining nontechnical but very important elements of the constraint set that will fit an innovation to the existing procedures, status relations, and other attributes of that part of the organization which the innovation affects.[7] Compromise is bad only if one is inflexibly committed to the innovation, rather than the results it is intended to achieve. In problems of fitting the innovation to the system, the technically qualified experts are the novices, and cannot match the knowledge base of the system members.

When two groups with different but equally relevant expertise are interested in the implementation of an innovation, a clear basis for conflict exists. If one thinks of resolving this through "participation," an implicit assumption is that one group (with power) is allowing another group (without power) to participate. But relevant knowledge is a basis for power, and it is more reasonable to think of resolving the conflict through negotiation. A rough equality of power and interest in the outcome, and a symmetry in the relation between groups is acknowledged in calling a process a negotiation.[8] We offer below several examples of this distinction between participation and negotiation.

In the initial development of an information system for department heads, it was necessary to define units of output for each department. Department heads participated in providing information that allowed such output units to be defined. The developed information system required department heads to use forecasts of output to make staffing adjustments for a future four-week period. At this point negotiations began, for department heads criticized the requirement, pointing out they had inadequate information from payroll. This "rather minor detail" led the research team into a forest of problems which has taken nearly twenty-four months to clarify, and to develop (but not yet implement) a reliable and timely reporting system for department heads.

The operating room supervisor in one of the hospitals found it unpleasant to contemplate a shift in scheduling procedure that would reduce the ability of the operating room to control its own scheduling. Initially, the supervisor was able both to ignore the proposed scheduling revisions and involve some surgeons in the issue. Discussions with surgeons helped neutralize that potential source of resistance, and the use of the hospital administrator's authority legitimated the research team's proposal. In about three months the four-sided (admitting office, operating room, surgeons, research team) negotiation was completed, and the basically unmodified component of the scheduling system that affected the operating room was accepted and used. We should emphasize that our concept of negotiation is in no way limited to people sitting on two sides of a table arguing. The setting may be a board room or a hallway, it may start with a formal presentation or be concealed in a general discussion of problems, it may have two clear "sides" represented or may have a whole series of interests being asserted or defended, it may be restricted to verbal exchange or, as in the case of the operating room supervisor, be communication through action. The example below also illustrates how effectively action, in this case by admitting physicians, can be used to communicate a negotiating position.

The final illustration comes from the implementation of the original admitting/discharge model.[9] In this hospital physicians in a medical staff meeting participated in (approved) the final design of the patient scheduling system. When implemented, however, physicians who were asked to delay admissions began admitting patients to another hospital, a bargaining tactic which so impressed the administrator that he considered eliminating the whole program. The controller, drawn into earlier negotiations because the innovation used computer facilities under his control, supported a compromise which would reduce the financial benefits of the innovation but minimize the number of admission delays experienced by physicians. The outcome of this, and a rather similar negotiation with physicians about the manner of securing discharge data estimates, was a substantially modified system which had cost savings much less than the initial design, but a level of fit for the key actors which allowed it to exist. In fact, the savings were not clearly greater than the operating cost of the system, and with less psychic investment in the innovation the research team might well have suggested its abandonment. In our experience, however, we find it nearly as difficult to abandon an innovation we have labored to produce as it is for hospital personnel to abandon work methods they have come to accept as their occupational reason for being.

We should like to emphasize that in each of the illustrations, and others that could have been given, technical experts were qualified to apply current state of the art knowledge to the achievement of specific goals, and system members were qualified to adapt these proposals to the unique sociotechnical system. The experts' problem can be stated as someone else's resistance to change, but that is misleading. The true issue is whether, and in what form, an innovation will be introduced in a hospital.

The negotiations cause pain in both parties. The pain experienced by system members is well recognized; it is also experienced by technical experts. In the case of the department head information reporting system, the original innovation was discussed, explained, illustrated, and otherwise sold to a rather passive group of department heads. Only when it was experimentally introduced did the department heads begin to point out problems. When those problems were acknowledged, roles were reversed and department heads were change agents, anxious to unfreeze the research team from allegiance to the original idea and forcing them to accept the need for adaptations. These adaptations were developed and brought back, again challenged by department heads and again renegotiated, with the Bureau team facing the unpleasant possibility that funding would end before results were in. The experts experienced the pain that comes when good ideas, carefully thought out, tested, and refined in discussion, committed to paper and asserted in talks, publicly presented as evidence of competence and accepted as such, are threatened by the very people who must make them work if the experts are to make good on their promises.

The symmetry in this relation of technical experts and system members is important to understand and often ignored. Unless those who design the change recognize that system members are also experts, properly credentialed to require change in the outsider proposals, then expert efforts will be directed toward manipulation of the system members, forcing them to accept ideas, and in other ways denying the valid basis of system members' expertise. Among academicians this is called (incorrectly and pejoratively) "overcoming resistance to change." Only when the symmetry in the relation is recognized is it possible to recognize that successful system member inputs are the assertion of additional constraints to the original set, and to evaluate that new constraint set which the innovation must now be designed to fit.

Recognizing the symmetry of the change process permits system members to adapt the innovation to fit their system; it also forces both technical experts and system members to repeatedly distinguish between the purpose of an innovation, and the mechanism (the innovation itself) designed to achieve it. The system member faces greater difficulty than the expert in giving up a focus on means and refocusing on ends, though the problem exists for both. Inevitably, genuine negotiations turn to issues of what will work, and finally to why do anything. The honest confrontation of this latter question is fortunately difficult to avoid in the negotiations, and is a central part of refocusing on goals. The negotiation/renegotiation process between technical experts and system members pictured in Figure 9–2 encourages a constant review of purpose, and thus protects the attainment of purpose for which the innovation was designed.

Neither experts nor system members speak with one voice. The status quo in either group is in reality an often delicate balance of opposing interests that many may find unpleasant, but none finds intolerable. Internal negotiations are a continuing process in any complex organization, and have been made a central part of several theoretic models of the firm.[10] An important part of the attitude change process is to establish mechanisms for bargaining between system members which are appropriate to the social system of the organization. Open discussion is always a preferred method, but both the status system of the hospital and the occasional existence of deep mistrust or hostility may make it impractical. We have found it helpful to assign individual members of

FIGURE 9–2

THE NEGOTIATING PROCESS

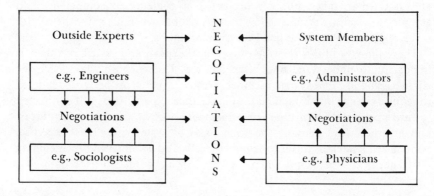

our group to be contact persons with key system members, both to keep them fully informed and also to develop alternative methods of hammering out compromise between system members when open negotiations are initially not possible.

A brief summary may help reemphasize the focal role we give to the negotiation/renegotiation process. Recognition of the symmetry of the change process between change designers and system members encourages honest negotiation and renegotiation. This process, by acknowledging the expert role of the system members, permits their meaningful participation in the design process, and this allows them to:

• Clarify the consequences for them of adopting the innovation; therefore to know whether they will gain or lose something of value.

• Fit the innovation to the system by requiring the change designers to accept the additional constraints needed and modify the innovation to meet them.

• Rethink relations between means and ends, and thus become open (unfrozen) to the possibility of new means being more appropriate. The negotiation/renegotiation process, in short, deals with the causes of resistance to change that apply to both system members and technical experts.

LEARNING TO PERFORM REQUIRED ACTIONS

Contrary to some beliefs about human nature, it is not the natural state of man to resist new ideas. It is natural to resist useless or troublesome information, and equally natural to be curious, problem solving, and anxious to experiment. The first step of learning is motivation, to be in a setting which evokes the second response set. It is sometimes (in our experiences often) necessary to provide this motivation by troubling people when they continue to use their present repertoire of skills. Providing feedback of bad current results often troubles people enough so that they wish to find new methods to achieve better results. Simply requiring a new task performance may trouble people enough to want to learn how to perform it. Fortunately, most persons have aspirations which already exceed their achievements, and the problem is to show them that alternative methods will narrow that gap. For example, two key physicians in one of the hospitals were already troubled by excessive lengths of stay: it was only necessary to show them that a proposed change in the admitting process could reduce length of stay for some patients by as much as one day, and their interest was assured. It was less easy to show admitting office personnel that maintaining several new records was important; their aspirations did not place high value on improved holiday scheduling or reduced cancellations, which in the past had been no part of their concerns. Thus it is often necessary to establish a setting in which new behaviors are required before there is sufficient motivation to learn them. The system actors may deal with a proposed change by ignoring or otherwise delaying it unless it is actually introduced. To provide teaching and to assume learning is to ignore the need for motivation. When motivation exists, learning is possible and teaching becomes relevant. The simple need to train in specific behaviors is the most important aspect of this step. Unthinking adherence to a practice is not good but is bliss compared to the chaos of an "it will become clearer as you go along" approach to training. Refreezing is a central requirement of successful change, and few things hinder it more than significantly increased error rates, angered employees, irate doctors, and similar results which a badly operated new system produces.

In the introduction of a department head information system directed toward staffing control, the three training requirements appeared to be:

• What department heads should expect to receive (forecasts, cost reports, etc.).

• What they should do (compare with prior period report and with budget, determine current and expected staffing, adjust forecast to expected local and specific causes of variation in future volume).

• What search process and decision rules they should use (with lower expected volume: review scheduled overtime, check with nursing administration to see if an employee can be loaned, etc; select an alternative that balances hours with expected requirements).

These requirements are applied in different ways to department heads and higher levels of administration, and to those in the hospital who would be generating the information and interfacing with the computer. The tendency to "train by results," telling system members to achieve a result rather than training them to perform a task, is perhaps natural (it substantially reduces what the trainer must understand) but leads inevitably to problems. System members, when asked to perform in ways that are new to them, become heavily dependent upon the outside experts to provide them with precise information on what to do next in order to perform the new functions. Since many of these requests for what to do may be considered unimportant details by the expert, he may not readily have the answers. Operating people then become less secure, and may also wish to return to previous procedures. The outside expert must have thought about as many of the questions regarding the required actions by the operating people as possible to be able to answer promptly and with authority questions regarding the actions necessary to implement the system. We are currently experimenting with simulation of the admitting process to see whether it is possible to offer direct experience with the search and decision component of training. This method may avoid the stress which accompanies experimenting in the live situation, arising from the anticipation of the real consequences of poor decisions.

Whether by classroom instruction, on-the-job training, simulation, or other methods, the key to the skill acquisition step in learning is the concentration on specifics. This is both because tasks cannot be completed with generalities but only with specific behaviors, and because confidence grows fastest as specifics are mastered and how-to knowledge becomes recognizably complete.

There is a fine but significant distinction between knowing how to do something and actually being able to do it. It is the distinction between swimming with and without a supporting hand, the distinction between knowing and using a skill. Often it is not certain whether a skill has been acquired until live application begins. A complicating factor in this step when implementing new control systems or similar organizational changes is that only rarely are the recently acquired new skills both appropriate and complete. As we have earlier indicated, negotiations continue during the initial introduction. Therefore, modifications continue to be made in the innovation, and necessarily in the required behaviors.

The first trial of the new behaviors is not only a key step in the learning process, it is also a key one in determining how well the initial requirement of a technically complete solution is met. An example is in an early implementation of the admission scheduling system. In this case, the admissions officer was given a computer output and instructed that when the physician called he was to admit patients subject to the constraints of admission given to him through the computer output. The problems arose when the physicians' offices called to have patients admitted and were also asked by the admissions personnel to give an estimate of the length of the stay of the patient. This was the first time that this type of information was ever requested. The reactions of the physicians varied: some physicians were willing to give estimates; others asked what the estimates really meant; and others flatly refused to give an estimate. In addition, the technical experts did not anticipate that in many cases the physicians' secretaries did the calling. During the introduction of this system, there were repeated questions by the admissions personnel as to how to handle these situations. The implementation of the system was hurt because the research team had not anticipated many of the questions and did not have answers readily available. In later implementation more thought has been given to this stage, and to the need for gradual transition from constantly present to readily available support, and from there to eventual disengagement of the technical experts from the ongoing process.

Meeting this third requirement of having system actors to perform the required actions is closely akin to the Lewinian change model. In Table 9-1 below we summarize this relation.

TABLE 9-1

STAGES OF THE CHANGE AND LEARNING PROCESS

Frozen	— Precondition	— Stability
Unfreeze	— Motivation to learn	— Rethinking goals, considering alternatives
Move	— Skill acquisition	— Learning new methods, feelings of insecurity
Refreeze	— Skill application	— "I like it! It really works!"
Frozen	— Postcondition	— Stability

HANDLING NEGOTIATIONS

What we have called the negotiation/renegotiation process is important in meeting all three criteria for successful implementation. Its formal purpose is to make the required refinement in the substantive content of the innovation to turn the technically optimal into the organizationally feasible solution. The sequence of repeated negotiations gives time and opportunity for attitudes to change, and the nature of negotiation makes learning the new skills natural and necessary. We conclude this chapter with some issues we have identified in making negotiation work.

THE NEED FOR INTERNAL COMMITTEES

An innovation which affects many sets of actors requires either many sets of negotiations, or more complex negotiations between technical experts and system members with potentially conflicting modifications to propose. It is in such cases that internal committees have their greatest value. System members' ability to influence the change designers is maximized by giving organizational recognition to such a group. Most important, an explicit arena is identified for the internal negotiations that are required to allow each system member to unfreeze and gradually move toward acceptance of the new consensus required by the (modified) innovation. We have said earlier that the technical experts must sometimes assist system members in making these internal negotiations genuine. The nursing department in one hospital had difficulty developing such a group, though the need was clear. Our practice is gradually turning to the initial identification of key members, and attempting to treat them as an entity. Where mistrust is high this is not feasible at the start, for people who mistrust each other will not communicate honestly. Dealing with groups also means delay in scheduling discussions, but on balance it is better to build groups and accept delays than to fail in developing a group of the key members which permits honest negotiation.

THE NEED TO NEGOTIATE WITH THE RIGHT GROUP

The centrality of an innovation to a member and his ability to determine its success will determine the importance of involving him in the negotiation/ renegotiation process. An innovation which touches everyone in the organization could have negotiation costs which far outweigh its estimated benefits. Given perfect knowledge about the centrality and power of each member, negotiations would be limited to that group of members which would result in the highest net advantage of the innovation. Perfect knowledge does not exist, and decisions must be made which make assumptions about the centrality and power of each member; negotiations would be limited to that group of members which would result in the highest net advantage of the innovation. In introducing the admitting system, for example, no effort was made to involve each admitting physician directly, and in one of the study hospitals only two representative physicians were involved in initial meetings. They were present in the discussion with the executive committee of the medical staff, and at the medical staff meeting in which approval was requested from all admitting physicians. By contrast, in the staffing control innovation, all cost center heads were directly involved. In practice, we discover additional system members as they become powerful at different stages of the innovation. (This element of a successful implementation program came to our attention in the evaluation of service unit management programs.)[11]

THE NEED FOR OPEN COMMUNICATION

We have alluded to the internal negotiation which takes place in the hospital as a feasible solution is being generated. Internal negotiation also occurs among the technical experts. Sociologists and engineers, for reasons mentioned at the beginning of this chapter, do find issues on which communication is difficult. Yet curiously this is not the most important problem. If the sociologist is the one who has developed an innovation and is carrying it to the hospital setting, it may be the engineer who helps him recognize that system members have the right, and the power, to force changes upon him if the changes make the innovation fit the system better. Much internal negotiation has taken place in the quite supportive environment of our Bureau research group.

THE NEED FOR PROTECTING SYSTEM MEMBERS

The fact that in our own group changes were negotiated in a basically friendly environment has helped us recognize that negotiations need not be antagonistic, and that once system member involvement is secured, the negotiation process in the hospital can provide a nonthreatening environment in which real issues can be faced, including uncertainty about ability to perform and questions about goals. ("Does cost really make that much difference? After all, most patients are covered by insurance.") One of the desirable methods of securing the joint products of the negotiation/renegotiation process is to implement early on a pilot basis, and then to proceed with modifications and training. The explicitly tentative, experimental setting is itself a protection from organizational criticism, and from a sense of failure when things go badly. Our experience is that additional protection sometimes is required when the results of an innovation are strongly desired by a powerful system member (the hospital administrator). In such cases the experts have either joined with system members to resist excessive pressure, or developed in advance with the administrator the necessary protection from an early demand for results.

The Common Need to Change the System

A fortunate, though problem-causing, byproduct of negotiation is the uncovering of clearly bad practices. Three examples will suffice. A part of the evidence adduced by a system member to prove that a department's output could not be forecast by conventional techniques was the (accurate) assertion that some physicians who rotated through the department would significantly increase the number of tests requested when they personally were receiving the fees. Another department challenged the possibility of developing an output measure by the (again accurate) assertion that many of the supplies issued were not recorded in departmental records. Finally, much trouble in resolving inconsistencies between different sources for manhour reports was eventually tracked down to a reporting practice that showed, for example, 100 overtime hours as 150 hours worked. The reporting of on-call hours and pay was equally confused. The elimination of such practices is of course desirable as an end in itself, but their identification through the negotiation/renegotiation process gives further evidence that system members are indeed experts at identifying what has to be changed in the hospital environment, as well as in the innovation, before the latter can be fit into the system and frozen into place.

The Need to Recognize that People Need Time to Change

One great advantage in acknowledging the negotiation/renegotiation process is that we have become more sensitive to time as a variable. We recognize that for others, like us, time needs to pass for ideas to become acceptable. An order can be followed in seconds; an idea cannot be accepted so quickly. In one hospital the controller was not enthusiastic about the admitting system for two months. Yet when the first challenge came from the physicians, he was among its strongest supporters. By treating negotiation as a part of the implementation process we have recognized that time is needed for attitudes to change, as clearly as it is needed to design the technically correct method.

THE NEED FOR MANAGERIAL RESOURCES

We occasionally find administrators who cannot accept an obvious corollary of our experience, that if the three requirements (excellence of the innovation, supportive key participants, and their ability to act) are really requirements, then we have specified a demand on managerial resources that cannot be avoided. In the study hospitals the Bureau research staff made up some of that required resource, but outsiders have limitations as well as advantages, and the absence of internal hospital resources to support the change process has caused significant delays in several of the innovations. We now believe that a hospital with a thinly staffed management structure may find it nearly impossible to introduce significant structural changes without major damage to the morale and effectiveness of the institution.

The resources requirements are varied. Technical assistance in data processing, sophistication in adapting forecasting models, assisting in budget preparations, advice on dealing with recalcitrant or insecure subordinates, technical training, facilitating open communication during internal negotiations—these are some of the skill requirements which can be supplemented by outsiders. But the competence and depth of a strong department head group cannot be replaced by consultants, for the possiblity of using task forces or ad hoc committees to be the internal change group cannot come from outside the organization. It rests on having management personnel with the competence to perform in such a group, and with backup that allows them the time to do it. Our interest is in the implementation of control systems, not the introduction of new management structures, yet we must say that a hospital which wishes to improve its control or any other system should first invest in its human organization.

SUMMARY

Our experience in implementing change in the study hospitals has taught us that three requirements are sufficiently important and identifiable to warrant their use as a focus of review and evaluation by those concerned with the implementation process. The first requirement is the excellence of the innovation itself. Our present feeling is that excellence is best reached by starting with a complete and technically optimal method for reaching a given purpose, and modifying it to meet local conditions only after that optimal definition is made. The second requirement is a favorable attitude on the part of key participants. This has required us to think carefully of which participants are key, and what demands they will make on the innovations. Third is the ability of the participants to take the required actions; and there we have learned to accept training, whether achieved through programmed instruction, simulation models, formal lectures, the provision of incentives, hands-on guidance, group discussion, feedback of results, or any other training method, as a key obligation of the change designers.

PROCESS

It has become clear to us that it is dangerously easy to slip over into a manipulative mode in our relations with system members, and that an explicit acceptance of a negotiation/renegotiation model helps avoid that danger. It becomes the key process by which the technically optimal solution is transformed into an organizationally feasible solution, and also becomes the key process in identifying and dealing with the (usually sound) reasons of system members for opposing the innovation. The learning which takes place in a negotiating as opposed to a manipulating or persuading context has proven to be more lasting and effective, though it by no means replaces the need for explicit training programs when the major modifications in the innovation have been hammered out in the negotiating process. We have also come to recognize and deal more explicitly with the need for internal negotiations, both within our own research group, and among the key participants within the hospitals.

TIME DIMENSION

The negotiations have produced innumerable illustrations of the Lewinian proposition that organizational change is a process made up of attitudinal changes in individuals and groups. These changes take time, and a later step in the process (refreezing) cannot take place until the prior step (moving) has been passed. Therefore it is a gross error to ignore the probable time require-ments for such attitude change. It is erroneous to assume that if resources are allocated, the intended change will take place. An intensive training session is a resource allocation, not the achievement of a step in the attitude change process. Needless to say, without the skilled human resources which can train, facilitate communication, find compromises, provide technical and social support, and perform the other tasks necessary to meet the three require-ments, the prospects for successful change are very poor. . . .

NOTES

1. Adapted from Fred C. Munson and Walton M. Hancock, "Problems of Implementing Change in Two Hospital Settings." *AHE Transactions*, December 1972, pp. 258–266.
2. K. Lewin, "Group Decision and Social Change," in G. E. Swanson, T. M. Newcomb, and E. L. Hartley (eds.), *Readings in Social Psychology, Second Edition*, New York: Henry Holt, 1952, pp. 459–473.
3. L. Coch and J. R. P. French, "Overcoming Resistance to Change." *Human Relations*, I, 1948, pp. 512–533. J. R. P. French, Jr., J. Israel, and D. As, "An Experiment on Participation in a Norwegian Factory," *Human Relations*, XIII, 1961, pp. 3–19. Rensis Likert, *New Patterns of Management*. New York: McGraw-Hill Book Co., 1961, chapters 4 and 8. George Strauss, "Some Notes on Power-Equalization," in Harold J. Leavitt (ed.), *The Social Science of Organizations*. Englewood Cliffs, NJ: Prentice-Hall, 1963, pp. 40–84. Dorwin Cartwright, "Power: A Neglected Variable in Social Psychology," in Warren G. Bennis, Kenneth D. Benne and Robert Chin (eds.), *The Planning of Change*. New York: Holt, Rinehart and Winston, 1962. James Q. Wilson, "Innovation in Organization: Notes Toward a Theory," in James D. Thompson (ed.), *Approaches to Organizational Design*. Pittsburgh: University of Pittsburgh, 1966, pp. 193–218. Rensis Likert, *The Human Organization: Its Management and Value*. New York: McGraw-Hill Book Co., 1967, chapters 3 and 4.
4. Chester Barnard, *The Functions of the Executive*. Cambridge, MA: Harvard University Press, 1962, chapter 11. Wilson, "Innovation in Organization."
5. E. L. Trist and K. W. Bamforth, "Social and Psychological Consequences of the Longwall Method of Coal-Getting." *Human Relations*, IV, 1951, pp. 3–38. Joan Woodward, *Industrial Organization: Theory and Practice*. London: Oxford University Press, 1965. Likert, *The Human Organization*.
6. Robert K. Merton, "Bureaucratic Structure and Personality," in Robert K. Merton (ed.), *Social Theory and Social Structure, revised edition*. New York: The Free Press of Glencoe, 1957, chapter 6. Herbert A. Simon, "On the Concept of Organizational Goal," *Administrative Science Quarterly*, IX, 1964, pp. 1–22. Richard M. Cyert and James G. March, *A Behavioral Theory of the Firm*. Englewood Cliffs, NJ: Prentice-Hall, 1963.
7. Peter F. Drucker, "The Effective Decision." *Harvard Business Review*, January–February 1967, pp. 92–98.
8. Dorwin Cartwright, "Influences, Leadership, Control," in James G. March (ed.), *Handbook of Organizations*. Chicago: Rand McNally, 1965, pp. 1–47.
9. Galen P. Briggs, Jr., "Inpatient Admissions Scheduling: Application on a Nursing Service." Doctoral dissertation, The University of Michigan, 1972.
10. Cyert and March, *Behavioral Theory*. James D. Thompson, *Organizations In Action*. New York: McGraw-Hill Book Co., 1967, chapters 9 and 10.
11. Richard C. Jelinek, Fred C. Munson, and Robert L. Smith, "SUM (Service Unit Management): An Organizational Approach to Improved Patient Care," A study report for the W. K. Kellogg Foundation, 1971.

<table>
<tr><td>10</td><td># Understanding Change in the Hospital[1]</td></tr>
</table>

10 | Understanding Change in the Hospital[1]

Kurt R. Student

The Bureau of Hospital Administration's four-year activity would be incomplete without some attempt to understand the implementation process itself. We do not seek to add one more model to the growing literature of organizational change, but have the more modest goal of developing a paradigm which helps the reader of the case studies in this section to understand some of the underlying factors in the implementation process as described in our cases. In attempting to understand our own work, we have identified five factors which appear to have been most important in our work at Able and Baker, and they are explained and illustrated in the material below.

THE SETTING FOR INNOVATION

There is some evidence in the cases that the best environment for innovating is different from the setting for maintaining high morale, high quality, or high efficiency. The goal of innovation requires a shaking up, the goals of morale, quality, or efficiency a settling down. This observation is not original; Morison noted it in his study of the American Navy, and himself quoted Admiral Mahan's earlier observation that no military organization can change itself; it must have assistance from the outside.[2] More recent work by Greiner, Haire, Kaufman, and Thompson supports this basic view of a favorable setting for innovation: there must be dissatisfaction, and the only

Reprinted from *Cost Control in Hospitals*, John R. Griffith, Walton M. Hancock, and Fred C. Munson, eds., "Understanding Change in the Hospital," by Kurt R. Student, by permission of the Health Administration Press, Ann Arbor, Mich., 1976.

reliable source for such dissatisfaction is the external environment.[3] In Able, two critical aspects of the external environment were a force for stability rather than change. Able physicians lost the benefit of admission at will in the new admitting scheduling system, and Martin Hospital was available to permit them to punish Able for making the change. Second, Able's trustees were significantly less interested in cost savings (only a small part of which would have benefited the Able service area) than they were in good relations with the medical staff. The potential for support within the organization was present, but such support was not sufficient to overcome the problem of an environment that was pleased with things as they were.

Baker presented a very different setting. Here a new administrator had been brought in with a clear purpose of raising occupancy, and the medical staff was faced with admission delays because of a bed shortage. Dissatisfaction was present and Baker did not need to change by itself; others were quite willing to help it.

The Pace of Introduction

There was an inevitable tendency for the Bureau to set timetables for the various activities which accompanied the presentation and introduction of their proposals. So long as a step was mechanical and required no acceptance by hospital personnel this was no problem. When acceptance by hospital personnel was required it gradually became clear that a process was at work which could not be scheduled by the calendar. Recent research by Robert Zajonc bears directly on this point.

Contrary to the popular maxim that familiarity breeds contempt, Zajonc and his colleagues hold that familiarity breeds comfort. The research deals with the effects of repeated exposure to a stimulus.[4] This work has produced interesting and unexpected results which are directly applicable to an understanding of the dynamics of the implementation process at the study hospitals. Although the nature of the experiments has varied widely, the results have been the same; the more often a person comes in contact with something or someone, the more favorable he tends to feel toward them. Zajonc observes that the exposure effect works best in connection with someone or something one has never seen before, toward which one's feelings are neutral. He notes that if one has had a childhood aversion to turnip greens or green snakes, new exposures are not likely to change it.

In our work at Baker, we experienced several examples of Zajonc's exposure effect in our implementation activities. An example was the experience of introducing early admission testing (EAT) for adult medical patients. When the innovation was first introduced there were mixed attitudes among the medical staff. One internist embraced the idea enthusiastically, but the initial response of most of the general practitioners and internists who admit medical patients was either neutral or somewhat negative. The admitting nurse reported that very few physicians furnished EAT orders willingly. Almost always, she had to call the physician's office, often again and again, before she was able to arrange for a patient's tests. The physicians resented these calls, claimed they were a nuisance and an interference with their practice. They did not want to be asked by telephone for a patient's tests while they were busy in their office seeing other patients. Initially few physicians cooperated with EAT. It is noteworthy that surgeons at Baker (and internists at other hospitals) routinely furnish the admitting nurse preoperative tests for their patients at the time admission is arranged. Initially only a few physicians dedicated to the concept of EAT arranged for their patients to receive these tests. Laboratory and radiology, in cooperation with the Bureau, developed the methodology to handle these special patients and word about EAT began to spread slowly throughout the hospital. A few more physicians agreed to try the innovation, and the admitting nurse began to report more cooperation and less difficulty in getting EAT orders from physicians. After some time, the remaining physicians decided, apparently, that the concept of EAT would not "go away" regardless of their attitudes. Nothing that we can detect changed in the system except the familiarity of it. Six months after the first EAT patient, the admitting nurse reported that EAT had become "routine" for almost all of the physicians who admit medical patients. With very few exceptions, EAT orders are routinely furnished and the physicians now consider EAT as a part of their standard hospital-based practice. Quite clearly, a professionally sound innovation had met initial negative response but had been successfully implemented in part as a result of the exposure effect dynamics.

The character of the innovation has an important bearing on whether exposure can be expected to play a role in the implementation process. This is illustrated in the differences between the EAT system and the physician-supplied discharge estimating system. Both innovations required physician cooperation; the former could use the exposure effect, but the latter could not. The feasibility and benefit of EAT were established by a small group of initial participants; over time, other physicians were exposed to the system, became familiar with it, and also became participants. The discharge estimating system, on the other hand, required initial participation by a large percentage of the total medical staff. As with EAT, a few physicians did supply estimates conscientiously after the system's start-up. However, too few estimates were received to base admission decisions on this system, and the manual system continued. Those few physicians who cooperated initially became discouraged; others who were more skeptical never were exposed to a successful system, and the Bureau was unable to overcome their skepticism and elicit their cooperation. Exposure was able to contribute to the success of the EAT system, but it was of no consequence in the physician discharge estimating system due to the different character of the latter innovation.

The pace of introducing an innovation is related to the technical as well as the human readiness of the hospital to accept the next step of an innovation. A six-month delay in getting daily census reports from the Able computer arose from an inadequate assessment of the difficulties of computer program adaptation, the resolution of a prior billing problem, and the securing of an adequate number of hours from trained personnel. Early identification of these problems would have required questioning the judgments of competent and senior personnel, and such questioning carries some risk of antagonizing people whose support is needed. The risk would have been taken had the technical preconditions for implementation been fully recognized. Such recognition is easy in retrospect, but to recognize it when it is needed, a remarkably detailed knowledge is required of the technical requirements of the innovation and the existing systems and data sources it will utilize. When introducing the admitting scheduling system at Baker several early warnings that the admitting office did not have the trained resources to manage or implement the system were heeded, and the prior (and somewhat frustrating) investments were made in improving that resource before firm dates were set for start-up.

INFLUENCE

Participants accept change more readily if they shape both the change itself and the process of implementing it. Externally imposed change can be expected to meet resistance unless those who must accept the change and make it work have had their "say" or exerted their influence.

All of the Bureau's innovations, the admissions allowances, the EAT system, the budgeting system, and the nurse scheduling system, have been influenced by the hospitals' participants. In the opening chapter of this section we termed the expression of such influence the "negotiation/renegotiation" process. Illustrations of this process appear throughout the cases, one of the clearest examples being the implementation of the surgical admission allowances. The initial allowance was based on historical data and attempted to keep the balance between surgical admissions and medical admissions the same as it was prior to the Bureau's intervention. This way of setting the allowances neglected to take account of the increase in occupancy which resulted from the system. The surgeons viewed this as unfair and unacceptable. The surgical department formed an ad hoc committee to advise the administration. The administration agreed that the surgeons should share in the greater number of admissions, and the allowances were revised to reflect changes in the length of the waiting times. The changes were relatively modest, amounting to a scarely noticeable change for each surgeon. Nonetheless, the surgeons had exerted influence and power which resulted in change; thereafter the revised allowances were accepted. Fortunately, they were accepted by the medical department as well as by the surgeons. Had the allowances not been changed, it is unlikely that the admission scheduling system could have been implemented.

A common explanation for the effectiveness of participation is that it reduces external control and allows the satisfactions available from the exercise of self-control to be secured directly. It allows participants to "prove" through high performance that the participative solution was a sound one. The reasoning is persuasive and has empirical support.[5] It is worth noting, however, that successful examples of participation such as the Scanlon Plan experiences do not eliminate control, but rather provide a setting in which expertness replaces authority, irrespective of who has it.[6] Authority is the typical source of influence in a static organization; the cases suggest that expertness is bound in the same close relation to successful innovation. The cases make clear the Bureau held no monopoly on expertness, particularly in devising the modifications necessary to make the budgeting, nurse scheduling, payroll-based reporting system, or other innovations viable. Participation in the discussions which modified the different innovations allowed persons who could identify problems in detail to bring this knowledge to bear on an innovation and on the strategy for its implementation. Admittedly, the power to direct (authority) was also important, as was the unquestioned power of the physicians to use or ignore the early admission testing program.

The number of influential participants in a hospital makes the mechanisms through which influence is applied of particular interest. The physician role in supporting or resisting change is often salient, but it is apparent for others as well that the mechanisms which allow participants to use their power base to stop an innovation also allow them to be co-opted. Whether because of the exposure effect, rational assessment, or the alchemy of participation, detractors may become supporters of innovation. The same widespread sources of influence which make the hospital a difficult setting in which to introduce innovations provide, paradoxically, fertile opportunities to generate support for them. The power of the idea, its inherent soundness, becomes a significant factor, and those who have shaped it use their influence to help bring it to fruition.

The conclusion from the cases is not that expertness is the only relevant source of influence. The significant point is that successful implementation was most often achieved when expertness was acknowledged to be the most relevant source of influence in framing and modifying the innovation, and participants with other sources of influence then used it to support the implementation.

Soundness of the Innovation

All of the innovations proposed in the study hospitals were worthwhile ideas; not all of them were brought to an acceptable state of technical and organizational soundness. The manpower input decision (MID) lacked technical soundness. It was not thoroughly developed, and inadequate resources were devoted to shortening the turnaround time from receiving raw data to presentation to department heads, and in developing the decision criteria and methods of applying them that would cause the MID to have an impact. The discharge estimating system both at Able and Baker was technically sound, but never achieved the modifications necessary to stabilize it within either organization. Nursing personnel were key actors in ensuring the success of the estimating system because of their role in securing estimates from the physicians. Yet the amount of criticism and conflict they experienced was directly proportionate to the energy they exerted in securing the estimates, and this organizational anomaly was never resolved.

The cases show rather clearly that key participants do test the soundness of an innovation, and also the degree of support it will receive from other key participants in the system. Outside groups such as the Bureau staff can expect some skepticism regarding proposals for change and some informal testing to see whether the proposal is a soundly conceived and seriously supported one. Change agents are often viewed as being unable to understand the "real world." When proposed changes have already been successful elsewhere, a common reaction nonetheless is: "We're different—it won't work here." Consequently, the external change agent, as well as his proposed changes, can expect to be tested. He must win the respect and approval for his proposals with each client system, each department head, each participant, anew.

The Bureau experienced such a testing by the Baker personnel. Almost all of the personnel tested the Bureau's representatives for their specific knowledge about Baker, its organization, its history, its way of doing things. Underlying all of our initial contacts was the unasked question: "Do these guys know what they're talking about?" The testing was not always so innocuous, however. Several physicians tested the reliability of the admission scheduling system by bypassing it and bringing their patients in as emergency admissions. Three physicians were brought before the executive committee of the medical staff; one was suspended for a month as well as being placed on probation for a year.

The operating room supervisor tested the admission scheduling system for weeks before beginning to cooperate fully. When surgical admissions were to be based on fixed day-of-the-week allowances rather than her judgments, she lost some of her power vis-à-vis the surgeons, and she did not implement the allowances correctly when she first received them. As the Bureau implemented a more complete data collection system, it became obvious that surgical admissions were not being based on allowances. When confronted with these data, the operating supervisor claimed there was a misunderstanding about when to implement the allowances. She then agreed to begin using the allowances; again she did not do so. Clearly, she was testing the system, as well as the power she had over her activities. After some time, the administrator sent a clearly worded memo to her with copies to the chief of the surgical department and to the admitting office ordering her to implement the allowances immediately. Shortly thereafter, the number of daily surgical admissions matched the allowances, and there were no subsequent problems with the operating room supervisor's administration of the surgical allowances.

From the point of view of the participants, testing is a common sense way of confirming whether the request for change is serious or not, and whether the organization has the required resources available to implement the proposed change. Typically, such testing is the way in which participants with relatively little power (or with little power they wish to use) can determine whether they can sabotage the change simply by ignoring it. The manner in which the Baker department managers thwarted the implementation of the manpower input decision (MID) illustrates this strategy. The department managers did not resist the introduction of the MID concept, and they cooperated with the Bureau in setting the initial MID levels. However, they ignored the planning reports based on the MID, they did not alter their usual staffing methods, nor did they make an effort to help the Bureau improve the reports. The hospital administration and the Bureau were unable to commit the resources necessary to make the MID concept effective, and eventually it was abandoned.

In a sense, testing is possible because the newness of a method permits variation from it that will be troublesome to those close to the innovation, but not to others in the organization. This can be viewed as permitting a silent but effective communication between two actors, the one by his actions asking "Do you really mean it?" and the other by his reactions answering "No, not really," or "Yes, I do." It is probable that many such communications were being watched with interest by other participants in the study hospitals, and that how they responded to the innovation was affected by the outcome of the test.

STRESS

The stress factor includes both individual stress and organizational tension. The two are similar in character, but we use organizational tension to refer to "climate," the generalized stress experienced by many or all of the members of a unit or department, while stress refers to the feelings of a single individual.[7]. We have described exposure, the exercise of influence, and the opportunity for testing as three processes which can help participants accept new ideas. Paradoxically, the experience of stress can also have favorable consequences for change although stress, by definition, is a painful experience. Individual stress occurs when an individual's adaptive resources or capacities fail to make a functional response to a situation. Whether a situation produces stress or a neutral emotional state depends on what the situation means to the individual; what is stressful for one person will not inevitably be stressful for another.

Closely akin to individual stress is an organization climate of apprehension and insecurity that is generally shared by participants when situations arise for which no adequate coping mechanisms exist. This can occur when the work process of a unit is changed to demand greater technical efficiency. Increased efficiency will usually require greater interdepartmental interaction and more effective coordination. Interdepartmental problems surface faster and require faster solution. As work processes become more demanding, greater management controls are implemented. These new controls tend to uncover inefficiencies which previously went undetected, and thus organizational units come under greater administrative scrutiny. In short, organizational tension occurs when slack is reduced and when the members of a department or unit are asked to work differently and more efficiently.

The probability that interventions like the Bureau's will cause stress is directly related to the amount and degree of behavioral change required for the adoption of the innovations. The relationship between stress potential, behavior change, and change method is presented in Figure 10–1. As this figure suggests, the potential for stress increases as one moves from a desire to alter customary organizational interaction patterns to shifting role behaviors, to changing values and orientations, to the most stubborn variable: changing basic motives.

While stress was an expected consequence of the Bureau's intervention at Baker, the localization of stress in the role of single participants was unexpected. Stress was experienced very clearly by the director of nursing at Baker, by the admitting officer at Able, and by others as well. Individual stress is in many cases dysfunctional, but it does cause those who experience it to look for ways of escaping the stressful situation. Experimenting with new behavior is one possible escape, and it is in this sense that stress can facilitate change. As we pointed out in the opening chapter of this section, stress is often

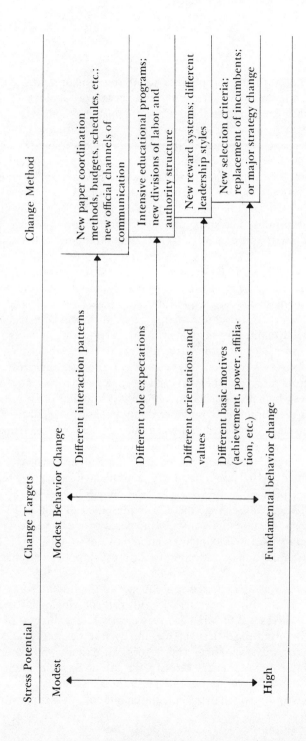

FIGURE 10–1

RELATIONSHIP BETWEEN STRESS POTENTIAL, CHANGE TARGETS, AND CHANGE METHOD

Stress Potential

Change Targets

Change Method

Modest

Modest Behavior Change

Different interaction patterns

New paper coordination methods, budgets, schedules, etc.; new official channels of communication

Different role expectations

Intensive educational programs; new divisions of labor and authority structure

Different orientations and values

New reward systems; different leadership styles

Different basic motives (achievement, power, affiliation, etc.)

New selection criteria; replacement of incumbents; or major strategy change

High

Fundamental behavior change

Adapted from Lawrence/Lorsch, DEVELOPING ORGANIZATIONS: DIAGNOSIS & ACTION, © 1969, Addison-Wesley, Reading, Massachusetts, Figure 6, Page 87. Reprinted with permission.

experienced when persons experiment with new behaviors; in that setting stress increases the tendency to revert to old methods.

It is worth noting that Bureau personnel also experienced stress, and responded in predictable ways. When their committment to the success of the innovation was high, it encouraged them to experiment with modifications that promised to improve the chance of implementing the change. This was not always the case, and the occasional hostility and antagonism directed at Bureau personnel sometimes caused the research staff to reduce contact with the hospital and thus avoid the unpleasant situations created. Such behavior rarely facilitated the progress of the innovation, for it avoided dealing with the problems which were creating the antagonism. The close, though sometimes tension-filled relations that were maintained in the testing of the patient classification system, and the early preparation of the admitting office for the admitting scheduling system required heavy investments of time and energy but resulted in closer and more open relations in the long term. They also resulted in successful innovations.

The report on the Baker nursing department makes clear that the Bureau's work had direct impact on the nursing department and its director. As a result of the administrator's intervention, the nursing units no longer controlled their own workload by making admissions decisions: these decisions were shifted to the admitting office. The discharge estimating system also increased the department's work, and brought nursing personnel into increasingly acrimonious interactions with the medical staff. A new organizational structure, the communication group, required the participation and cooperation of the nursing supervisors. This group gave the participating nursing supervisors new responsibilities and reduced the organizational importance of the director. Some problem solving and decision making which she had previously handled alone was now being made on an interdepartmental basis. This new group also resulted in exposing some of nursing's intradepartmental problems which might otherwise have gone undetected. The EAT system created a new class of patients requiring better coordination between nursing and housekeeping so that beds would be ready for EAT patients. Finally, the admitting nurse was shifted to the admitting office where she was no longer responsible to the director of nursing, but to the business office manager. When as a result of the Bureau's activity the admitting nurse's role was expanded, the director of nursing and the admitting nurse both began to report increasingly stressful interactions.

The administrator also reported experiencing stress as a result of the dramatic way in which the surgeon's dissatisfaction with the initial surgical allowances developed. The administrator quickly consulted the chief of the surgical department and the surgeons' ad hoc committee was formed to study the situation and to "help the Bureau raise the allowances." This committee effectively neutralized the immediate situation and provided a mechanism for handling the grievance. The administrator later reported his major concern was that the surgeons would go outside the formal organization and bring the matter to the executive director or members of the board. A man as experienced as Baker's administrator would be quite used to conflict, yet the possibility of effective bypassing by the surgeons concerned him deeply, for he feared the consequences of a breakdown of the formal mechanisms for handling grievances.

Organizational tension, like stress, can act indirectly as an attention focusing mechanism. The experience of the Baker nursing department suggests that as the department searched for ways to cope with tension being caused by the several changes, they developed communicating channels (such as the communication group) and clarity about existing problems (such as the criteria for patient transfer) which provided fresh perspectives on the innovation.

Our experience in the study hospitals suggests that individual stress and organizational tension inevitably develop in a change process and that this stress has both functional and dysfunctional consequences. The presence of stress prior to change may signal the need for change. In this case, stress is functional and will elicit initial cooperation if the proposed change is perceived as a means of reducing the stress. During the change process, some stress is also functional because it will speed the acceptance of change. Individuals experiencing moderate stress will adapt to the required change, thereby relieving their stress. However, excessive stress is dysfunctional and disabling. If stress goes too high, withdrawal behavior and/or aggressive behavior results, and organizational performance suffers. We conclude this discussion of the cases with an example which draws from three of them and shows rather clearly how stress can operate both for and against change.

In early 1972 change programs in Baker hospital were moving ahead on several fronts. The early budgeting procedures were being replaced by more extensive department head involvement, an early admission testing (EAT) experiment had begun, the formal admission scheduling system had just been installed and surgical allowances were being negotiated, the program of securing discharge estimates was being pushed, work on nurse scheduling was picking up, a project identifying delays between request and receipt of radiological exam results was just concluding, discussions with nursing administration concerning a reorganization that would create greater accountability at lower levels of the department were going on, and data on absenteeism and payroll accounting procedures were being collected in two separate and somewhat unrelated projects. In a word, things were busy at Baker. In Mid-May of 1972, overt hostility toward the Bureau surfaced within nursing, x-ray, and among the surgical staff. By mid-June all cause for concern seemed past, and the Bureau experienced an era of good feeling that was as unexpected as the earlier hostility. In retrospect, the reason for hostility is obvious; many of the individual activities in nursing, radiology, the admitting office, and the business office were not "in" these locations exclusively, but were in other parts of the hospital as well. No single project was enough to cause the eruption, but the interaction of several was, and the resulting tension and stress found a focus in the Bureau and its activities. One of the surgeons suggested the climate nicely when he told a nurse not to worry about discharge estimates, the Bureau staff would be out of Baker soon.

The reasons for the rapid resolution of stress are less obvious. A significant one is a somewhat exogenous event. The Bureau's nursing research program was making preparations for its hospital management summer course scheduled for June 5-9. The course was to focus on five years of research and evaluation of service unit management (SUM) and nursing organization. The Baker director had asked to attend some weeks before. The administrator's willingness to sponsor her at this particular time reassured the director about the importance of her role at Baker.

Her week in Ann Arbor brought her in contact with other directors and associate directors, hospital administrators, unit managers, and others who had had extensive experience in implementing change in nursing departments. These contacts were a stimulating experience for Baker's director. For the first time in some years, she had the opportunity to come into direct contact with some of the changes taking place in nursing; the course seemed to give her a new perspective on the problems she had been experiencing at Baker. Specifically, it seemed to alter her attitudes toward the possibilities for change in her department. The effect appears to have been more general than specific, for example, in a new openness toward nursing reorganization issues, a greater understanding of the value of hard data in planning change, and a willingness to question some prevailing nursing department practices.

Perhaps the crucial factor in resolving the stress was an immediate move by the Bureau staff into a negotiating mode for the surgical allowances. Revisions here, combined with strong support from the administrator's own superior, had the effect of mollifying the irate surgeons and strengthening the confidence of the administrator that he could still count on front office support when it was needed.

A third factor was really a payout on some earlier negotiations which had involved a number of key participants. Various nursing supervisors and other hospital personnel who had taken part in the communication group meetings were, like the nursing director, developing new orientations toward some of the changes, and the inclusion of suggestions from them in part of the nurse scheduling study produced a favorable attitude.

The reasons for the sudden appearance of favorable attitudes included a large component of coincidence. The significant point is that the stress and tension produced a setting for the director to benefit materially from her attendance at the seminar, for the nursing supervisors to value highly their inputs to the scheduling study, for the administrator to do the same with his support from the executive director and, not the least, for the Bureau to approach the surgical allowance negotiations with a distinctly conciliatory attitude.

Our summary and discussion of the cases have not distilled any single rule, which if adhered to would invariably have brought success to the hospitals' change efforts. Perhaps this is because we failed to see the rule; perhaps it is because there are sets of conditions, but no single condition, which ensure success to a change effort. We hold to the latter view, and hope that the documentation of our work will assist others in determining the necessary and sufficient conditions which will make their own efforts successful.

NOTES

1. A revised version of this paper entitled "Understanding the Implementing of Change" was published in *Hospital Progress*, June 1974.
2. Elting Morison, "A Case Study of Innovation," *Engineering and Science Monthly*, April 1950.
3. Larry E. Greiner, "Patterns of Organization Change," *Harvard Business Review*, Vol. 45, No. 3, May–June 1967, p. 122. Mason Haire, "Biological Models and Empirical Histories of the Growth of Organizations," in Haire (ed.), *Modern Organization Theory*. New York: John Wiley & Sons, 1959, pp. 288–290. Herbert Kaufman, *The Limits of Organizational Change*. Birmingham, AL: University of Alabama Press, 1971, pp. 41–67. James D. Thompson, *Organizations in Action*. New York: McGraw-Hill Book Co., 1967, pp. 66–82.
4. Robert B. Zajonc, "Attitudinal Effects of Mere Exposure," *Journal of Personality and Social Psychology*, No. 9 (Part 2), 1968, pp. 1–27. Robert B. Zajonc and Donald W. Rajecki, "Exposure and Effect: A Field Experiment," *Psychonomic Science*, 17, 1969, pp. 216–217.
5. See for example the research reviewed in Rensis Likert, *The Human Organization*. New York: McGraw-Hill Book Co., 1967, pp. 13–46.
6. Frederick G. Lesieur, *The Scanlon Plan: A Frontier in Labor-Management Cooperation*. Cambridge, MA: The Technology Press, 1958.
7. The interested reader is referred to the following for a more complete discussion of stress: S. Levine, and N. A. Scotch (eds.), *Social Stress*. Chicago: Aldine, 1970; and R. L. Kahn, D. M. Wolfe, R. P. Quinn, J. D. Snoek, and R. A. Rosenthal, *Organizational Stress*. New York: John Wiley & Sons, 1964.

11 | Crisis Points in Unit Management Programs

Fred C. Munson

The introduction of service unit management (SUM) in a hospital produces significant changes in the social and technical organization of the patient unit. These changes in turn cause strains, which sometimes are so severe that they threaten the success of SUM itself. This paper provides a framework for understanding the strains, so that hospitals interested in introducing SUM can take steps to minimize them and to lessen the chance of failure. The data will come from 14 hospitals, five of which succeeded and nine of which failed in introducing SUM. The proportion of actual successes in the total SUM population is much higher; we could have chosen from more than 200 success stories and from far fewer identifiable failures.

Service unit management is a shift in the structured organization of the patient unit that (1) reallocates tasks, (2) changes reporting relations, and (3) is done for identifiable purposes. The reallocation of tasks can be understood most clearly if one thinks in terms of five groups of activities that take place on a patient unit.

- Professional patient care, made up of patient teaching, patient monitoring, the preparation of care plans, and patient care activities that require professional judgment in their completion.

- Other patient service, which includes a rather extensive range of patient-

This work is a part of the Patient Unit Management Project of the Bureau of Hospital Administration, School of Public Health, the University of Michigan, Ann Arbor, supported by the W. K. Kellogg Foundation, Battle Creek, Mich. Other members of the study team who have helped in this portion of the project and in its presentation here are Robert Smith, Barbara Horn, Johann Parker, and Douglas Campbell.

serving activities, including feeding, washing, bed making, and many activities for relatively well patients that for the more seriously ill would be professional patient care.

• Unit service activities, such as repairs and maintenance, hall cleaning, waste removal, stocking supplies and securing equipment, and assisting visitors.

• Operation of information systems, including the preparation of reports, requisitions, records, schedules, and other writings (or talking, as in the calling in of a stat order or the arranging of a patient appointment); includes activities that are separable from the performance of associated activities.

• Coordination of patient care and unit activities.

In practice, the head nurse role has concentrated mainly on the fourth and fifth classes of activities (operating information systems and coordinating), the ward clerk has concentrated on the third and fourth (unit service and information systems), ancillary departments have concentrated on the second and third (patient service and unit service), aides and orderlies on the second (patient service), and professional nurses on the first, second, fourth, and fifth (patient care and service, plus the head nurse functions). Unit management is a structural change that shifts elements from the second, third, fourth, and fifth classes of activities from the nursing and ancillary departments to new personnel (the unit manager and the unit aide), adds the existing ward clerk position to that group, and puts the whole in a new department, service unit management. Some SUM introductions do little more than shift a portion of the coordination activities to a unit manager; other introductions shift major parts of classes two through five to unit management. A major variable to be identified in the 14 hospitals is the transfer of tasks that has taken place.

Some hospitals, recognizing that close coordination of SUM with nursing will be required, establish unit management as a department reporting to nursing. Other hospitals give greater weight to the administrative skills and the administration support required by the new department and place it under a nonnursing administrator. Although the reporting channel is less important than the degree of task transfer, the organization structure for the new department is an important variable to be identified for each of the hospitals.

The final characterizing feature of a service unit management program is its purpose. Why did the hospital adopt it? To save money? To increase nursing satisfaction? To facilitate a major redefinition of nursing roles? One of these three reasons is usually the key explanation. Occasionally, a fourth reason, a desire to give better patient service, is the key reason for introducing unit management. There is no doubt that the reason for introducing unit management does affect the way it is introduced, and thus it is identified for each of the study hospitals.

[Table 11-1] provides a 14-hospital summary of the three SUM program characteristics (activities transferred, reporting relations, and purpose). The activities column shows the situation in each program at its most complete development, and the department location column shows both where SUM started and where it is (or where it was when the program failed). The purpose column shows initial expressed purpose but cannot show changes in purpose, the degree to which the purpose was understood, or which members strongly held the purpose identified. Study hospitals are identified by the letters A through N, assigned in chronological order of introduction of SUM.

SIX STAGES ARE IDENTIFIABLE

The 14 hospitals we studied appeared to go through six common stages:

• *Stage 1*—Introduction of the idea to the system. This stage starts with first consideration of the idea and ends when a formal decision is made to introduce SUM fully or on a pilot basis.

• *Stage 2*—Preparation period. This stage includes the selection and training of initial unit personnel and the training or informing of other members of the hospital. It ends when the first unit manager goes on the floor to work.

• *Stage 3*—Unit adjustment period. This is the shakedown period, usually including a gradual transfer of additional duties, an identification of problem areas not seen initially, and some friction between the ever more self-confident unit managers and the ever less tolerant floor nurses.

• *Stage 4*—Expansion period. This stage blends into the unit adjustment period and includes the expansion of unit management to its designed coverage, often extending coverage to other shifts as well as to other parts of the hospital. It often is characterized by much unevenness in the degree of nurse-manager cooperation on different units and by unsolved problems of coordination with one or more ancillary departments. This period typically ends with a change in leadership of the unit management program.

• *Stage 5*—Reorganization. Problems that have been growing in the unit adjustment and the expansion periods are faced at the hospital level, and structural adjustments are made to deal with them.

• *Stage 6*—Adaptation. The program adapts to its environment, either growing slowly along designed paths and stabilizing and securing its designed role, or slowly declining to insignificance and final disappearance.

These six stages are not clear-cut in all 14 hospitals, but they are identifiable, or *should* be identifiable, in most of them. If a hospital proposes to introduce service unit management (or a similar structural innovation), it will do well to give each stage the attention it deserves and not to set absurd time constraints on itself.

TABLE 11–1
CHARACTERISTICS OF SERVICE UNIT MANAGEMENT (SUM)
PROGRAMS IN 14 STUDY HOSPITALS

Hospital	Year of introduction	Activity groups* with major task transfer to SUM	Location of department (first/last)	Primary purpose
A	Pre-1961	5	Administration	Relieve nursing
B	Pre-1961	2,3,5	Administration	Improve patient care
C	Pre-1961	5,4,3	Nursing/ administration	Permit nursing redefinition
D	1961–64	4,3,5	Administration	Relieve nursing
E	1961–64	5,4,3	Administration	Relieve nursing
F	1961–64	5,4	Administration	Compensate for nursing shortage
G	1965–67	4,5	Administration/ nursing	Relieve nursing
H	1965–67	5	Administration	Permit nursing redefinition
I	1965–67	4,3,5	Administration	Relieve nursing
J	1965–67	5	Nursing	Relieve nursing
K	1965–67	5,2,4,3	Administration	Permit nursing redefinition
L	1965–67	5,4,3	Administration	Relieve nursing
M	Post-1967	4,5	Nursing	Unclear
N	Post-1967	5,4,3	Nursing	Permit nursing redefinition

*Activity groups listed in order of importance in the program:
1. Professional patient care
2. Patient service
3. Unit service activities
4. Operating information systems
5. Coordination of unit activities

TABLE 11-1, *continued*

Hospital	Locus of key inputs to start decision	Initial commitment†	Unit manager equivalent in status to	Failed in stage
A	High	MML	Nursing supervisor	5
B	High	HML	Nursing aide	6
C	High and medium	HHM	Head nurse	5‡
D	High	MHM	LPN	3‡
E	High and medium	HHH	RN	—‡
F	High	HHL	RN	5‡
G	High and medium	HML	LPN	6
H	High and medium	HMM	Nursing supervisor	5
I	Medium	LHM	LPN	3
J	Medium	LML	LPN	3
K	High and medium	HHM	LPN	—‡
L	High and medium	HMM	RN	4
M	High	MLL	RN	3
N	High	HHL	RN	4

†Initial commitment to program of administration/nursing administration/floor nurses (H=high, M=medium, L=low).

‡Difficulties only; hospital continues with SUM.

The best setting for the preparation stage came when three conditions were present: (1) both nursing and administration were involved in initial consideration of unit management, with involvement also of middle-level personnel such as nurse supervisors, medical staff, and the executive housekeeper; (2) the initiation stage included discussion on both purpose and substance, that is, on the need for unit management and on the tasks it might be given; (3) the discussion period was long enough for the discussion to move into many parts of the hospital. These are not guarantees of success; Hospital L took six months, involved nursing at the supervisor level and representatives from the medical staff, and still failed. Hospital F went from first consideration to decision in three days and continues to have a unit management program. Nevertheless, the chance to consider and to digest the idea by persons who could make the program succeed or fail did seem to set the stage for more thorough preparation in the following stages.

FAILURE AT UNIT ADJUSTMENT STAGE

None of the hospitals we studied gave up service unit management during the initiation or preparation stages, though obviously there are hospitals that have considered service unit management (the initiation stage) and have decided against introducing it. Two hospitals, however, the 700-bed teaching Hospital J and the 300-bed Hospital M, gave up their programs in the unit adjustment stage.

In Hospital J, the nursing department decided to try a new position that would report to the nursing supervisor and would be responsible for handling supplies and other contacts with ancillary departments. The unit manager was to serve four units, was to be paid midway between the LPN and the RN, and would manage supplies and interdepartmental relations but would not supervise other employees. The first manager left in six months; his replacement left in five months, and she was not replaced. Both managers said they felt they were glorified messengers. Hospital J failed because initiation and preparation were done within the nursing department alone, with little involvement of middle- and lower-level nurses. Its purpose was to relieve nurses, but little thought was given to the process of making the manager role "livable" for those who had to occupy it.

In Hospital M, the administrator encouraged the director of nursing to consider service unit management. Several months later the director of nursing retitled one (apparently superb) ward secretary as unit manager and hired a college graduate to work in a second unit. Criticism of the newcomer by nurses and other ward secretaries forced abandonment of the experiment within a year.

Hospital I, also a large teaching hospital, gave much more thought to the design of its program than had either Hospital J or Hospital M. The initiative for it originated in the nursing department, which was successful in interesting an administrator to the extent of his accepting responsibility for the program. Other members of administration were opposed to the principle of split responsibility on the patient unit, however, and the program began with administrative responsibility but lukewarm support, which was expressed in a great concern for evaluation of results but a minimal interest in program design, recruitment training, or facilitation of SUM-nursing problem-solving behavior at the unit level. Managers were not well trained, and nurses grew increasingly resentful of the managers' inability to cope with problems that they had understood would be handled by unit management. Managers reacted by avoiding such confrontation, and at the end of a year nursing administration suggested that the program be abandoned and that administrative secretaries be assigned to the nursing supervisors on the two floors instead.

Hospital D faced a similar crisis in the first year of its program. A proposal to dump the program was on the agenda of an administrative committee, but a new administrator who recognized the potential value of the program discussed and illustrated the problems that service unit management could help correct. Instead of terminating the program, the committee asked the new administrator to take a more active role in shaping it. This she did, bringing it through both the unit adjustment and the expansion phases.

FAILURE AT THE EXPANSION STAGE

Hospital L and Hospital N, teaching hospitals of 400 and 700 beds respectively, both passed the unit adjustment phase satisfactorily but gave up SUM during the expansion phase. In Hospital L, the program involved significant transfer of unit service, information system, and coordination functions to the service unit management department, with the unit manager, who was equal in status to the nursing supervisor, covering one floor and supervising a ward secretary and unit aides in each unit. Physicians and floor nurses were informed of the plans, but despite these efforts to communicate there apparently was little understanding of the program. Nurses felt genuinely threatened, in part because the unit management program was designed to be independent of nursing and because managers were taught to perform tasks, not to serve nurses. Quite possibly the period of tension would have passed, but a serious financial pinch triggered a physician group to recommend the elimination of the unit managers. The recommendation was accepted, and Hospital L lost its program before the expansion phase was really complete.

Hospital N had the most sophisticated and rational program design of any of the 14 hospitals studied. Seven levels of tasks permitted opportunities for growth within the program, and careful division between shifts permitted effective use of night personnel. By midsummer of the first year of operation, the hospital had full 24-hour, seven-day-a-week coverage, and though marked tension existed on the units the program was well under way. In the fall, however, a sudden exodus of 10 to 15 unit managers and secretaries to return to college hurt the effectiveness of the program seriously, and several months of inadequate coverage by hastily trained replacements ensued. Early the following year, a physician committee recommended that unit managers be removed, that secretaries be reduced in number, that the saving be used to hire more nurses, and that remaining staff report to the head nurse. This recommendation was not vigorously resisted by the administrator, and it spelled the end of the program well before the initial tensions of the expansion stage had been resolved.

In both Hospitals L and N, floor nurses clearly won a major victory by drawing on physician support, and the plan of returning the nurse to the patient was abruptly halted. In both cases also, a somewhat exogenous event—a financial crisis in one case and the loss of a dozen key persons in the other—triggered an attack on the program when it was clearly vulnerable.

FAILURE AT REORGANIZATION STAGE

If a hospital weathers the crisis that may occur in the expansion stage, the next major stage is reorganization. In one sense reorganization is the peaceful resolution of tensions and inconsistencies that have become apparent during the unit adjustment and the expansion stages. In Hospital A, the unit management program had not secured the strong support of the nurses. With unit managers short and nursing dissatisfaction high, the nursing department proposed a reorganization that would extend the role of the nurse supervisor into some of the coordinative responsibility of the manager. Though expressed as a nursing reorganization, it effectively made the unit manager a secretary to the nurse supervisor, and the program gradually faded into oblivion.

Hospital H, a major teaching hospital, chose to introduce and to pay its unit managers at the nurse supervisor level, with the managers assigned almost exclusively to the coordinative function. The problems that had plagued nurses now plagued the unit managers, and, as the managers tried to solve the problems, rather hostile relations developed with some service departments. The situation prompted top administration to reconsider the underlying causes of the problems, and a decision was made to undertake a fundamental restructuring of the hospital. The unit manager program was allowed to die, somewhat to the disappointment of the nursing supervisor, who had appreciated the reduction in errands and nuisance jobs.

Hospital C's reorganization was clearly the smoothest and most peaceful of those studied. The hospital had weathered an early storm in the expansion period that had nearly wrecked the program, but a strong emphasis on manager training, an effort to have managers define success as anticipation of nurse requests, and a major nursing administration commitment to getting nurses back to patient care helped the program get back on its feet. Some seven years after it started, the unit management program in Hospital C was transferred to administration. This reorganization took a carefully nurtured segment of the nursing department into administration, providing more natural promotional lines for unit managers and more effective opportunities to sort out problems and opportunities with service departments. Today Hospital C has one of the most stable and effective unit management programs we have studied, with an exceptionally clear sense of its obligation to provide a setting where professionals may practice nursing.

Hospital G's reorganization was less peaceful. It followed a strongly administration-oriented introduction that finally led to the dismissal of the chief of unit management and to his replacement by a former supervisor of escort messengers in the nursing service. Unit management itself was placed under a former nurse who had taken an administrative position. The reorganization reduced the status of service unit management and seriously weakened the morale of the unit managers. Turnover, especially among the college-educated unit managers, became a problem, although the acceptance of the program by floor nurses increased.

Hospital F's reorganization came close to eliminating unit management. The hospital had set something of a record in going from conception to implementation in two weeks, and other stages also were speeded up. Reorganization one year after inception put unit managers under the direction of a senior assistant who in turn reported to the chairmen of the various divisions, such as medicine, surgery, or radiology. Thus, a central focus of unit management was lost, and for a time the program really disappeared, as it had in Hospital A. For two years the unit managers continued to be responsible primarily for supplies, equipment, and the nominal supervision of ward clerks. Gradually, more chairmen added senior assistants, and at the end of the period a resurgence of interest in the program led administration to reestablish a chief of unit management, with responsibility for coordinating the work of the senior assistants and with more direct hiring, training, and support responsibility for the unit managers. At the same time, plans were introduced for unit managers to take over direct supervision of some of the patient service functions. Unit management in Hospital F is now quite stable. It is not certain why Hospital F's unquestionably bad introduction did not cause it to fail. An important factor may be the director of nursing's commitment to a redefinition of the nursing role: her nurses were being offered real alternatives to the telephone, the nurses' station, and the medication cart.

ADAPTATION AND OTHER OUTCOMES

Only two hospitals, B and G, reached stage six before failing, and one of these is a doubtful arrival. Hospital B was an early experimenter with unit management and was alone among the hospitals in giving primary emphasis to the goal of improving patient care. The program was set up and run entirely by administration, with the strong support of nursing, which approved administration's explicit decision to look for unit managers who could accept comfortably a clearly subordinate role to the nurses. The chief of unit management was a skillful manager and was strongly supported by a senior administrator.

Serving nurses well and bothering no one, the program was to some degree invisible until the administrator left and the chief of unit management retired. The new chief was a poor choice. Some bad practices that had developed were not corrected, nor was the high esprit de corps maintained. Relaxation of early hiring standards produced a cadre of aides and managers of very uneven quality. The seriousness of the situation became clear three years after the new chief had taken over. A decision was reached to break up the department, placing aids under housekeeping and managers under nursing. A series of events led to unionization, and Hospital B's unit managers are now members of Local 1199.

Hospital G came through its reorganization with nursing support more secure but with an internal problem that remained quite serious. It became increasingly difficult to hold unit managers, and nurses gradually adjusted to providing more or less regular supervision to ward clerks and aides when unit managers were not replaced. At one point there were no unit managers to cover the 15 patient units under the program. Since then, the program has been transferred to the nursing department, a nurse supervisor has been put in charge of it, and active recruiting of unit managers has begun. The program has been strengthened by the addition of an assistant unit manager on each unit, leaving unit managers to cover five units each. Hospital G shares with Hospitals J and M the distinction of restarting a program after initial failure.

Hospitals D, E, and K all have reached the adaptation period successfully. Hospital D has a large program that provides patient and unit services. Although it faced considerable resistance from nurses in its expansion period, there is now clear support from floor nurses for the program, though equally clear criticism of its shortcomings. Hospital D has not been able to find a satisfactory relationship between SUM and nursing although recent changes in leadership of both departments offer new hope for solution.

Hospital E has had a similar problem, and its SUM department has been the recipient of sharp and quite threatening attack from floor nurses. An articulate group of floor nurses has seen SUM as an organized attempt to place nurses in a subordinate status to the floor managers. Recent reorganization of the nursing department may help overcome this conflict, though the outcome is still unclear.

Hospital K consistently has been willing to use its relatively comfortable financial position to facilitate the introduction of SUM. It has used SUM aides in a way that is pleasing to nurses, and together with Hospital N had some of the most careful technical planning in making task allocations between nursing and unit management. (Unlike Hospital N, it did not have a major problem in the expansion stage.) Hospital K currently has a stable and successful program.

Why have hospitals failed in introducing SUM? Three hospitals, I, J, and M, were clear neither on purpose, nor on the pain, energy, or money involved in successful implementation. They failed quickly; Hospital D also would have failed but for the intervention of an individual who caused a refocusing, and effectively a restarting, of the program. Two hospitals, L and N, had bad luck, but the bad luck was really an external event occurring in a setting that already had influential groups anxious to dump unit management. Neither Hospital L nor Hospital N had satisfied floor nurses that SUM was a step in the right direction.

Hospital C nearly foundered during expansion, and Hospital G also faced difficulties, both situations being resolved when an aggressive (and in Hospital C's case, clearly incompetent) leader of the program was replaced, thus defusing a growing distaste for the program by floor nurses. No SUM introduction got to the reorganization stage without aggressive leadership in the early stages; those that went beyond that stage found it necessary to shift to a more collaborative, less driving form of leadership. Yet leadership alone could not solve the fundamental problem of SUM, that it took from nurses a part of their identity. This loss was desirable for nurses only if it permitted a new identity to be shaped, but that reshaping did not happen spontaneously. In hospitals where the redefinition of nursing roles was (or became) a major goal in nursing administration (Hospitals C, D, F, H, K, and N), all but two continue with a strong unit management program.

A Paradox Emerges

A small paradox is evident in our study hospitals. Programs that "take over the scut work and leave nurses free to nurse" are easy to start because they please nurses initially, but they are hard to maintain. Programs that seek to manage a setting in which professionals can practice patient care are more threatening initially, because they start with the assumption that nurses should change, but they have more intrinsic vitality—if they survive.

The study team remains convinced that careful thinking through of purpose, preparation of affected staff, and adequate allocation of resources to the pilot program all are important in the successful introduction of SUM. We are convinced also that strong leadership is necessary in the early stages.

The study team is intrigued by a possiblity not clearly seen before, that SUM can remain in existence by failing to have a significant impact on the delivery of patient care—that it can, so to speak, succeed by failing. Unit management can have a significant impact on patient care only if an independent event takes place, the acceptance of patient care management as a separable and an acceptable role by floor nurses. SUM makes this possible; it does not make it happen. Some of our hospitals dropped SUM because the program literally had "left the nurses free to nurse," and too little attention had been given to the consequences of that freedom. The most difficult challenge comes not in the structuring of unit management, but in the associated and necessary restructuring of patient management.

12 | Introducing Structural Change: Service Unit Management (SUM)

George F. Wieland
Robert A. Ullrich

When management acts to introduce a structural change such as SUM, problems may be created at a number of points in the organization (Smith 1971). . . . At the *individual level*, the manager must be particularly concerned with employees' feelings of security. He or she will need to anticipate potential reactions of head nurses, who may view their administrative skills as having been rendered obsolete and their status as having diminished accordingly. At the extreme, ambiguities arising from the transition period and attendant insecurities may lead to conflicts, to disruptions, and to staff turnover.

New patterns or relationships will be created at the *unit level* by the creation of the service unit manager's position. Existing patterns of interaction and status will be altered. Left to themselves, these alterations may produce undesirable consequences; for example, the head nurse may use the time he or she once spent on administrative matters to supervise licensed practical nurses more closely. This change in the relationship between superior and subordinate may result in a decrease in the latter's job satisfaction.

Problems also arise at the *system level*. The service unit manager will replace the head nurse as liaison with other hospital units. Consequently, relations between nursing and other departments will change. In addition, the service unit manager will need to forge new relations with other units in order to discharge his or her boundary role.

Adapted from Robert A. Ullrich and George F. Wieland, *Organization Theory and Design*, rev. ed. (Homewood, Ill.: Richard D. Irwin, Inc., 1980) Chapter 15. © 1980 Richard D. Irwin, Inc.

It is possible to eliminate the causes of some of these problems in the planning phase of the change effort. The process whereby unfreezing is achieved and motivations mobilized can be structured to minimize resistance and anxiety. Here, of course, the whole area of participation in planning is relevant. Individuals who will be most involved and affected can participate in planning for change. Those whose involvement will be merely tangential ought to have the opportunity to provide input. Finally, various other individuals will need to be kept informed, at least.

Training can also pave the way for change. The research by Smith showed lack of training to be a source of serious problems—especially in the case of the service unit manager. When he or she was inadequately trained for the tasks associated with the role, nurses and others were reluctant to relinquish their control and pass their authority on to the newcomer. Where justified, this concern implied the service unit manager's striving for undeserved status. The training advocated here should focus on the development of interpersonal skills as well as technical competence. If he or she is sensitive to potential conflict areas and competent to deal with them, the service unit manager will be free to perform the technical aspects of the job more easily. This is equally true for the head nurse and ward staff.

PHASES OF CHANGE PROCESSES

DEVELOPMENT OF THE ROLE

According to Smith (1971), the change process can be divided into three phases, each concerning problems relevant to the three levels discussed above. The first phase concerns *development of the role*, the second *unit integration*, and the third *system integration*.

Problems facing the head nurse are acute, since he or she must not only learn a new role, but unlearn an old one as well. The former role consisted of stabilized sets of role expectations together with skills and attitudes consistent with the former. This integrated set of skills, attitudes, and behaviors is disrupted by the change, and the nurse will be required to learn new responses to events on the ward.

Smith suggests three approaches to preparing the head nurse as well as other nursing personnel for the anticipated changes. First, they can be made aware of the problems associated with role changes—the need to unlearn and suppress old behaviors before new behaviors can be learned. Second, they can be provided emotional support throughout the period of transition. Admittedly, this is difficult, but at the very least, nurses should be provided opportunities to express their feelings and be reinforced as they demonstrate progress in adapting to their new roles. Third, the most important, is to provide the nurses with role models which they can emulate. It is not enough to inform them of tasks that will no longer be required and to assume that they will use their free time effectively. What is required is a model, or description, of the new role—one that is integrated and makes sense in terms of the nurses' training, skills, and function in the hospital.

Studies of other kinds of organizations also indicate the importance (and usual lack) of role models and support in moving into new roles. New educational programs, for example, may attempt to change the teacher's role from lecturer to resource person. Teachers can be unfrozen by learning the shortcomings of the lecture method and of the possible harm it does as it creates dependency in the student. Teachers can be persuaded to adopt new roles, but these experiments frequently meet with failure. If the new role is not clearly defined, the teacher will not *know how* to be a resource person. If adequate training in the role is not provided, the teacher will lack the *skills* of a resource person. Even when these are provided, the teacher will need additional resources in the form of materials and supplies as well as psychological support.

UNIT INTEGRATION

As progress is made in the first stage (as roles are learned), new problems come to the foreground. In the second phase of the change process one finds interrole conflict. What was formerly a single role (head nurse) has now become two separate roles (head nurse and service unit manager). Other individuals must therefore reorganize their roles vis-à-vis the two major changes. This is descriptive of the integration phase.

Smith describes how the new arrangement (the creation of roles that are highly interdependent and physically close) creates potential for conflict. Role conflict emerges as individuals solve the problems of learning their new roles. Power plays are symptomatic of role conflict. Typically, management and nursing will attempt to influence their superiors to pressure the rival group to conform to specific role expectations; for instance, management may court the hospital administrator's support in laying claim to an area of authority that is also claimed by nursing. Distrusting one another, the two groups resort to power plays, defensiveness, and rigidity, rather than confront the disagreement directly. Cooperation may be perceived as a sign of weakness and subservient status.

The change agent must be aware of the potential for role conflict and, in this situation, reinforce the individuals' perceptions of equal status. It is particularly important that role overload be avoided at this point in the change process. Overload is likely to heighten the intensity of existing conflict.

Excessive work-related demands cause the individual to suffer tension and frustration which frequently lead to aggression and aggravate existing difficulties in interpersonal relations. Furthermore, excessive tasks absorb organizational slack which could have been used to explore and remedy sources of conflict.

Another potential source of conflict is found in differences between the nurses' and managers' roles. The orientation of the nurses' role is professional while the manager's is efficiency-seeking. Thus, managers are likely to value stability as a means to steady state efficiency, while nurses value flexibility as a precondition to individualizing health care according to the patient's needs. The change agent may alleviate this source of conflict by devising performance measures that evaluate the ward as a total entity, as opposed to constructing separate measures of management's and nursing's performance. Thus, attention is focused on a superordinate goal. Pressures to suboptimize performance are reduced to the extent that incumbents of each role perceive cooperation as essential to goal attainment.

SYSTEM INTEGRATION

The third phase of the change process, system integration, becomes salient as problems encountered in unit integration are stabilized. At this point, the manager becomes caught between the demands of nursing (which he or she has come to view as legitimate in the second phase) and those of other departments such as housekeeping, dietetics, or the lab. Typically, these departments do not adapt automatically to changes on the ward. According to Smith, their unresponsiveness has its roots in their ability to maintain the status quo without suffering undue consequences; for example, lab employees can continue old ways of behaving toward people on the ward. They will still contact nurses when problems arise with respect to a patient's test, rather than follow the new lines of communication. Consequences of this behavior will be borne on the ward, but not in the lab. Thus, even after relationships and roles are established on the ward, they will be threatened by elements of the system that have not articulated with these novel roles.

This is probably the lowest point in the change process. The act of solving problems on the ward level has created new problems elsewhere in the hospital, which impede the service unit manager's effectiveness. One possible remedy for problems of system integration is the temporary assignment of an assistant administrator to oversee relationships between service unit management and the various ancillary departments. A second remedy is to establish a task force, comprising department heads and representatives of service unit management, to establish guidelines for interaction. Either way, formal authority is brought to bear in one form or another on recalcitrant department members.

It is entirely possible that problems arising in the third stage of the change process may never be solved. Alternatively, it may be that as one set of problems is resolved another is created. Hospitals, indeed, all complex organizations, are systems. Changes to one part of a system must be met with adaptation in the remainder of the system for interdependencies to remain viable. Furthermore, each of these changes is temporary in the sense that each can be altered by feedback and adaptation. Thus, phase three may never come to an end. As radical as this notion may seem when made explicit, we suggest that it is one with which most of us are familiar and comfortable. Organizations and societies are never freed of their problems by acts of humans or nature. Rather, they alleviate the severity of those most intolerable and, in so doing, create new ones.[1]

REFERENCE

Smith, Robert L. Management of change. In Jelinek, Richard C., Munson, Fred, and Smith, Robert L. (Eds.) *SUM (service unit management): an organizational approach to improved patient care.* Battle Creek, Mich.: W. K. Kellogg Foundation, 1971. Pp. 57–78.

NOTE

1. Of interest is whether the introduction of service unit management improved patient care and reduced its costs in the eight hospitals surveyed. It turns out that the quality of nursing and nonnursing patient care improved overall. However, there is no evidence that the change reduced personnel costs. Job satisfaction increased for both professional and nonprofessional employees. One might conjecture that because of this labor turnover will be reduced, constituting one form of cost reduction.

   One interesting finding is that while the change provided head nurses more time to devote to improving the quality of patient care, the greatest improvements were made by nonprofessionals. Nurses generally failed to take full advantage of the opportunities provided by the service unit management system. This may have been due to the failure of many of the hospitals to provide adequate training and support for nurses whose roles changed. In short, one major conclusion of the present study is that service unit management is productive but can be made even more productive if sufficient attention is paid to the implementation of the nurses' role.

| 13 | Systems Intervention: New Help for Hospitals |

Norman S. Stearns
Thomas A. Bergan
Edward B. Roberts
John L. Quigley

When the chief of medical services at the Lawrence Quigley Memorial Hospital announced his decision to resign, the hospital director knew he could expect trouble in finding a replacement. Salaries at the Chelsea, Massachusetts hospital complex were simply not competitive. Without a highly qualified chief of medicine, the quality of the hospital's medical residency program would drop. Should the residency program be withdrawn, the hospital would soon be unable to recruit staff physicians interested in teaching opportunities in spite of the hospital's low salaries. The hospital might be forced to drop some services. Inevitably, patient care would suffer. To head off this spiral of decline, the director suggested to the board of trustees that Quigley Memorial set up a "systems intervention" project. He explained that systems intervention is based on the assumption that all units within an organization are involved in the organization's problems—causes, effects, and, ultimately, solutions. The board supported his proposal.

Within four months, a systems intervention task force composed of senior hospital staff, a consultant, and key persons from outside the hospital had set in motion a course of action that strengthened Quigley Memorial's residency program, and enabled the director to recruit five new staff physicians, to improve coordination of inpatient and outpatient services, to heighten staff

Reprinted from *Health Care Management Review,* Vol. 1, No. 4, "Systems Integration: New Help for Hospitals," by Norman S. Stearns, Thomas A. Bergan, Edward B. Roberts, and John L. Quigley, by permission of Aspen Systems Corporation, © 1976.

awareness to problems in the delivery of ancillary services, and—not the smallest of achievements—to convince the chief of medicine to withdraw his resignation.

DYNAMICS AND TECHNIQUES

Systems intervention is a process that uses systems dynamics[1] and behavioral science techniques[2,3] to overcome barriers to change. By involving those key players who could prevent change in the process of planning and directing change, the systems intervention process goes right to the heart of the issue that ordinarily stymies hospital administrators—the rivalry and personal conflict among "autonomous" departments and service chiefs.

SYSTEM FLOW DIAGRAMS

Systems intervention relies on system flow diagrams. These visual models help policy makers to analyze current problems, to see how the problems have evolved over time, to design potential solutions, and, most important, to understand the implications of each possible solution for each affected department of the hospital. Models focus on (1) the relationships among services within the hospital, and (2) the behavioral factors that are central to both problems and solutions. In the process of developing their own models, participants come to understand the root causes of personal and professional conflicts and can discuss these conflicts within a structured context. Structure provides safety; it promotes openness and a new sense of mutual trust.

TEAM COMMITMENT

Once they perceive avenues for change together, key hospital leaders are committed to the "team" approach. This commitment does not end with the preparation of a list of recommendations. It continues into the implementation, monitoring, and reevaluation stages of problem-solving activities, and can lead to a new awareness of the hospital as an organic unity.

BARRIERS TO CHANGE

SEPARATISM

Most hospitals are organized into separate departments along functional lines; e.g., medicine, surgery, outpatient, nursing, laboratory. The delegation of substantial power and authority to each department chief instills in each a sense of autonomy. Within each department, this sense is heightened for staff by an intense, and exclusive, identity with their immediate peer group. Few staff members in any one department understand how other departments operate. Separatism is nourished by a common assumption that other departments are competing for scarce resources—money and people—and by a history of interdepartmental rivalries. There is seldom agreement among departments on the causes, or even the nature, of problems that affect them all, and certainly not on the solutions. Half-hearted and, therefore, unsuccessful attempts to work together to solve problems breed frustration and resignation—"it can't be done." Long-standing problems are often dealt with only when they become too critical to put aside, and then usually by a handful of administrators, rather than key members of all affected groups.

PRIMARY RESPONSIBILITY

The facts of life are that all the functions within a hospital are interrelated and interdependent. But few hospitals have a permanent structure for solving problems that takes this interdependence into account. It is rare to find a committee composed of department heads who see their *primary* responsibility as working *together* to solve the hospital's problems.

SYSTEMS INTERVENTION KNOCKS DOWN BARRIERS

Four tactics are basic to systems intervention: the formation of *a broad-based task force of key hospital staff; a focus on specific problems;* the preparation of *flow diagrams;* and an *orientation toward implementation.* Task force members must have sufficient authority among themselves to insure that a consensus would be tantamount to an authorization for action. A specific focus provides a structure within which to resolve personal and organizational problems. Flow diagrams promote a dynamic view of a problem situation by showing past changes over time; they also provide a framework for future change by projecting the impact of change on all affected departments. Since flow diagrams, or models, show the attitudinal and behavioral changes that must accompany changes in activity, the task force can prevent conflicts *before* they occur. And finally, task force members are encouraged to participate in every stage of change, to oversee as well as to recommend new policies and activities. This is the most crucial aspect of systems intervention. The people most likely to resist change take responsibility for seeing that it happens.

SYSTEMS INTERVENTION IN ACTION

In the remainder of this article, we shall demonstrate how the systems intervention process works by describing how the Lawrence Quigley Memorial Hospital complex (QMH) put it to work.

The Quigley Memorial complex consists of a large general medical and surgical outpatient department, a 305-bed domiciliary unit, and an inpatient unit that includes 100 acute medical and surgical beds and 200 extended-care and chronic-care beds. All patients are veterans who are not directly charged for the services they receive. The hospital is supported financially by the Commonwealth of Massachusetts. Medical and surgical services at the hospital are staffed in part by residents from two Boston community hospitals with medical school affiliations: St. Elizabeth's Hospital and the New England Deaconess Hospital. (St. Elizabeth's Hospital also provides clinical and laboratory services to support its residency program.) The two residency programs are vital to the operation of Quigley Memorial's medical and surgical services. Thanks to the presence of residents, QMH can operate with fewer salaried physicians, and, despite its low salaries, can recruit full- and part-time physicians.

When Quigley Memorial's chief of medicine decided to resign, the hospital director chose to address the major issue—how to make QMH more attractive to full-time and part-time physicians. Toward this end, he solicited suggestions for ways to improve the medical residency and patient care programs. From a source within the hospital, he received a document entitled: "A Proposal for Development of an Expanded Patient Care and Teaching Medical Service." This proposal called for a restructuring of the medical service, more emphasis on teaching, and development of a new program called "Teaching Teachers to Teach." Key staff people who reviewed the proposal were favorably disposed, but they argued that it would put an unbearable strain on certain supporting services (e.g., nursing, laboratory, and radiology). Further discussion revealed that relations among members of these services were already strained to the breaking point. It was clear that *no* plan to improve the medical service would succeed unless something was done to deal with this basic barrier to change.

What happened next is described below in tandem with the basic steps of the systems intervention process.

STEP 1. DEFINING THE RULES

Before a systems intervention project is launched, it is essential that the key actors—the hospital director, the consultant (who may be a systems intervention expert from within the hospital), the task force chairman (in some cases, the hospital director), and potential task force members—reach agreement on three subjects. These are (a) the project's objective; (b) the initial problem focus; and (c) the steps involved in the project (i.e., *all* the steps, herein discussed, essential to the systems intervention process).

Once the QMH trustees approved a systems intervention project, a consultant was appointed and the key staff people were able to reach an agreement in all three areas. The objective was to improve the medical residency and patient care programs. The immediate task was to evaluate the specific proposal received by the hospital director.

STEP 2. FORMING A TASK FORCE

The systems intervention task force must be broad-based. This means that membership must include all senior staff people, and others from outside the hospital, who have the power to prevent change in the areas directly involved in the problem under consideration. At Quigley Memorial, the task force was composed of the medical director, the chief of medicine, representatives from the surgical services, the director of the outpatient department (OPD), the director of the nursing service, and representatives from St. Elizabeth's Hospital and its teaching affiliate, Tufts Medical School.

STEP 3. CONDUCTING THE RESEARCH

In order to analyze the problem at hand, the systems intervention consultant must interview all task force members, and may also decide to question other persons whose knowledge and opinions are germane. (In addition, the consultant may prepare and distribute questionnaires.) He or she then prepares a list of the problems and an issue-by-issue synopsis of interviews (and survey results). Although the consultant need not check the validity of data received from interviews and questionnaires (unless conflicting information is received), he or she must inform all those who are asked for information that data will be discussed openly at task force meetings.

At QMH, the consultant began his interviews immediately after the first task force meeting. He asked questions relating to (a) the interviewee's role in the hospital and the relation of his or her function or department to other areas in the hospital; (b) current problems confronting Quigley Memorial, their causes, and possible solutions; (c) other internal and external trends and changes that might affect the hospital; (d) the proposal for expanded teaching programs, the interviewee's view of changes needed to implement the proposal, and the potential benefits and drawbacks of the proposal and associated changes. The consultant then prepared an issue-oriented synopsis of all his interviews with hospital staff and members of the larger community.

STEP 4. PREPARING THE FLOW DIAGRAMS

After the interviews are conducted, the consultant prepares a set of cause-and-effect diagrams that describe the current problems, how the situation has evolved over time, and the possible opportunities for change. As more information is gathered, and as the task force, on the basis of these initial diagrams, changes its perceptions or redefines problems, the consultant prepares new diagrams that express the relationships among actors and issues. The QMH consultant presented his initial diagrams at the second task force meeting. These are shown here as Figures 13-1 to 13-5.

Figure 13-1 sets out the factors affecting the quality of the hospital's residency program and illustrated that the expanded-teaching proposal might help the hospital to attract new physicians, as well as improving residents' motivation. It also demonstrated that the poor quality of some supporting services and a decline in the hospital census could undermine an expanded

FIGURE 13-1

FACTORS AFFECTING THE QUALITY OF QMH'S RESIDENCY PROGRAM

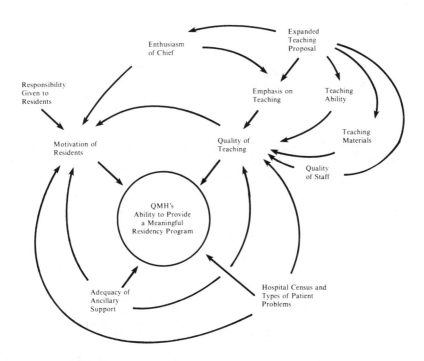

teaching program. The proposal for the new program did not address these problems. Figure 13-2 revealed that services dependent on technology at QMH were not competitive with other hospitals' services. This technology gap affected staff in these services, and residents were unsatisfied. St. Elizabeth's Hospital, as a result, might decide to terminate its residency program and withdraw its supporting services. Figure 13-3 showed that the hospital's low salaries and inadequate support services had weakened its ability to recruit staff physicians. If these problems continued, staff turnover would increase and the residency program would suffer. An expanded emphasis on teaching, however, could revitalize QMH's acute services, especially if ancillary services were improved. Figure 13-4 suggested that the several problems together could cripple the hospital's ability to function, unless steps were taken to intervene in the "vicious cycle." Figure 13-5 brought the outpatient department into the hospital picture.

FIGURE 13-2

A MORE COMPLETE VIEW OF SOME OF THE FACTORS INFLUENCING
THE ADEQUACY OF ANCILLARY SERVICES AND THE
QUALITY OF TEACHING

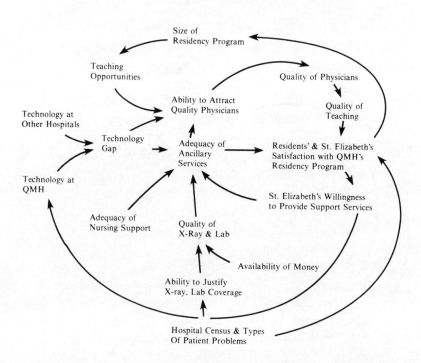

FIGURE 13-3

ATTRACTIVENESS OF QMH TO PHYSICIANS AND
THE NEED TO HIRE PHYSICIANS

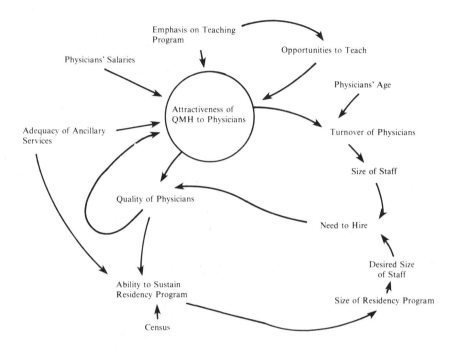

STEP 5. DISCUSSING THE DIAGRAMS

Once the consultant has prepared models that diagram the dynamic, cause and effect relationship among problems, the task force members have a framework for discussion. The diagrams enable them to redirect their attention from individual problems to the situation as a whole. They may then decide to narrow, expand, or shift the problem focus of their project.

At the second task force meeting, members discussed the diagrams prepared by the consultant. They focused on the inadequacies of certain ancillary services, the lack of equipment in some services, and the need for more professional personnel. They agreed that the specific problems were:

- lack of round-the-clock laboratory and blood bank services,
- limited availability of X-ray services and radiologists,
- inadequate pulmonary and coronary-care equipment,
- the hospital's inability to recruit full-time physicians in the OPD, part-time

physicians in the inpatient units, and registered inhalation therapists, laboratory technicians, and nurses (particularly RNs with specialties),
- disagreements among OPD staff and medical and surgical staff regarding admission criteria and procedures, preadmission tests, and the use of medical service residents in the OPD, and
- long delays for patients using the area Veterans Hospital for diagnostic procedures.

Task force members were especially sensitive to problems in the OPD, as shown in Figure 13–5. Most patients at Quigley Memorial are admitted through the OPD, which, for its part, depends on the hospital for laboratory, X-ray, and other services. During the year prior to the task force project, the number of physicians in the OPD had declined and the volume of OPD patients had dropped as a result. Figure 13–5 demonstrated that if this trend continued, the OPD would soon be unable to provide adequate service to its patient population, and that there would be fewer hospital admissions as a result. A decline in the hospital census would, in turn, make it even more difficult to maintain an adequate level of ancillary services, to justify the

FIGURE 13–4

OVERALL RELATIONSHIPS AFFECTING THE
EVOLVING SITUATION AT QMH

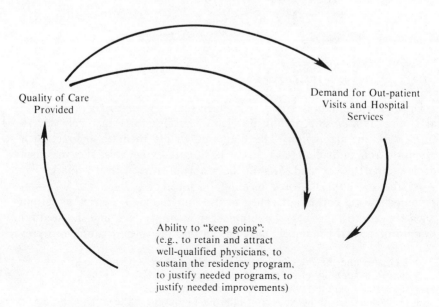

FIGURE 13–5

INTERDEPENDENCIES BETWEEN OPD AND HOSPITAL SERVICES

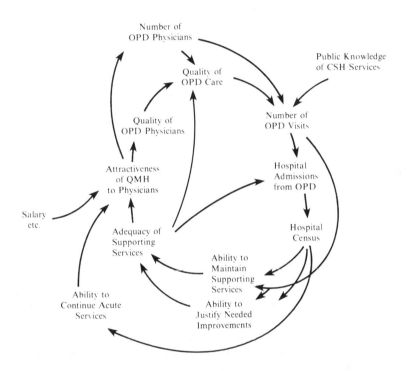

purchase of equipment needed for chronic and acute patients, to support a residency program, and, therefore, to provide quality hospital care as a back-up to the OPD. This would further diminish the hospital's ability to recruit physicians for the OPD and the inpatient units.

The fact that all these problems were interrelated suggested, on the one hand, that deterioration in every crucial area of the hospital affected the rest of the hospital, and, on the other, that improvement in any one area would upgrade other areas. For example, improvements in ancillary services would improve the quality of care and the quality of the residency program, thus making it easier to retain and recruit physicians of high quality. This, in turn, would improve the residency program and would persuade St. Elizabeth's Hospital to maintain the program and to continue to provide supporting services.

STEP 6. DISCUSSING DIFFERING PERCEPTIONS

The systems intervention consultant helps the members of the task force discuss differences of opinion about the interpretation of data and variables in the models, and to handle personality conflicts. Questions about validity of data may refer to material facts (costs, numbers of people, spatial dimensions, etc.) or behavioral perceptions. Material facts are easy to check. Validation of behavioral perceptions may be less "clean-cut," but this is the *sine qua non* of the systems intervention process.

In the discussion that followed the presentation of the consultant's models, task force members at Quigley Memorial agreed that the problems revealed were critical. They also admitted that these problems had been the major source of conflict among hospital departments, and, in the past, among the task force members themselves. The chief of medicine said these problems had influenced his decision to resign. The diagrams convinced them that each department, not just Medical Services, would benefit if the problems were solved, and that it would take the cooperation of all task force members to solve them. Despite their past disputes and their apprehension about working together, they agreed to these key points.

STEP 7. SHARPENING THE FOCUS

Once the first diagrams have been analyzed and discussed, task force members may ask the consultant to collect additional information and, if necessary, to prepare new diagrams. This may happen several times during the course of a project. The task force may also decide to authorize the development of a computer simulation model, based on the diagrams, to enable them to analyze problems involving a larger number of variables. On the basis of new diagrams and/or a computer simulation model, the members may decide to redefine the project by concentrating on fewer problems or expanding the ground to be covered.

As a result of its initial findings, the QMH task force decided to focus on the specific problems that were adversely affecting patient care, relationships among departments, and the quality of the residency program. This was a significant redefinition of objectives. Before the end of their second meeting, task force members developed a list of specific problems to be addressed, made recommendations for analyzing and solving them, and established priorities. Members also distributed responsibility among themselves for following up on these priorities.

STEP 8. STUDYING POTENTIAL SOLUTIONS

After task force members have become accustomed to using models for analyzing the causes and effects of current problems, it is a small step to the use of models for studying the impact of each proposed solution to a specific problem. Members will find that they have become proficient in preparing and using these models for further discussion and analysis. During their third and fourth meetings, QMH task force members examined several specific problems and potential solutions. Each of these meetings was task-oriented. Diagrams were prepared beforehand that showed the causes and implications of each problem; other diagrams helped members to analyze the impact of proposed solutions. As before, the visual models helped to structure discussion and to defuse hostilities. Participants at these meetings discovered that they could discuss differences of opinion without rancor. Discussions almost always led to a consensus of opinion on how to solve commonly recognized problems. Some members found that the recommendations they most ardently championed could not be implemented without causing new problems and were willing to seek new answers.

STEP 9. PREPARING AN ACTION PLAN

As soon as the task force members have reached a consensus on how to solve the problems they have been studying, they should prepare a plan that will translate recommendations into actions. This plan should be shown to a broad range of staff within the hospital, and, where necessary, modifications should be incorporated into the final report. During its fifth meeting, the QMH task force consolidated its findings, developed preliminary recommendations for change, drew up plans for implementing recommendations, identified areas needing further research or analysis, and assigned responsibility for following up on these activities among themselves. The draft report they prepared included recommendations for solving current problems, proposals for development of several new specialized programs, and several portions of the original proposal for a "Teaching Teachers to Teach" program. Task force members next discussed the draft with the hospital director, and held a sixth meeting to make appropriate revisions. They then distributed the report throughout the hospital and, after a short time, held a staff meeting to discuss their recommendations. They found that most of the resistance to their proposals came from key staff who had not been invited to participate in the task force, confirming the importance of involving all persons who are important to the implementation of change into the systems intervention process *from the beginning*. After this broad review, the task force made further revisions and submitted a final report to the hospital's Medical Executive Committee and the board of trustees. This report emphasized the interdependencies among hospital departments and the need for cooperation to effect change. Both groups approved the report.

STEP 10. CONTINUING THE COMMITMENT

Task force members should begin to implement their recommendations as soon as they receive the necessary approvals, and even before where approval is not in doubt. All members must take responsibility for monitoring progress and taking whatever actions are necessary to follow each proposal through to its successful conclusion. As often as necessary, task force members should reconvene to analyze and resolve unforeseen setbacks. It is this continuing commitment, beyond the preparation of a "final" report, that will make accomplishment of project goals possible.

The achievements mentioned at the beginning of this article suggest that Quigley Memorial is already beginning to reap the benefits of its commitment to the systems intervention process. It is a process that can be used successfully by service chiefs, hospital directors, and other administrators with major organizational responsibilities.

NOTES

1. Forrester, Jay W. "Market Growth as Influenced by Capital Investment," *Industrial Management Review*, Volume 9, No. 2, pp. 83–105.
2. Beckhard, R., *Organization Development: Strategies and Models*, Reading, Mass., Addison-Wesley, 1969, p. 100.
3. Kolb, David A. and Frohman, Alan L. "An Organization Development Approach to Consulting," *Sloan Management Review*, Fall, 1970, pp. 51–65.

III

Psychological Changes
and Organization
Development:
The Behavioral Approach
to Improving
Organizations

Introduction

This section introduces the psychological or behavioral approach to organizational change and improvement. In this view of organizations and their improvement, people are the key elements. Technology and structures are operated by people, and without people, there would be no organization. If psychological characteristics, such as attitudes toward cooperation and being open to criticism and to new ways of working, can be improved, then innovations and improvements in structures and technology will follow, if necessary, from the improved behavior of organizational members.

The first reading in this section (Chapter 14) summarizes theory and practice in the area of organization development, or OD, as the main psychological approach to change is termed. A theoretical introduction to OD is provided in terms of the unfreezing-changing-refreezing model for changing individual and group behavior. This is followed by a theoretical account of the process by which an OD consultant effects change in individuals and groups.

ORGANIZATION DEVELOPMENT

The prototype technique in OD is sensitivity training or T-groups, an approach to changing interpersonal relations by improving deeply held, emotional attitudes regarding collaboration, openness, and trust between organizational members. Research and practitioner experience are cited to suggest that less deep (i.e., shallower, less emotional and more cognitive) approaches to improving work relations may be more effective in some circumstances. This reading deals with OD as generally used in a variety of settings; later readings (Chapters 15-16, 18-21) describe OD in specific health care settings.

The discussion in Chapter 6 shows how valuable physician participation in management might be, but it also provides some basis for being skeptical about the efficacy of organization development in hospitals and other health care organizations. In Chapter 15, Weisbord writes about this and other problems, entitling his article "Why Organization Development Hasn't Worked (So Far) in Medical Centers."

Weisbord provides objective evidence on the freedom of physicians from organizational and managerial constraints. When he asked medical center physicians to whom they were responsible in dealing with patient care, 55 percent said "no one" or left the item blank. Organization development is meant to increase interdependency, so it is no wonder, as Weisbord says, that physicians see OD as a threat.

SUCCESSFUL ORGANIZATION DEVELOPMENT

According to a few accounts, OD has worked in some medical settings. Chapter 16 reports success at the Martin Luther King, Jr., (MLK) Health Center, which is aimed at providing comprehensive family-based ambulatory care for some 6,000 individuals in a ghetto setting. The consultants focused on the primary health care teams composed of physicians, nurses, and family health workers (indigenous community members). The fifteen hours of training for each team covered many of the potent interventions of OD: diagnostic interviewing and feedback, process facilitation, role negotiation, and training in giving feedback and sharing of feelings. The reaction of the teams is described as "generally positive." One family health worker said, "I feel more important. The importance of everyone's job has been explained, and I am more efficient. As for other team members, they are more considerate, more willing to give" (p. 66).

An attempt was also made at training internal OD consultants, who were members of the central, bureaucratic MLK office. Apparently, while the participants in the training personally benefitted, the trainees and their new skills were not subsequently used in any organized fashion. The OD consultants responded to this failure by saying "management too needs to be trained in how to effectively utilize this new resource" (p. 100).

PSYCHOLOGICALLY DEEP AND SHALLOW INTERVENTIONS

Why is OD apparently effective in the setting of the ambulatory, community health care team, but not in the medical center setting? One key to providing an answer is described in Chapter 14—Harrison's "depth" dimension in change interventions. "Shallow" interventions such as changes in managerial procedures (e.g., replacing an old report form with a new report form) are essentially cognitive and not threatening in a personal way, while OD is "deep" and involves emotions. The shallow change strategy will change structures that are "outside" of the individual psyche. These are impersonal matters of "information" that do not require psychological readjustment, changing a person's motivations, values, or sense of self. On the other hand, OD is generally a psychologically "deep" intervention strategy, although the specific techniques may be used to intervene over a wide range of depth, from moderate (e.g., changing one's work style from a centralized control of subordinates to a more decentralized sharing of information in weekly meetings, allowing input during planning sessions) to rather deeper (e.g., changing deeply held attitudes about the nature of others as people, changing the degree of trust and openness one displays toward others) to quite deep (e.g., exploring and dealing with one's basic anxieties, feelings of worth, and sense of being).

Individuals tend to resist deep interventions, but, suggests Harrison, if a relatively powerful consultant is operating in the small training group setting (where the clients have abdicated their formal roles), he or she can overcome the clients' resistance. In terms of the classic OD paradigm, the consultant can use his or her power: (1) to "unfreeze" old behaviors, (2) to help the client model new behaviors ("change"), and (3) to "refreeze" or reinforce new, more appropriate behaviors.[1]

In short, to intervene at a "deep" level, as in OD, the consultant usually must have power over the client. In the medical center, the physicians are very powerful; they have the expertise needed by the organization and they are not dependent on others. If threatened, an individual physician can also call upon the collective power of the medical staff to resist OD efforts. In contrast, in the community care setting, a physician is rather dependent on other team members and their expertise. The physician is only one part of an inter-dependent team with the goal of providing comprehensive care, and he or she needs the help of the others on the team.

A SHALLOW PSYCHOLOGICAL INTERVENTION: SURVEY FEEDBACK

The next reading (Chapter 17) provides a description of a relatively shallow or cognitive (not deeply emotional or personal) OD technique, survey feedback. Research evaluating survey feedback, sensitivity training, and other OD techniques as used in 23 different organizations shows survey feedback to be effective in achieving improved interpersonal behavior, including leadership, communication flow, and collaboration. This technique is described in detail here, not so much as a panacea but as exemplifying the kinds of approaches to OD that may be effective under some circumstances. Survey feedback is a relatively flexible technique; it can be used for relatively deep interventions as well as (more usually) shallow interventions.

Used as a relatively shallow, but still a psychological, intervention, survey feedback will go beyond a discussion of the "facts" of the survey. The group discussions will explore the attitudes and feelings behind the findings. It will question, for example, whether poor coordination between two departments is due to feelings of "superiority" and the withholding of information, to impersonal attitudes and resentment because contacts are infrequent and only on an "emergency" basis, and so on. The OD facilitator will help the group members examine their feelings about these matters and help them explore ways they can test alternative explanations and develop more appropriate modes of interaction. Subsequent discussions will consider such issues as whether the new patterns of behavior are effective and how further problems might best be handled.

The next reading, by Margulies (Chapter 18), provides an account of survey feedback used in a health care setting. This apparently successful OD intervention in a health maintenance organization (Kaiser-Permanente) seems to support the view that physicians may resist very deep OD interventions like sensitivity training but can accept psychological interventions that are a little more shallow. A questionnaire survey on organizational climate was followed by data feedback, discussions, and then the designing and implementation of concrete operational improvements. Areas of focus included freer communications, improved relationships between those from the "hospital culture" and those from the "clinic culture," better relationships between physicians and managers—especially providing the physicians with more of a managerial orientation, better interdepartmental cooperation, and more clarity on responsibilities and authority.

This OD effort has apparently achieved some initial success in part because the physicians in this setting, a health maintenance organization, are less powerful than those in the medical center. The physicians at Kaiser probably have more power to resist than do those in community health care teams, because they are in relatively familiar hospital or clinic settings and they have colleagues for support. But they have less power than those in the medical center or usual hospital setting because they are employees, with a contractual and integrated relationship with their organization, not permitting the independent behavior more common in the medical center or hospital.

In addition, the Margulies project was apparently successful because it was a relatively shallow intervention, an effort which would not arouse much resistance from physicians as well as other organizational members. Physicians were less likely to use whatever power they had, because the intervention was not as "deep" or as threatening as most OD efforts involving emotional issues in small group settings. In part, this was because the interventions were by means of relatively impersonal questionnaires and feedback reports.

Even more important, however, is the fact that a great emphasis was apparently placed on what Margulies terms "concrete operational improvements"—structural matters such as reassignment of staff, procedural changes such as new kinds of reports to patients or a new orientation program on the role and function of other departments. Such a relatively shallow focus on managerial problems, rather than deeper interpersonal or individual problems is not so likely to arouse the power of physicians to resist.

Weisbord's analysis of OD in the medical center setting supports this point about the importance of using relatively shallow interventions where the clients have considerable power to resist deep interventions. He suggests that OD consultants and managers should work with physicians on matters such as budgeting procedures, clarifying goals, planning resource management, and generally involving physicians in managerial activities.

MANAGEMENT BY OBJECTIVES

The next two readings (Chapters 19 and 20) describe management by objectives (MBO) as used in the hospital. These chapters could appear in Part II, since MBO is often an attempt to rationalize and facilitate managerial action. First, the goal or goals for the organization as a whole are decided upon and clarified by those at the top of the organization. Then, the objectives or goals of those at the next lower level are decided upon so that they serve as the means to goals at the higher level, and so on, down the hierarchy. In this way, the work of the organization is more clearly structured and better coordinated.

However, by giving subordinates an opportunity to propose their objectives, and to participate with their superiors in setting goals, motivation may be enhanced (Beck and Hillmar 1972). Depending on how the joint goal-setting meetings are handled, and also how follow-up and subsequent performance appraisal are treated, more or less of an impact may be made on "people" variables, such as motivation, cooperation, communication, and supportive interpersonal relations.

In other words, MBO is quite flexible. Like the survey technique, MBO can be a technique that is essentially cognitive, improving information and providing a structure for articulating work efforts in a more rational fashion. On the other hand, the MBO meetings, like the feedback meetings in survey feedback, can be used as an OD technique, to unlock motivation or enhance collaboration.

The first of these two readings on MBO (Chapter 19) describes the technique essentially as a means of improving managerial action, improving the rational structure of coordination in the hospital. Then, in Chapter 20, two change agents describe an MBO effort that was modified and made more effective by emphasizing psychological change techniques. The initial application of MBO, while acceptable and apparently successful at top management levels in the hospital, was rejected by physicians at the ward level.

Then, in addition to labeling the approach to change differently—not "better management" but "better patient care"—the change agents emphasized that the ward teams were themselves to decide the focus of the improvement efforts in their own particular settings. Emphasis was on participation rather than on matching procedures to higher-level goals, as in the rational and structural approach to MBO. Ward team meetings were used to engender enthusiasm and commitment, and from these psychological changes subsequently flowed changes in the patterns of patient care (including an apparent 10 percent savings in patient length of stay).

Evaluation Research

The final reading (Chapter 21) in this section presents some excellent evaluation research on a failed effort at OD training in a hospital emergency department. Some psychological characteristics changed. Departmental members were more satisfied with their work, pay, and coworkers, and they had more positive views about the opportunities to try out new ideas and the freedom to use their own judgment and make their own decisions. But the aim of the experiment, improved communications behavior, apparently was not obtained. The authors conclude that a training intervention may change attitudes, but this is likely to be temporary, unless real and supporting changes are made "by the organization" (read: by management). In the terms we have used, psychological changes may be relatively fragile unless coordinated with managerial actions to change structures and technologies.

The findings of this last study are thus of some interest, but an even more important aspect of the research is the use of a rigorous evaluation methodology, with experimental controls, to assess whether the change intervention really did work. This study is almost unique in the field of OD in providing a rigorous evaluation which allows the prospective purchaser and user of such techniques to form his or her own relatively objective opinion of their value.

Reference

Beck, Arthur C., Jr., and Hillmar, Ellis D. OD to MBO or MBO to OD: does it make a difference? *Personnel Journal*, 1972, *51*, 827–834.

Note

1. Harrison argues, however, that the use of high consultant power ultimately fails when the "changed" clients are reintegrated in the organization. Colleagues undo the changes which they see as incompatible. In this regard, longitudinal data on the durability of changes at MLK would be of interest.

14 | Organization Development

George F. Wieland
Robert A. Ullrich

THEORY IN ORGANIZATION DEVELOPMENT

Warren Bennis (1969), one of the best-known proponents of organization development (OD), describes it as an educational strategy intended to bring about planned organizational change. While numerous strategies (techniques) are advocated, all are related in that they seek organizational change through changes in "people" variables such as values, attitudes, interpersonal relations, and organizational climate. This is in contrast to some of the change strategies described earlier that deal with structure, technology, and the physical environment. The primary focus on people variables arises because those who developed and presently work in the field are, for the most part, psychologists. To these people, the individual and small-group aspects of a situation are most readily understood and appear most amenable to change.

The second basic characteristic of OD, according to Bennis, is that it attempts to solve *problems* that are experienced by members of the organization. The changes sought are not advocated by an outside consultant. Rather, they are in response to needs felt within the organization. As examples of problems typically addressed by OD, Bennis cites communications problems, intergroup conflicts, leadership issues, questions of identity, problems of satisfactions and inducements to work, and questions about organizational effectiveness.

A third characteristic of OD is its reliance on educational strategies emphasizing *experienced behavior*. Data feedback, sensitivity training, confrontation meetings, and other kinds of experiential learning methods are

Adapted from Robert A. Ullrich and George F. Wieland, *Organization Theory and Design*, rev. ed. (Homewood, Ill.: Richard D. Irwin, Inc. 1980) Chapters 15 and 16. © 1980 Richard D. Irwin, Inc.

used to generate publicly shared data and experiences upon which the organization can plan and act.

A fourth characteristic is that change agents are, for the most part, external to the client system. Bennis argues that an external change agent can be more objective than an employee in his assessment of an organization. Furthermore, he can affect the power structure in ways that are unavailable to internal change agents.

A fifth essential aspect of OD is the *collaborative* relationship between the change agent and the client system. Bennis defines collaboration as comprising mutual trust, joint determination of goals and means, and high total influence.

The sixth point is that change agents share a *social philosophy* (or a set of values) about the world in general and especially about organizations. Practitioners tend to believe that realization of these values will lead to the development of more humane, democratic, and efficient systems.

NORMATIVE GOALS IN ORGANIZATION DEVELOPMENT

The values of change agents in OD stem from *humanistic psychology*, and are in contrast with those arising from the so-called Protestant ethic (e.g., rationality, task orientation, and so on). According to Bennis, goals arising from these values include the following:
1. The improvement of interpersonal competence.
2. The reinforcement of values that legitimize feelings and emotions.
3. The increased understanding of behavior in groups.
4. The development of more effective work groups and team management.
5. The development of more effective methods of conflict resolution, namely, replacing bureaucratic methods with more open approaches.
6. The transition from rational to organic systems.

In short, then, OD is ideally a:

long-range effort to improve an organization's problem-solving and renewal processes, particularly through a more effective and collaborative management of organization culture—with special emphasis on the culture of the formal work teams—with the assistance of a change agent, or catalyst, and the use of theory and technology of applied behavioral science, including action research. (French and Bell 1973, p. 15)

PROCESS CONSULTATION

Another leading OD proponent, Schein (1969), emphasizes the role of *process* in organization development programs; that is, the change agent studies organizational processes (ways of behaving) in order to help his client become more aware of the way in which he or she behaves and affects others. It is this awareness and understanding that enables the client to improve organizational effectiveness.

Schein argues that studying interpersonal and group events enables the change agent to help the manager define his or her own problems and decide what further help he or she needs. The *process consultant*, as Schein terms the change agent, examines work flows, interpersonal relations, communications, intergroup relations, and the like and *works with* managers in diagnosing problems and the processes from which they arise. Schein feels that the consultant can seldom learn enough about the client organization to know which improvements are best for the particular group of people involved, given their unique traditions, histories, and personalities. The process consultant's job is to help the managers help themselves—to help them diagnose their own problems, generate alternatives, and select a solution that is suited to their own unique circumstances. As a result, clients also become aware of potentials for group conflict, anxieties that may prevent or distort communication, unspoken organizational assumptions and beliefs, consequences of various managerial styles, and alternative ways of communicating, providing leadership, and including communication and cooperation among individuals and groups.

Schein suggests that process consultation be contrasted with two alternative models: (1) the consultant as *expert advice giver* and (2) *patient-physician* model. In the first model, the client defines his or her needs in terms of knowledge or services that are lacking and engages a consultant to provide them. This assumes that the client can diagnose needs accurately, communicate them effectively, and identify change agents who are competent to deliver the appropriate information and services. Furthermore, the model assumes a known cause-and-effect relationship between the consultant's activities and the elimination of the problem to which they are addressed. These are tenuous assumptions that can lead the client to purchase consultations that ultimately prove unsatisfactory. Many consultants' reports gather dust in some forgotten file because they are not what the client wanted. Even worse, consultants can generate unnecessary conflict between groups that will benefit or suffer losses if the recommended action is undertaken. Furthermore, where recommendation actions are inconsistent with the organization's culture, progress may be fleeting and changes reversed over time. For these reasons, Schein advocates collaboration between change agents and clients wherein the client system learns to diagnose and remedy its own problems.

In the second model (patient-physician), the client hires consultants who diagnose the organization's ills and recommend a program of "therapy." Difficulties arise when individuals and departments resent and resist the consultants' probing or reject the diagnosis or therapy. Again, Schein's advocacy of process consultation is based on his belief that collaboration in diagnosis and problem solving will alleviate the causes of these difficulties.

As Schein sees it, the change agent must pass on *skills* and *values*, not knowledge. He helps the organization learn from its processes and the problems they generate and how to solve these problems using internal, rather than external, resources.

Schein's view of OD provides an amplification of the philosophy of practitioners in general. However, we shall now examine some of the more common models in use for understanding the change process.

BEHAVIORAL EQUILIBRIUM

Lewin's (1952) *unfreezing-changing-refreezing* model provides a useful vehicle for understanding change processes. According to this model, behavior is determined by the net effect of an elaborate set of contemporaneous forces. A crude analogy, if you will, likens these forces to fields of magnetic flux within which an iron particle is trapped. In some configurations of flux, the particle will move. In all static configurations, it will eventually come to rest at a point where each force on the particle is met by an equal and opposite force.

It is helpful to view behavior in terms of analogous forces. Theoretically, we can postulate forces that move individuals to change their behaviors, but we must also recognize similar forces that resist deviations from habit or the status quo. Some of these forces emanate within the individual and include needs, attitudes, feelings, and habits. Others flow from second and third parties who respond to the focal individual's behavior with rewards or punishments.

The focal individual experiences these forces as he or she perceives them. While perceptions may be valid or not, Lewin argues that they are real to the individual, who responds to them regardless of their actuality; that is, imagined threat is experienced as realistically as actual threat and is responded to accordingly. Thus, the forces described by Lewin are psychological forces.

It is probably impossible to comprehend all of the forces acting on an individual in a unique situation. No wonder human behavior seems unpredictable. Yet, we admit that behavior is fairly predictable within reasonable limits. This is most often true when dealing with groups of individuals whose norms are well understood. The study of group dynamics follows Lewin's early work. Particularly, studies of group norms and group pressures follow his original theoretical directions. We shall examine Lewin's work in terms of group work norms and behavior. For this purpose, we shall define norm and norm-following behavior, respectively, as: (1) a set of expectations for behavior held by group members and (2) the fairly regular behavior resulting from these expectations and the positive and negative sanctions used for their enforcement.

Lewin's model can be applied to a group norm specifying level of worker productivity. Where such norms exist, the individual's behavior will conform fairly closely since deviations in either direction may be met with negative sanctions. Yet, there are forces on the individual that, by themselves, would cause him to deviate in one or the other direction.

First, group pressures limit deviation in either direction. Slight deviations are met with mild sanctions, such as half-joking, half-critical comments from fellow workers. Major deviations evoke more severe sanctions; for instance, the informal group leader may rebuke the offending worker, other group members may threaten action, and, ultimately, physical violence may erupt. The latter sanction is a rare, but not unknown, penalty for violating important group norms.

Several motives can cause a work group to establish and maintain norms such as the one discussed here. First, output above the norm is likely to signal to management that it has established unrealistically low output requirements. One likely consequence is that the requirements will be restudied with the result that workers eventually find themselves working harder for the same hourly wage. This can be especially threatening to older members of the work group who would have difficulty keeping a faster pace of work. Output below the norm is also sure to attract management's attention. A consequence to be anticipated in this event is increased pressure from supervision.

We have looked at two kinds of forces limiting deviation from the norm and serving to maintain behavioral equilibrium. In addition to forces emanating from the work group are those solely within the individual; for example, fatigue serves to limit the individual worker's rate of productivity. Counteracting this force to some extent are psychological forces that stem from the need for achievement or the Protestant ethic. Work-related aspirations, anxieties about the state of the economy and employment security, and pressures and inducements applied by the organization may also enter into the balance.

According to Lewin, the net effects of these forces are stabilized behavior and social equilibrium. However, the resulting equilibrium is dynamic rather than static and, thus, is termed *quasi-stationary equilibrium*. It is dynamic in the sense that it can be altered by a number of possible changes in the balance of forces.

UNFREEZING BEHAVIOR

For convenience, Lewin terms forces hindering movement from the existing equilibrium *restraining forces*. Opposing forces which direct behavior away from the status quo are called *driving forces*. Now, in order to cause change, one must upset the balance of driving and restraining forces; that is, *unfreeze* the quasi-stationary equilibrium. There are, of course, three ways to unfreeze the situation: (1) increase the driving forces, (2) decrease the restraining forces, or (3) accomplish some combination of the first two strategies. We shall examine these change strategies in order.

Driving forces can be increased through manipulation of positive and negative incentives; for example, management may inform the work force of impending layoffs that can be avoided only by increases in employee productivity. Alternatively, an incentive payment scheme can be implemented. The success of neither approach is guaranteed. In the first case, workers are led to fear that their present level of productivity will result in punishment in the form of unemployment. Even so, they may think that in yielding to these pressures they will encourage management to seek further changes in the same manner. In the second case, workers may fear that increased productivity motivated by incentive payments will lead management to restudy the job (Whyte 1955). Both attempts appear to produce additional restraining forces inadvertently.

Thus, increasing driving forces can produce or increase restraining forces, especially as movement is made away from the previous equilibrium. In the event that the increased driving forces are of sufficient magnitude to overcome existing and newly created restraining forces (which is not true in all cases), behavior may reach a state of equilibrium at a new level. Whether or not a new equilibrium level is reached, the individual will experience greater tension. This occurs because both driving and restraining forces have been increased. Were this not the case, behavior would change endlessly in the direction of the driving forces. Obviously, this cannot occur, for fatigue, if nothing else, will restrain behavior ultimately.

Increased tension of this sort creates additional dynamic potentialities in the situation, which imply greater instability and unpredictability. A minor fluctuation in one of the major driving or restraining forces may create widely fluctuating behavior. Large forces are not maintained effortlessly and are more likely to change than are smaller forces. This produces a tendency toward instability. In psychological terms, the individual experiencing pressures from two directions is in a conflict situation. He or she will expend considerable energy monitoring the conflicting pressures and making tentative moves, first in one direction, then in the other.

Because of this, it appears more reasonable to unfreeze behavior by removing restraining forces. In the previous examples, we described restraining forces arising from labor's distrust of management. To continue the example, we note that these forces can be reduced by assurances that such distrust is unfounded. This may, of course, require effort over and above giving assurances. Trust between workers and management must be established, possibly by some tangible evidence that such restraining forces are unwarranted. Other avenues of progress include redesigning work to reduce worker fatigue, reformulating group norms, and so on.

In the event that management is successful in reducing or removing certain restraining forces, existing driving forces may be sufficient to change behavior in the desired direction; that is, forces already in the situation, such as need for achievement, can drive performance higher and in so doing unfreeze the situation. Furthermore, the new equilibrium will contain less tension since a smaller set of opposing forces results.

From this observation, we find the two major advantages of the second change strategy over the first. First, it takes less effort to remove forces than to add them. Adding driving forces may create opposing restraining forces. Thus, further driving forces may be needed. Reducing restraining forces permits existing forces to effect change. Second, given the same degree of change, the latter strategy produces a more psychologically healthy and, in managerial terms, more controllable situation than does the former. This occurs because the reduction in forces yields lower tension, more stability, and greater predictability.

The third strategy, increasing driving forces while reducing restraining forces, is probably the most advantageous of the three. The addition of driving forces can provide further impetus for change in the desired direction. Furthermore, the unfreezing effect may be more pronounced as positive motivations are increased. Theoretically, the increased tension experienced at the new equilibrium may be justified by the arousal of positive motivation. Not all tension is undesirable or unpleasant.

CHANGING BEHAVIOR

The second stage in Lewin's model is the *changing stage* which we have already begun to discuss. Unfreezing sometimes elicits change as the addition and reduction of forces drive behavior away from the initial point of equilibrium. However, this is not always the case. Despite a reasoned alteration of the force field, new forces may come into play as existing ones are manipulated. We might think of this in terms of people's willingness to tolerate uncertainty and ambiguity rather than move in directions they do not wish to travel.

When unfreezing does not produce adequate change, management is left with the task of analyzing and reshaping the force field. Returning to our former example, we may find that production has increased somewhat but is limited by employee fatigue. Management will deal with this restraining force, perhaps by redesigning the job or employing superior equipment. These actions, in turn, can evoke additional restraining forces. We resist change "in principle" because it can lead to unanticipated consequences and requires additional effort. Thus, the change process must be supported by psychological as well as material improvements. In our example, workers will need assurances that change will not work to their detriment.

REFREEZING BEHAVIOR

Typically, behavioral changes gained even through the expenditure of considerable resources and effort dissipate over time; for example, the manager whose attitudes and behavior have changed as a result of recent management development activities may return to old habits shortly after his or her return to the organization from the classroom. This occurs when the *refreezing stage* of the change process has been dealt with inadequately.

Following change, a new quasi-stationary equilibrium must be established by an appropriate, balanced configuration of driving and restraining forces. The unfreezing and change stages of the process usually are facilitated by psychological support and inducements applied by the change agent. These forces tend to disappear once change has been accomplished and management loses interest in the problem, assuming that its remedy has been found. Indeed, the maintenance of these forces over the long run may prove infeasible. Yet, as they are removed they must be replaced by other forces if the new equilibrium is to be maintained. Failing this, behavior may return to its former state.

Change programs are likely to be accompanied by something akin to the "Hawthorne effect" arising from the attentions of management and other novel influences that may disappear once the process of change appears to have been completed. The refreezing stage is advocated in recognition of this phenomenon. Basically, this stage consists of the systematic replacement of temporary forces with more permanent ones. In some cases, the technique used to create change can be continued as a vehicle for its maintenance; for example, if the change program was structured around the survey feedback technique, the same technique can be employed to investigate problems and performance arising from the new equilibrium point. In other cases, it may suffice to formalize the change situation through revisions of rules, regulations, and procedures. These activities can lend organizational authority as well as legitimate sanctions to the new state of equilibrium and, thus, maintain it temporarily until norms evolve to sustain it in a more permanent fashion.

CHANGE AND THE LARGER ORGANIZATION

Thus far we have restricted our view of the change process to individuals and small groups. Lewin's model can also be applied to problems of organizational change—to the diffusion of change from one group to another, and from subsystem to subsystem throughout the organization. If one subsystem is unfrozen and changed, other related parts of the system will be affected. Furthermore, the effect of subsystem A on adjacent subsystem B is likely to produce a countereffect wherein B affects A. We noted the managers' tendencies to revert to habitual behavior on reentering their organizations following management development activities. This may be due, in part, to their inability to sustain newly learned attitudes and behaviors as members of subsystems that expect their former behavior of them. Specifically, the returning manager's altered behavior affects his or her group and, perhaps, other adjacent groups as well. But, these subsystems have not undergone corresponding changes that would enable them to incorporate the manager's newly acquired behavior successfully. Consequently, they fail to reinforce this behavior and, in some cases, sanction against it. These acts can shift his or her behavior back to its prior form.

Similarly, changed work groups can experience frictions with other groups with which they no longer "fit"; for example, our workers, who now produce at a higher rate, pass their increased output downstream to other groups in the productive process. These interdependent groups, feeling pressured by increased supplies of work in process, may react adversely, having been inadvertently unfrozen. Whyte (1955) describes a change program that was curtailed by this phenomenon. Employees working at one station of a production line were encouraged to organize their own work and to enrich their jobs by combining delimited individual tasks into a group operation. The increased motivation thus tapped caused an increase in productivity. However, the increased productivity of one group entered the work flow of the next group in the process. Unfortunately, the second group could not be reorganized as the first had been to handle the increased work required of them. In Lewin's terms, the second group became unfrozen by the output of the first. Restraining forces in the situation prevented them from adapting to the new driving forces (increased work in process inventories). Ultimately, they were successful in resisting change, and the experiment with the first group was discontinued.

Of course, pressures and discomfort experienced by adjacent subsystems can provide an entree for change agents as they attempt to move their change efforts through the organization. The change agent's potential to help with uncomfortable, unsettling problems can elicit cooperation from other subsystems, paving the way for additional changes that are congruent with changes made in the initial subsystem. Furthermore, by decreasing the resistances of adjacent subsystems, refreezing (maintenance of change) in the initial subsystem is enhanced.

A PROCESS FOR CONSULTANTS

The intervention of a consultant complicates the change process somewhat. Lippitt and colleagues' (1958) amplification of Lewin's model clarifies the role of the consultant in aiding clients to bring about organizational change.[1] The first of seven phases in the change process described by Lippitt is *the development of a need for change* and is the essence of Lewin's unfreezing stage. The second phase, *the establishment of a change relationship,* creates the basis for all subsequent phases of the change process. The third through fifth phases have to do with change itself; phase three is *the clarification of the client system's problems,* phase four is *the examination of alternative means and ends and the choice of those to be implemented,* and phase five is *the transformation of intentions into actual change efforts.* The sixth phase concerns *the generalization and stabilization of change* and is comparable to the refreezing stage of the Lewin model. Peculiar to the consultant's role in the change process, the seventh phase directs effort toward *ending the relationship.* This phase is essential since dependence on the consultant throughout the change process must be dissipated prior to his departure if change is to be permanent.

DEVELOPING A NEED FOR CHANGE

Stress or disruption within a system or between the system and its environment must be translated into actual problem awareness (desire for change) before the process of organizational change can begin. Oddly enough, this does not occur naturally in all cases. In some instances, management is unaware of existing problems. In other cases, awareness has not advanced to a level at which problems are conceptualized and, thus, meaningfully viewed as needing (and amenable to) change; for example, existing problems can be seen as inevitable. Alternatively, they may be viewed as being prohibitively expensive to correct. However, even when awareness of problems is accompanied by knowledge of potential sources of help, an additional form of resistance must be overcome. Seeking help is admitting to failure, in a sense. It admits to problems beyond the capabilities of management.

Now, it is quite likely that these elements in the first phase of the change process will be resolved in the absence of a consultant. Even so, the change agents may find that the problems they are asked to address are symptomatic of others of which management is unaware. In this instance, the change agents will eventually work at several phases in the process concurrently, progressing on one problem and developing the need for change on others.

ESTABLISHING CHANGE RELATIONSHIPS

Initial relationships between the consultant and client serve as levers for subsequent change in the organization. For this reason, the second phase can be critical to the consultant's role in the process of planned change. First impressions are important. Consultants, as professionals, must be competent and trustworthy. Furthermore, they must *appear* so to members of the client organization. The change agents must convey evidence of their skills and knowledge and the ability to employ them successfully. At the same time, they should appear similar to clients—as people who will understand their roles and problems and respect their organization's needs and values.

A critical element of the second phase is *clarification* of the consultant's relationship to the client. Each party must learn of the effort and participation expected by the other. This is admittedly difficult, coming as it does before a thorough diagnosis of the organization's problems. The change agent must communicate realistic, though general, goals for the change program as well as a realistic assessment of the effort that will be demanded of his or her client. The issue of depth of intervention should also be raised at this point to establish joint norms regarding appropriate and inappropriate areas in which to pursue change.

Because organizations comprise a variety of subsystems, the change agents need to clarify their relationship vis-à-vis each subsystem with which they will work. Although this cannot be accomplished in any detail at this preliminary stage, the consultants will at least "touch base" with important sources of power. In light of the tentative nature of arrangements at this point in the change process, the consultant and client may agree to a "shake down" period of finite duration, giving both parties an option to withdraw from the relationship should this appear warranted by events of the trial period.

CLARIFYING THE PROBLEM

The substance of this phase of the change process will be determined by techniques employed by the consultant. One format will be used for survey feedback approaches while other formats will accompany techniques such as management by objectives (MBO). In general, the format will be collaborative regardless of the particular techniques employed. The client possesses information which the consultant needs. The consultant has a range of diagnostic skills that can aid the client. Wherever possible, we advocate that the consultant help the client learn these diagnostic skills so that collaboration can occur. For instance, using the survey feedback technique, the client may be called upon to design and implement means for data collection and analysis with the help of the consultant (see, for example, Wieland and Leigh 1971).

The diagnostic phase also serves to unfreeze further the client's organization. Analysis of data may show that problems are more numerous and more threatening than had been expected. The need for change may be seen as more pervasive or as affecting more subsystems than was originally thought. At this point, the change agent may guide the process of diagnosis to prevent the client from becoming overly impressed with his or her problems, fatalistic about them, or convinced that their solution can only be achieved by experts such as the consultant. Numerous problems can be brought to light by the diagnostic phase. Balance is achieved as alternative change strategies are considered for each problem as it is brought to light. Rather than an inventory of problems lacking solutions, the process yields an assortment of problems in various stages of resolution as management considers alternative actions and definite intentions to change in specified ways (Lippitt et al. 1958).

CHOOSING FROM ALTERNATIVES

At this point, the fourth phase has begun. Evaluation and choice are, ostensibly, cognitive, rational processes, but the actual process is likely to deviate from these expectations to one degree or another. Satisficing behavior (i.e., accepting an adequate solution) may supersede optimization by necessity. One or at most two custom-made solutions may be considered rather than a broad array of feasible alternatives.

Equally important as the cognitive aspects of alternative selection is a motivational process accompanying this phase of the process, for at this point the organization must marshal commitment to act and carry out the programs of change selected. This is accomplished in large measure by the collaborative nature of the change process as the client develops commitment to the solution he or she helped design.

TRANSFORMING INTENTIONS INTO CHANGE EFFORTS

As we indicated earlier, many client-consultant relationships terminate at the conclusion of the previous phase when alternatives are selected and described in report form. This is unfortunate when it occurs, for the present phase is at the heart of the change process, so to speak. It is at this point that the consultant's expertise can be critical to the entire process of change. As we indicated in discussing Lewin's model, the change agent's expertise can be of value in aligning an adequate configuration of forces and maintaining a favorable imbalance in the force field throughout the change period. In a sense, the consultant helps the client progress through a series of cycles in the change process in which: (1) preliminary moves are made, (2) gains are consolidated and compared to desired outcomes, and (3) depending on the nature of this comparison, further consolidation is effected or further changes are sought.

STABILIZING CHANGE

The sixth phase of the process concerns diffusion of change throughout the client organization. As we indicated in our discussion of Lewin's model, a change in one subsystem often necessitates corresponding changes in adjacent subsystems. In helping the client achieve this, the consultant serves a second purpose, namely, providing an external and fairly objective evaluation of progress. Added to the client's own evaluation, the consultant's opinion can provide reinforcement for the efforts and results obtained.

Stabilization can also be achieved as the consultant helps the client diffuse change to adjacent subsystems. As converts to a better way of life reinforce their own conversions by proselytizing new converts, so do managers reinforce their newly learned skills and behaviors by helping others acquire them.

ENDING THE RELATIONSHIP

When change is realized and stabilized, the consultant's role has been discharged. To the extent the change agent involved the client in participation and transferred his or her skills to the client's organization, difficulties in terminating the client-consultant relationship will have been reduced. But they still may be substantial. By seeking expert help, the client began a process through which he or she became dependent, although perhaps not as dependent as might have been the case had the consultant behaved differently. The consultant attempts to reduce this dependence as the change program draws to completion. If he has been successful in transferring skills to the client's organization, the problem may entail little more than reinforcing the client's confidence by demonstrating his competence.

TACTICS FOR CHANGING PEOPLE

TRAINING GROUPS

Many different programs and techniques have been used to change people variables in organizations. Here we shall describe the efficacy of several of the basic ones, starting with the prototypic OD intervention, training groups.

Laboratory training groups (or T-groups and sensitivity training groups as they are called) have been one of the most common elements of organizational development efforts. Rush (1969) gives evidence of the widespread use of T-groups in noting that a 1968 study of some 240 companies indicated that one-third used sensitivity training.

THE OBJECTIVES OF TRAINING GROUPS

T-groups have been used for a quarter of a century, ever since the National Education Association joined the Research Center for Group Dynamics of the University of Michigan in holding experimental laboratories at Bethel, Maine. These laboratories were designed to teach the processes involved in social change. As the name *sensitivity training* implies, contemporary laboratories are designed to make participants more sensitive to: (1) their own behavior; (2) their conscious and unconscious motivations; (3) the ways in which their own behavior is perceived by, and affects, others; (4) the behavior of others and its underlying motivations; and (5) the processes that help and hinder group functioning.

Sensitivity training differs from other educational endeavors in that it is not designed primarily as an intellectual exchange between the teacher and learners. Rather, the group's behavior, including members' emotional responses, is the subject of study. Actual behavior in face-to-face interactions constitutes the process from which learning occurs. It is claimed that sensitivity training works by making participants aware of the determinants of group and individual behavior. This awareness, furthermore, paves the way for improvements in the participant's control of his or her own behavior and interaction with others.

THE SETTING AND ROLE OF THE TRAINER

T-groups are often conducted in settings remote from the participants' organizations—where distractions and props such as habitual roles, furniture arrangements, various kinds of technologies, books, reports, and the like are absent. It is claimed that a setting of this sort allows the participants to involve themselves totally (physically, intellectually, and emotionally) in the task of studying their behavior in the group.

T-groups are normally led by trainers who neither lecture nor engage in typical leadership functions, but serve instead as observers and nondirective resource persons. After the usual ten or fifteen persons have gathered in the group setting, the trainer may give a brief introduction, stating the group's task. Typically, the introduction is bland and rather uninformative and suggests merely that participants will engage in learning about the behavior of individuals in groups. There is no agenda and nothing else to structure the group. The trainer generally retires to the "sidelines" without instructing participants further.

Task-oriented managers who are accustomed to meeting for specific purposes become rather frustrated in a situation that lacks both structure and assigned roles. Groups begin in a number of ways. Some start with a lengthy silence which is broken by an individual's attempting to structure the task of the group. Other groups begin when a member introduces himself or herself to the group and invites others to do likewise. In some cases, conflict arises when several participants vie for the leadership role. Frustration also develops as participants attempt to deal with the lack of agenda. Some group members become anxious, some hostile, others apathetic.

At some point, the trainer will comment that the group has already begun to learn—that members are behaving and reacting to each other's behavior. He or she may articulate some of the feelings and behavior observed. At any point, he or she may ask participants to examine what is occurring. Occasional pointed questions help members become aware of the dynamics of the group's behavior.

With the help of the trainer, group members learn to speak their minds and express their feelings. Openness and honesty are encouraged. Norms of trust, openness, and helpfulness emerge as participants report how they perceive and react to behavior in the group.

It is also claimed that participants learn about the dynamics of group behavior and individual behavior within groups in this manner. Furthermore, self-understanding and the opportunity to "work through" feelings and experiment with new, more appropriate behaviors are considered attributes of training groups.

RESEARCH ON THE EFFECTIVENESS OF TRAINING GROUPS

Several reviews of research on sensitivity training have appeared (Campbell and Dunnette 1970; Campbell, Dunnette, Lawler, and Weick 1970; House 1967). Campbell and associates suggest that 30 to 40 percent of trained individuals are reported to exhibit some sort of perceptible change. Typically, changes are perceived by colleagues in terms of increased sensitivity, more openness to communication, and increased flexibility in role behavior. It should be mentioned that most of these studies lack control groups. Furthermore, the raters usually know who has attended a T-group and who has not, and thus a bias may creep in. Furthermore, Campbell and associates emphasize that while the individual's behavior may change, it is not clear that these changes lead to better job performance. In fact, one study (Underwood 1965) shows that trainees display more positive changes (rated in terms of effects on job performance) than controls, but also more negative changes.

Suppose that a manager undergoes positive changes as a result of his T-group experiences. We must ask how effectively these changes are utilized "back home" to improve organizational performance. Much of the criticism of T-groups centers around this question of whether or not changes in the manager's behavior transfer to the work role and improve performance on the job.

The returned T-group veteran frequently is unable to articulate what has been experienced and how he or she has changed for the better. This inability to communicate affects the manager's ability to enlist the cooperation of other employees in behaving differently (i.e., more appropriately). Furthermore, it probably signifies the manager's inability to maintain whatever changes he or she achieved. To the extent that the individual is unable to think about what has happened and how he or she is different, there may be a lack of control over the changed potentialities.

A recent, generally sympathetic review (Margulies et al. 1977) of T-group research admits a "lack of evidence supporting the long-range impact of off-site stranger labs on organizations" and reviews only on-site labs. Careful attention to the research designs and methods shows that most studies were not well controlled. An exception, Friedlander's (1967) study, did show improved morale (and perhaps also improved organizational climate), but no change in organizational performance. Several other studies used T-groups along with other change techniques, resulting not only in improved morale and organizational climate, but also in improved performance. Unfortunately, the research designs in these studies, for the most part, did not allow one to separate out the influence of sensitivity training from other techniques. Margulies and colleagues tentatively conclude that "morale and/or climate tend to improve" for those T-groups conducted in organizational settings.

TEAM BUILDING

Team building is a variation of sensitivity training that attempts to apply T-group processes to work settings. It is focused on organizational members who have some need for teamwork: they have a common supervisor, common organizational aims, interdependent work roles, or perhaps an assignment to a temporary task force. A variety of activities may fall under the rubric of team building (Huse 1975). Team members may discuss their common and individual goals with a view toward clarification and better coordination, and they may participate in setting team goals so as to improve motivation and commitment. These goals may concern the task of the group members, their roles (including leadership, power), or the interpersonal processes by which the group will work.

Other team-building efforts emphasize improving the culture or climate of the group; there may be a family-type T-group, where group members have some relationship on the job. Mutual trust, supportiveness, and openness in the context of the actual work of the group members is encouraged, so that interpersonal skills are improved and the team works more effectively ("conflict is confronted, problems are solved effectively, and good decisions are made"). Often the consultant will feed into the team-building meetings various data he or she has gathered on the interpersonal relations of the group.

Beckhard and Lake (1971) used team building to facilitate changeover to electronic data processing in a large investment and commercial bank. The nine managers in the mortgage department and the three in a group installing and operating the computer engaged in team building for a year. The members first went to a sensitivity training lab. Individuals then provided the consultant with anonymous accounts of the obstacles to the more effective functioning of the team, as they saw it. These data were fed back to the team at a weekend meeting, and the group then held discussions, set priorities, and began to work on the problems (such as supervisory style of the head of the group and relationships between the mortgage group and the computer specialists).

The group made a commitment to continue meeting monthly (without the consultant), to create task forces to work on its problems, and to have the supervisor of the mortgage group call a meeting of certain other managers outside the group so as to improve communications with others. The team met with the consultant again six months and a year later to discuss special problems and make action plans, but in the interim, smaller task forces from the team had been set up and were working effectively on problems, and no further meetings were thought necessary.

An independent evaluation of the team-building effort showed that the team had improved morale, increased productivity ratings, and showed apparently reduced turnover and absenteeism, compared to various other groups in the bank. Even four years later, the productivity of the mortgage group was rated by others as being higher than other groups. Unfortunately, the team building in this project was accompanied by other changes (e.g., installation of the computer) so a definitive conclusion about team building is not warranted. However, other similar studies of team building do provide consistent evidence for improvements in morale, climate, and (quality of) performance.

SURVEY FEEDBACK

Surveys using interviews or questionnaires are very common. The OD technique known as survey feedback uses the survey data to trigger discussion and open examination of problems among respondents. As in team building, natural groupings of organizational members form the membership for the meetings. A superior and his or her direct subordinates meet to compare and discuss data relevant to their respective responsibilities, such as the work satisfaction of the respective departments and the ratings of communication between superior and subordinate.

The OD consultant facilitates these discussions, providing additional data if necessary and explaining any technical problems with the data. Even more importantly, the OD consultant can help the group develop and move beyond a simple discussion of the data. He or she can facilitate the development of an open and trusting climate within the group, in which data on additional problems and conflicts can be volunteered, and in which individuals can examine their typical work styles and their feelings about others in the work place. In a fully developed OD intervention, the consultant can operate as a process consultant, working on team building within the "team" of the supervisor and direct subordinates. The consultant must also play a supportive role as each of the subordinates in a feedback meeting initiates a subsequent feedback meeting with his or her own subordinates, and these subordinates in turn initiate their own meetings, and so on down to the lowest level in the organization.[2]

As with team building, our knowledge of survey feedback suffers from an absence of rigorous research. The extant less than rigorous studies do show, as do the studies of team building, apparent positive change in the attitudes, morale, and culture of participating organizational members. In addition, some measure of the comparative efficacy of survey feedback as an OD technique is found in a massive study by Bowers (1971, 1973) who examined the effects of four OD practices on over 14,000 respondents in 23 organizations.

The four OD practices examined in the study were: (1) T-groups, (2) interpersonal process consultation, which is similar to Schein's process consultation described earlier, (3) task process consultation, which focuses on task or work objectives and the interpersonal relations associated with their attainment (a form of team building), and (4) survey feedback. In addition, two control groups consisted of one which received no treatment whatsoever and a second ("data handback") in which members were sent tabulated survey data in envelopes.

Pre- and postsurveys were undertaken to measure changes in 16 indices of organizational behavior. These included measures of organizational climate,[3] managerial leadership, peer leadership, group processes, and employee satisfaction. It was found that the survey feedback technique was associated with significant improvements on almost all of the measures. Interpersonal process consultation was associated with improvements on about half of the measures. In contrast, task process consultation, no treatment, data handback, and laboratory training were associated with little, or negative, change. However, when the researchers controlled organizational climate, laboratory training showed positive results, suggesting that the preexisting organizational conditions (the climate already existing in the organization) can be an important factor in determining whether some OD interventions will take root and prove effective.

One caution about this particular research is that the questionnaire used in the survey feedback effort was the same instrument used to measure change from before to after. The discussions of the survey items and the data may have created changes in the responses in the second administration of the instrument, but perhaps less change in actual behavior (Passmore 1976).

An even more important problem is the general paucity of data (obtained by means of a rigorous research design) showing changes in organizational efficiency or output as a direct result of survey feedback or other forms of OD (Morrison 1978). However, there have been a few rigorously evaluated, successful OD efforts. In these efforts "structural" and "people" interventions jointly create improvements in output (e.g., Marrow et al. 1967) or the "people" interventions are carefully tailored to the client's specific needs (because the client organizations themselves select and conduct the intervention) to yield improvements in the efficiency and output (see, for example, Chapters 24 and 25).

CRITICISMS OF OD

In general, despite a number of negative features (among which are included anti-intellectualism, overselling of results, and overemphasis on conflict) we find that OD is of some merit. Strauss (1973), a long-time observer and sometime critic of "human relations," suggests that:

> ... compared to traditional management training, OD is generally more meaningful, certainly leads to far more involvement, and clearly runs less risk of being excessively stressful. Despite the difficulties of research, it is now reasonably clear that *under some circumstances* OD can lead to lasting organizational gain. (p. 16)

In addition to asking what conditions are prerequisite to positive outcomes from OD, one must ask about the comparative efficacy of OD, as opposed to alternative approaches to change, and also about the relative costs of such alternative efforts. Strauss, for example, suggests that ". . . it is often better to change the organization so that ordinary people can function well within it rather than to try to change the people themselves. Thus, I sympathize with those who believe that the purpose of OD should be to induce managers to step back, not just to reexamine their interpersonal relations and emotions, but to take a fresh look at the organization as a whole, its goals, and its relationship to its environment" (pp. 17–18). Organizations comprise not only people but also technology, structure, goals, management systems, and strategies. Attempts to improve organizations should consider all of these.

Critics of organization development also question whether the aims of changing people espoused by practitioners are always matters of choice. For example, Levinson (Sashkin et al. 1973) is critical of OD's reliance on confrontation techniques and advocates more thorough diagnostic processes which can suggest alternative change strategies. "Organizations indeed have changed significantly as a result of other (non-OD) consultants' interventions, as a result of supportive efforts without confrontation, and with many other devices; . . . this is not to say that I think confrontation is by definition bad, but only that it must be a technique of choice based on diagnosis" (p. 203). Strauss (1973) asks,

> If, as one authority on the subject insists, OD turns out . . . better decision-makers, would equal results be obtained from programs specifically designed to improve decision making (such as Kepner-Tregoe)? Dalton and Korman both argue that OD's key objective should be to raise self-confidence and esteem. If so, perhaps the answer is to provide training directly designed to alter levels of aspiration and aggressiveness—such as "rational training," the various programs designed by McClelland and Miner, or those packaged under the title of "Behavior Reinforcement". (p. 18)

In the long run, answers to questions regarding the relative efficacy of different approaches to organizational change will be provided by comparative research. Such research must deal with generic variables (the basic differences in these various approaches), and it is to several such generic variables that we now turn.

ALTERNATIVE OD STRATEGIES

THE CONSULTANT-TRAINER ROLE

One way of viewing the problems associated with changing behavior is in terms of its cognitive and emotional components (Wieland and Leigh 1971). As used here, cognitive refers to the aspect of a problem that is amenable to logic and rationality, to intellectual approaches. The emotional component is based on feelings, attitudes, and emotional reactions.

Some organizational problems may be essentially cognitive, requiring information for their solution. Clients may be ignorant and a simple provision of information or correction of misinformation may be all that is required of the consultant. Even if the problem is one of conflicting beliefs rather than ignorance, the change agent is likely to find that the communication of better information or expert opinion can serve to reorganize these beliefs. At the very least, it can be argued that this kind of change is easier to bring about than changes in people's feelings.

We sometimes believe that people are so rational that if one provides reasons for behaving differently they will do so, or if one supplies more and better information they will make better decisions. Emotions, feelings, and attitudes are not developed rationally or logically. Behavior and decisions based on emotions, therefore, are not likely to be altered by appeals to logic or reason. One's aversions toward snakes and spiders, for example, are not likely to be altered by knowledge that these are generally useful creatures, nor is one's behavior toward these creatures likely to change.

Emotions and feelings are difficult to change, but once altered they may become stable. Furthermore, it is believed that overt behavior is more closely linked to feelings and emotions than to ideas or thoughts. This is the reason psychoanalysts lead their patients to reexperience the emotional situations and stimuli that are sources of their apparent maladjusted behavior. By relearning emotionally, the patient comes to behave more adaptively.

Because of the phenomena described here, Seashore and Van Egmond (1959) advocate that the roles of expert advice giver and group trainer be combined. This combination they term the *consultant-trainer role.* The expert portion of the role enables the consultant to diagnose organizational problems and to make sure that important issues are raised. This, of course, does not always happen in T-groups. The training portion of the role enables the consultant to pass on the attitudes, values, and behavioral skills that are essential changes in OD.

DEPTH OF INTERVENTION

Viewed one way, the consultant-trainer role seems to combine two extremes. Harrison (1970) labels attempts to change a person's values (that are central to his or her sense of self) as *deep change strategies. Shallow change strategies* are those more formal and public attempts to change ideas, technologies, and the like. The operations research analyst, in redesigning tasks and roles to fit a rational model, uses shallow strategies. Psychological readjustments do not enter into his design for change. The Seashore-Van Egmond approach may be viewed as an attempt to combine deep and shallow kinds of change.

Harrison, though, argues that the depth of intervention ought to be as shallow as the problem permits. Intervention strategies can be arrayed on a continuum of depth. The choice of a particular change strategy will be determined by two criteria: (1) the depth to which one must go to locate information that must be exchanged in order to improve organizational performance, and (2) the level of intervention that is acceptable to the client.

At the shallow end of the continuum of change strategies one finds *cognitive* and *rational* problem-solving techniques such as those used in operations research, managerial accounting, and the like.

Somewhat deeper are the practices of *industrial psychology*, which include methods for employee selection, placement, and appraisal. Here the focus is on individual performance as it can be predicted by education, work experience, biographical data, personality characteristics, and other dimensions that are measured, but not changed. Using these kinds of measurements, industrial psychologists advise management on hiring, promotion, and dismissal decisions. Other change strategies at a comparable level include job enrichment and management by objectives. In neither case is personality change sought.

A still deeper, *instrumental* or "work style," approach to change is exemplified by the Blake and Mouton (1970) managerial grid. Using a two-dimensional rating scale, managers rate themselves and their colleagues on their orientations toward people and production. By analyzing their own ratings and those given them by others, managers are helped to alter their managerial styles, attitudes, and work-related behavior. Some managers are encouraged to give more emphasis to productivity, others to attend more to the needs of employees, and still others to increase their emphases on both. These changes in emphasis are manifested in increased delegation of authority, enhanced concern for employees' needs, better planning, and increased use of feedback in the control and support of subordinates. Change at this instrumental level is deeper than interventions made using MBO and similar techniques. Job enrichment and MBO alter task-related behavior and the objectives to which it is addressed. The Blake and Mouton approach attempts to change attitudes and social orientations as well, but only insofar as these are instrumental to effective task performance.

The next level down, according to Harrison, deals with *interpersonal relations* and is exemplified by some of the so-called human relations training programs. These change strategies bring to light the feelings, attitudes, and perceptions that individuals have about one another. The focus here is not only on instrumental behavior, but also on the quality of interpersonal experiences. T-group sessions which emphasize trust, openness, and authentic behavior are designed to produce changes at this level.

Finally, Harrison cites *intrapersonal analysis* as the deepest level at which change is commonly sought. Psychoanalysis is an example in which the patient's attitudes, values, and conflicts concerning his ability to function effectively, his identity, and existence are examined. Some of the most extreme T-groups operate at this level, such as marathon groups which probe to the very basis of the individual's psychological makeup.

DEPTH OF INTERVENTION AND CLIENT DEPENDENCY

Harrison suggests that the deeper change strategies make the client *dependent* upon the change agent. As we have indicated, deep changes are *difficult* to bring about and carry considerable risks for the client. Furthermore, it is hard for the client to *transfer* the benefits of these change efforts to other members of the organization.

If a change effort is shallow, the change agent will be able to teach his or her practices to the client; for example, when a consultant employs an operations research technique to solve a problem, the client will gain some understanding of the technique and its applications. In fact, should the client wish, he or she can learn to solve such problems and teach others what has been learned. At deeper levels, change efforts are less readily communicated. It is difficult for a trainer to explain what a T-group is going to be like to potential participants. Even after experiencing a T-group, the clients will be at a loss to explain what has happened to them. Furthermore, they may have trouble imagining themselves ever acquiring the skills to train others. The T-group experience does not equip participants to act as trainers.

Because of this, clients tend to become dependent on consultants using deep change strategies. This, of course, has its consequences. Dependency is costly since the consultant's role cannot be reduced as clients learn the consultant's skills. Furthermore, change will spread slowly in the organization. Unlike shallow change attempts, which can "snowball" as clients begin to impart their newly gained knowledge to others in the organization, deep change generally is limited to those who participate in exercises with the consultant. In general, dependence makes it difficult for the consultant and client to terminate their relationship. Clients may find they are "hooked" on the help of the change agent. As a result of this dependency, the change agent comes to have considerable power over clients. Being unable to provide, let alone understand, the process through which help is given, the client must depend upon, and even accept strong influence from, the change agent.

At this point, the reasoning behind one of Harrison's criteria for determining the depth of intervention should be apparent. Because "costs" increase with the depth of change sought, one ought to go no deeper than necessary. Ideally, the client and consultant will examine the situation in which changes are sought and agree on an appropriate depth of intervention; for example, it may be found that bottlenecks in the work flow can be eliminated by the applications of techniques from industrial engineering. Morale and productivity may be improved through the introduction of job enrichment schemes. Sources of conflict may be ameliorated through redesign of work roles. Each of these change efforts, although relatively shallow, may be sufficient for the problem to which it is addressed and may spare the organization the costs of deeper efforts.

The second criterion states that the depth of intervention should be limited by its acceptability. According to Harrison, the consultant must investigate the client system's norms, values, fears, and resistance to deep interventions. The consultant will need to ask: Do the clients resist discussing their management styles, personalities, or innermost feelings? How much of this sort of information can be discussed, examined, and acted upon legitimately? This varies considerably from one organization to another and among individuals within a single organization. It is particularly important for the change agent to ascertain whether there are group or organizational norms that are likely to be violated by a deep intervention strategy. For example, if there is a norm that one should refrain from discussing personal matters at work (such as one's feelings about the boss or the personalities of coworkers), then one would assume that deep strategies such as T-groups will effectively violate the norm.

Deep Intervention Strategies and Social Norms

Because deep change strategies tend to make clients dependent on consultants, the latter are able to influence the former; that is, the change agent can exercise power over the client to overcome organizational norms. Despite the existence of a norm of the sort described above, the T-group trainer can establish norms to the contrary. However, Harrison suggests that in doing this, the trainer is likely to become counterproductive. While the change agent may have considerable power vis-à-vis individuals and small groups, he or she does not have such power over the organization as a whole. In the larger organization, established norms are more powerful. Thus, individuals leaving the sheltered T-group setting will revert to their former behavior once their newly learned attempts to reveal their feelings and to change the feelings of others are met with sanctions or organization-wide norms to the contrary.

Harrison describes how change agents working at the interpersonal and deeper levels tend to adopt a resistance-oriented approach to change. Some consultants seem to take pride in confrontation, in dramatically violating organizational norms, and in pressuring organizational members into departing from them. He cites the marathon T-group as a case in point wherein the irritability and fatigue that attend prolonged contact and lack of sleep move participants to deal with one another more emotionally, personally, and spontaneously than they would normally.

Harrison's point is substantiated by the study of encounter groups by Lieberman and colleagues (1973). They found that the type of group technology (sensitivity training, gestalt therapy, transactional analysis, marathons, etc.) did not affect the individual outcomes achieved. In fact, what went on in the groups of the same type was usually not very similar, and groups supposedly of a different type often had fairly similar processes and outcomes.

What did make a difference in terms of outcomes, and especially casualty rates, was the behavior of the leader. Leaders who "pushed" the individual participants (regardless of the readiness of participants to confront their problems and deal with the perceptions of the group) produced high casualty rates.

The practice of inducing clients to behave in ways of which they would not approve otherwise is subject to question on ethical grounds. In addition, Harrison judges it to be ineffective since existing organizational norms will tend to reverse changes attained in this fashion.

This problem may be likened to that of the community developer in an underdeveloped nation who, by virtue of his or her personal influence over certain villagers, succeeds in convincing them to dig a well or build a school which, upon the developer's departure, quickly falls into disuse. In situations such as this, the change agent fails to integrate "improvements" into the social structure of day-to-day life. Although successful in solving an immediate problem (or perhaps in removing a symptom of a more basic problem), the community developer fails. In order to succeed, he or she must develop new norms supporting the use and maintenance of the improvements and overcome existing norms that impede this progress. In the absence of the latter activities, community development may even be counterproductive to the extent that it discourages future projects of a similar nature.

If the change agent is to work at a level of intervention that is deeper than organizational norms permit, he (or she) must create new norms, and this is no easy task. It is better, Harrison suggests, to establish the level of intervention at the *level of the system's felt need for changes.* Certain problems of communities and organizations are given high, conscious priorities by their members. Individuals and groups generally are willing to invest time and energy in dealing with these felt needs. Conversely, needs that are experienced solely by the outside consultant (experienced because of the consultant's values or his or her power to achieve specific kinds of changes) are unlikely to spur the cooperation of the community or organization. In short, the consultant must take the role of collaborator in the client's attempts to solve problems that are important to the client, and, in so doing, mobilize existing motivations.

Here, then, we have summarized the reasoning behind Harrison's second criterion for choosing an intervention strategy: intervene no deeper than the level at which the client desires change. In attempting to meet this criterion, the change agent will examine the norms of the organization to determine whether they will legitimize the depth of intervention he or she is considering. Furthermore, the change agent will devise change strategies that are clearly relevant to the consciously felt needs of the organization's members.

THE CONSULTANT'S DILEMMA

Unfortunately, it appears that these two criteria can be contradictory when applied in practice. The first criterion suggests intervention at a level deep enough to obtain information with which to diagnose the problem and subsequently rectify it. This level is sometimes deeper than the level at which an individual or a group is willing to invest energy and resources. Harrison refers to this discrepancy as the *consultant's dilemma*.

Ideally, the dilemma is resolved by intervening first at a level that generates support from organizational norms, the power structures, and the felt needs of members. As time passes and the consultant gains trust and support from within the organization, he or she can begin to intervene at deeper levels— levels at which particularly important forces may be operating. This, however, is no simple matter to accomplish.

Harrison encourages consultants to accept the client's felt needs and problems and to work on them at the level where the client can serve as a confident and willing collaborator. He generalizes from his own experience that the level of intervention most likely to permit collaboration and feelings of legitimacy falls somewhere between interventions at an instrumental or "work style" level and those at the interpersonal relations level. Deeper levels of intervention are likely to produce hostility, passivity, and dependence in clients.

OD AND STRUCTURAL INTERVENTIONS

There has been some change since the earlier days in OD when there was an overreliance on relatively "deep" sensitivity training, and when one often got the impression, as Warren Bennis (1968) put it, that "We're a one product outfit with a 100 percent fool-proof patent medicine." More "shallow" structural (or structural-technological) interventions in an eclectic approach to change are now common.

Huse and Beer (1972), for example, described their work in a small, nonunion plant which designed and manufactured medical and laboratory instruments. The team of four change agents (an outside consultant, an outside-the-plant but within-the-company consultant, the personnel manager, and a research assistant for interviewing and gathering data) relied partly on seminars and on survey feedback, but it also did considerable work-centered consulting as well as counseling. The team's basic approach was to make some recommendations and get organizational personnel to alter their problem-solving behavior. Success was then expected to lead to positive feedback and reinforcement, and also to a change in attitude toward OD. In all this, there was an emphasis on the here and now of the on-the-job situation and its problems. The team focused on changes in work arrangements and in work behavior. Ultimately changes in attitudes would follow.

The change agents saw both structural and interpersonal variables as important for effective organizational change. Job structure was changed, with the elimination of assembly lines and institution of enriched jobs in which a worker would be completely responsible for the assembled product.

Decision making was decentralized, mutual goal setting instituted, and the reward system changed to reflect merit and a new employee appraisal system. A series of formal monthly meetings was begun at every level in the plant in addition to a weekly meeting between the plant manager and a sample of his production and clerical employees. Confrontation meetings between departments were also held. Gradually, these meeting opened up, with increased two-way communication about various problems.

The interventions apparently were quite successful, with Huse and Beer reporting a variety of improvements: productivity increases, waste reduction, and absenteeism reduction. Plant management staffing was also reduced (from 5 to 3) as a result of the decentralization efforts, as was the number of inspection and quality control personnel.

A similar OD effort combining interpersonal and structural interventions was undertaken in a large retail food chain (Luke et al. 1973). Two years of sensitivity training for employees were followed by a structural change in which the level of management immediately above the grocery store level was moved out of the line to become staff, or "consultants," to the store managers. The idea was to reduce the close supervision of the store managers (and their specialists in meat and produce), to give them more authority, and to make the specialists directly responsible to store managers. Because the new consultant relationship would be very difficult for the former line managers to learn, they were given help in the form of sensitivity training, team building, and on-the-job counseling for consultant skills. Some of the more senior managers displayed resistance to this decentralization effort and the shift of managers out of the line to staff positions. They were losing power and subordinates and, furthermore, they did not believe that the store managers were competent enough to operate without close direction. Over time, however, most of the store managers not only adapted but thrived, as the control system cycle was changed from a weekly to a monthly check on their attaining sales and cost targets. A comparison of the change in performance of the experimental district (comprising 15 stores using the new consultant team) with 5 "control" districts showed that the change program was indeed successful. The experimental district moved from fifth to first in sales per work-hour and in efficiency measured by labor cost as a percentage of sales.

However, scattered in the report are some costs of the change program. Two of the 15 store managers, the two with the most years of service, were unable to manage on their own without direct supervision, and they had to be transferred out. Another manager had to be "demoted" to a lower-volume store which was easier to handle. The rest of the 15, however, "were doing at least an adequate job." A number of senior managers, especially those who lost staff and therefore power, were unhappy about the change program. The new consulting-team members had even more reason to be unhappy; they lost their line authority and the prestige that went with it. The change was also quite a risk for them, and while they did have the formal option to decline participation (the store managers did not), in fact they could not decline the new positions for which they had been hand-picked. Fortunately, the change program was effective, and all three of the new consultants received considerable prestige from the success.

Golembiewski, an experienced OD consultant, provides some suggestions about the role of structural interventions in OD: the outcome depends very much on how they are used (Golembiewski et al. 1974). He describes an extensive OD effort involving T-groups, team building, and confrontation meetings (for 400-plus employees at the top six or seven organizational levels) which had taken place over four years. OD values were apparently well institutionalized. Out of this setting arose the idea that a structural intervention, flexi-time or flexible hours of work, could further enhance OD values in the firm. Congruent with OD values, a bottoms-up approach was used to implement the change, and subsequent evaluation showed positive changes in attitudes as well as apparent decreases in overtime and absenteeism of participants, compared to controls.

Golembiewski and colleagues emphasize that the intervention worked in part, or perhaps wholly, because of the OD context. In another context—with an authoritarian management or a management attempting to undercut a union and to extract longer hours out of workers—flexi-time might not yield the results of this study. They aver that the OD values underlying the structural intervention determined its efficacy.

ARE STRUCTURAL INTERVENTIONS LEGITIMATE FOR OD?

These accounts of successful structural OD interventions point out the great potential importance of values in determining how one proceeds in organizational change. One must ask oneself, How important is the humanistic approach in which change comes about through collaboration and mostly from within the person? Or, to what extent do external, structural interventions represent legitimate and expedient means toward perhaps the same ends as more humanistic interventions? There often seem to be strong forces pushing the answers to one side or the other of a basic dilemma: does one maximize humanistic approaches within the fundamental constraints of organizational structure, or does one premise the ultimate constraints in terms of humanistic values, only then to change structures as permitted by these constraints?

A second area of dispute seems to revolve not so much around the conflict in ends, but around the relationship of means to ends. Some commentators seem to indicate that there is no major value difference in the way that much of what is called OD is usually practiced. Such OD relies on nonhumanistic, external forces and influences just as much as everyday management does. ("Management is making things happen, and so is OD.") We have already indicated above (in discussing Harrison's work) the great powers for premise setting and other forms of influence that an OD consultant may possess in the small-group and one-to-one situation. A recent critique of Chris Argyris' OD work exemplifies this argument (Sashkin 1977). Argyris (1976) has worked with presidents of several firms in a small-group setting (away from their organizational bases of power) to instill in them an appreciation for his "double-loop" model of how they ought to learn and to manage. Argyris' basic approach is cognitive; he uses his powers to control the premises of his clients. From Sashkin's viewpoint: "I do not see a great deal of humanness in Argyris' approach, and I find this troubling" (p. 278).

The defender of OD can respond that collaborative or mutual forms of influence are used. The individual fully "buys into" the relationship and thereby accepts certain limited forms of influence, much as the lower-level employee buys into an organization and accepts superiors' directives which fall within the employees' zone of indifference (Schein 1973). Furthermore, as the OD intervention proceeds and the consultants' influence is successful, individuals (and groups) are freed and enabled to grow, to apply their own internal powers and implement their own values. However, in the case of Argyris' approach to organizational change, as implemented by the presidents in his experiment, OD placed the most reliance on selection/replacement, on "firing the individual" (Sashkin 1977, p. 278).

Perhaps the best response to these criticisms is that OD practitioners aspire to be different. They are acting in the service of certain values which they hope to infuse in their techniques (means) as well as in their ends. There is a danger of technicism, of the techniques' obscuring the ends, but as long as the OD ideology is accepted as an indication of aspirations, not achievements, much unnecessary dispute may be avoided.

Perhaps what is needed in the OD endeavor is an attempt to articulate OD values better, and, especially, to consider the progression involved in the "development" of individuals and organizations. A first step has been taken by Lavoie and Culbert (1978) in mapping organizational stages of development into stages of individual cognitive and moral development. Interestingly enough, they argue that OD only works if focused at the next stage up from where individuals and organizations are. That is, OD develops individuals and organizations when it stretches them a little bit—but not too much. Even more important, they argue that most current OD interventions are inappropriately presented, at developmental levels much higher than those characteristic of most organizations and most individuals. It seems, then, that either OD must change to incorporate more lower-level interventions, which are structural, or else OD must leave the great majority of organizations to the attention of the traditional management consultant's basically structural interventions.

REFERENCES

Argyris, Chris. *Increasing leadership effectiveness.* New York: John Wiley & Sons, 1976.

Beckhard, Richard, and Lake, Dale G. Short and long-range effects of a team development effort. In Harvey A. Hornstein et al. (Eds.) *Social intervention: a behavioral science approach.* New York: Free Press, 1971. Pp. 421–439.

Bennis, Warren G. The case study—I. introduction. *Journal of Applied Behavioral Science,* 1968, *4,* 227, 231.

Bennis, Warren G. *Organization development: its nature, origins, and prospects.* Reading, Mass.: Addison–Wesley, 1969.

Blake, Robert R., and Mouton, Jane S. *The managerial grid.* Houston: Gulf Publishing, 1970.

Bowers, David G. Development techniques and organizational climate: an evaluation of comparative importance of two potential forces for organizational change. Technical Report. Office of Naval Research, 1971.

Bowers, David G. OD techniques and their results in 23 organizations: the Michigan ICL study. *Journal of Applied Behavioral Science,* 1973, *9,* 21–43.

Campbell, John P., and Dunnette, Marvin D. Effectiveness of T-group experiences in managerial training and development. *Psychological Bulletin,* 1970, *70,* 73–104.

Campbell, John P., Dunnette, Marvin D., Lawler, Edward E., III, and Weick, Karl E., Jr. *Managerial behavior, performance and effectiveness.* New York: McGraw–Hill, 1970.

French, Wendell L., and Bell, Cecil H., Jr. *Organization development: behavioral science interventions for organization improvement.* Englewood Cliffs, N.J.: Prentice–Hall, 1973.

Friedlander, Frank. The impact of organizational training laboratories on the effectiveness and interaction of ongoing work groups. *Personnel Psychology,* 1967, *20,* 289–307.

Golembiewski, Robert T., Hiles, Rick, and Kagno, Munro S. A longitudinal study of flexi-time effects: Some consequences of an OD structural intervention. *Journal of Applied Behavioral Science,* 1974, *10,* 503–532.

Harrison, Roger. Choosing the depth of organizational intervention. *Journal of Applied Behavioral Science,* 1970, *6,* 181–202.

House, Robert J. T-group education and leadership effectiveness: A review of the empirical literature and a critical evaluation. *Personnel Psychology,* 1967, *20,* 1–32.

Huse, Edgar F. *Organization development and change.* St. Paul, Minn.: West, 1975.

Huse, Edgar F. and Beer, Michael. Eclectic approach to organizational development. *Harvard Business Review,* 1971, *48,* 5 (Sept. – Oct.), 103–112.

Lavoie, Dina, and Culbert, Samuel A. Stages of organization and development. *Human Relations,* 1978, *31,* 417–438.

Lewin, Kurt. Group decision and social change. In G. E. Swanson, T. M. Newcomb, and E. L. Hartley (Eds.), *Readings in social psychology.* Rev. ed. New York: Holt, 1952. Pp. 459–73.

Lieberman, Morton A., Yalom, Irvin D., and Miles, Matthew B. *Encounter groups: first facts.* New York: Basic Books, 1973.
Lippitt, Ronald, Watson, Jeanne, and Westley, Bruce. *The dynamics of planned change.* New York: Harcourt, Brace & World, 1958.
Luke, Robert A., Jr., Block, Peter, Davey, Jack M., and Averch, Vernon R. A structural approach to organizational change. *Journal of Applied Behavioral Science,* 1973, *9,* 611–635.
Margulies, Newton, Wright, Penny L., and Scholl, Richard W. Organization development techniques: Their impact on change. *Group and Organization Studies,* 1977, *2,* 428–448.
Marrow, Alfred J., Bowers, David C., and Seashore, Stanley E. *Management by participation: creating a climate for personal and organizational development.* New York: Harper & Row, 1967.
Morrison, Peggy. "Evaluation in OD: a review and assessment." *Group Organization Studies,* 1978, *3,* 42–70.
Pasmore, William A. The Michigan ICL study revisited: an alternative explanation of the results. *Journal of Applied Behavioral Science,* 1976, *12,* 245–251.
Rush, Harolw M. F. *Behavioral science: concepts and management application.* New York: National Industrial Conference Board, 1969.
Sashkin, Marshall. Review of *Increasing leadership effectiveness* by Chris Argyris, *Personnel Psychology,* 1977, *30,* 273–280.
Sashkin, Marshall, Burke, W. Warner, and Levinson, Harry. Organization development pro and con. *Professional Psychology,* 1973, *4,* 187–208.
Schein, Edgar H. Can one change *organization,* or only *people* in organizations? *Journal of Applied Behavioral Science,* 1973, *9,* 780–785.
Schein, Edgar H. *Process consultation: its role in organization development.* Reading, Mass.: Addison–Wesley, 1969.
Seashore, Charles, and Van Egmond, Elmer. The consultant-trainer role in working directly with a total staff. *Journal of Social Issues,* 1959, *15,* 36–42.
Strauss, George. Organization development: credits and debits. *Organization Dynamics,* 1973 (Winter), 2–19.
Underwood, W. J. Evaluation of laboratory method training. *Training Directors Journal,* 1965, 19 (5), 34–50.
Whyte, William F. *Money and motivation.* New York: Harper & Bros., 1955.
Wieland, George F., and Leigh, Hilary. *Changing hospitals.* London: Tavistock, 1971.

NOTES

1. This model is based on a great variety of observations of work by consultants with individuals, groups, organizations, and communities and is a distillation of what seems to be effective in helping the client to change.
2. For further details on the practice of survey feedback, see Chapter 15 in this volume.
3. Organizational climate entailed such measures as the importance of human resources, communications flow, motivational climate, decision-making practices, and influence at lower organizational levels.

15   # Why Organization Development Hasn't Worked (So Far) in Medical Centers

Marvin R. Weisbord

*"You can feed her all day with the Vitamin A
and the Bromo Fizz
But the medicine never gets anywhere near
where the trouble is. . ."*

—*Frank Loesser, Guys and Dolls*

Understanding and helping improve medical organizations has become a passion for many behavioral scientists, including me. It is a passion matched only by that of health administrators to have their organizations improved. On my pessimistic days, our mutual frenzy reminds me of a story the late Saul Alinsky liked to tell. It concerns a bitch in heat parading up and down behind a screen door, while a neighbor's hound scratches to get at her.

"That's a laugh," says the bitch's owner. "Your hound's fixed. Even if he got in here he couldn't do anything."

"You don't understand," replied the neighbor. "My dog's a consultant!"

Though many of us have pawed through the screen door, we find medical centers particularly impregnable, at least with our present equipment. On the one hand there's a vast descriptive literature of health organizations.[1] On the other, there exists little practical data on how to use this knowledge

Reprinted from *Health Care Management Review*, Vol. 1, No. 2, "Why Organization Development Hasn't Worked (So Far) in Medical Centers," by Marvin R. Weisbord, by permission of Aspen Systems Corporation, © 1976. ADELAIDE'S LAMENT from "Guys and Dolls" by Frank Loesser, © 1950 Frank Music Corp. © Renewed 1978 Frank Music Corp. International Copyright Secured. All Rights Reserved. Used by Permission.

effectively. In my interviews with health center managers, I note a mounting despair over trying to organize what seems, increasingly, a bottomless pit.

If those who are not "hands on" providers of health services wish to have useful impact on the functioning of health delivery organizations, we must start by owning up that certain management methods, no matter how valued in other settings, are—by any standard of scientific objectivity—not working very well in medicine.

In this article, I want to provide, from the standpoint of a student of organizational behavior, a new diagnosis of what ails medical centers. Using this diagnosis, I will explain why one elixir for which I have had high hopes— organization development (OD)—is, for now, not even a good placebo. My central thesis is that medical centers, unlike industrial firms, have coordination problems not subject to rationalization even by "state-of-the-art" administrative practice. I think advocates of other management technologies will find this explanation relevant too.

I see three major reasons OD works better for industry than medicine:

1. Medical centers have few of the formal characteristics of industrial firms, where OD, like all management science, was first recognized, tested, and developed.[2]

2. Physicians and scientists are socialized to a form of rational, autonomous, specialized, expert behavior, which is antithetical to the organization of any but the most narrow individualized pursuits.[3]

3. Medical centers, therefore, require three different social systems, not one, as in industry. The links among the *task* system which administrators manage, the *identity* system which undergirds professional status, and the *governance* system, which sets standards, are extremely tenuous.

Therefore, it is hard to achieve a "good fit" between individual and organization. Medical centers represent what the late pscyhologist A. H. Maslow called "low synergy institutions"[4] — that is, while the systems are extremely interdependent, people do not act that way. This is the opposite of business, where productivity improves measurably when people learn to work together better.

OD is hard to use in low-synergy situations, because it is based on an assumption not widely shared in our culture: that it is possible, through trial and error, to discover *organizational* procedures that enhance both productivity and self-esteem. In industry, people recognize a common stake in this discovery, even while skeptical of its worth. In medicine, professionals believe in their bones that procedures an organization needs for its survival will be inimical to theirs.

We need a new, non-industrial model for what constitutes a good individual/organization fit in medical centers. Industry has not been a very good teacher, for professionals experience "business-like" methods as threatening to their self-esteem. Why should coordination be more threatening in medical centers than in business firms?

OD Is Industry Specific

Nearly all organization development theory and research derive from industry, which sponsored the seminal work of Argyris, Beckhard, Blake and Mouton, Herzberg, Lawrence and Lorsch, Likert, McGregor, Trist and many others. Firms like Esso Standard Oil, Texas Instruments, TRW Systems Group, Union Carbide provided clinical test sites for theories about the relationships between human satisfaction and productivity.[5] This is probably because OD is intended to help organizations balance, better than they often do, the need for structural constraints and the need for creativity. Such constraints exist to a greater degree in industrial organizations than elsewhere.

Structure is important because it is the creation of rational, systematic relationships which constitute the essence of an "organization." Organizations make it possible for people to do things they value and cannot do alone. But, no matter how innovative, organizations perform if—and only if—they achieve a balance among four key structural features, which restrain individual behavior:

- Task interdependence
- Concrete goals
- Performance measures
- Formal authority.

The co-existence of these structural constraints makes an organization sensitive to improvement through focus on its informal system, for people either carry out or subvert goals through their normative behavior.

Historically, industrial firms were structured following the theories of church and military thinkers. To them, authority, goals, and interdependence were central; today, bureaucracy as a structural mode pervades our society. In the 19th Century technologies and performance measures made possible the marriage of bureaucracy to production. Management, as a profession, was born.

Bureaucracy's strength lies in certainty and order. However, its practices, like many industrial products, do not age well. In no time managers discovered that bureaucratic processes have built into them an intractable rigidity. This works against optimal performance. More, at some point the constraints of order outweigh the benefits, restricting personal judgment so that output suffers—and along with it people's self-esteem and morale.

In industry, behavioral scientists using OD provide exactly the right medicine. We introduce counterbureaucratic values and practices, making it legitimate to do things not a part of everyday work. This includes examining group problem solving, how people express and act on feelings ("personal style"), norms, policies, ways of handling conflict—anything that might conceivably impact on the performance of work.

Organizational development methods go under names like "teambuilding," process consultation, intergroup problem solving, survey, data feedback. All of them help people understand, express, learn about, and free themselves from their more irrational constraints. They can then achieve a better balance among goals, authority, task interdependence, and measures. Having done it together, they are more likely to feel committed to making things work, and given recognition for their efforts, their morale improves.

HEALTH CARE PROFESSIONALS ARE SOCIALIZED DIFFERENTLY

Science-based professional work differs markedly from product-based work. Health professionals learn a rigorous scientific discipline as the "content" of their training. The "process"—not explicit—inculcates a value for autonomous decision-making, personal achievement, and the importance of improving their *own* performance, rather than that of any institution.

In consequence physicians identify much less with a specific institution and more with the culture of medical science. This constitutes a set of values, skills, and knowledge quite independent of any work setting. The rewards of major significance to them—respect, reputation—may come more from this larger arena than from their institutional affiliation.

MEDICAL CENTERS: THREE SYSTEMS, NOT ONE

Both health care and industry require financing; both have customers; each has inputs and outputs, environmental constraints, physical facilities, technologies, employment contracts, managers. At the same time, much important medical center activity does not seem connected to its administrative machinery.

Professionals are enmeshed in the three social systems—Task, Identity, Governance—that pull and tug at each other. Health administrators operate the least influential of the three, quite the reverse of the situation of the industrial manager.

The Task system refers to a specific work organization, which seeks to coordinate three tasks: patient care, education and research. The Identity system refers to the professional development, or career track, in medical science, on which the status and self-esteem of health professionals depends. The Governance system is the network of committees, boards, and agencies, within and without task systems, which set standards for the profession.

Each system has its own ground rules and membership requirements. Each is necessary to the others. Health center professionals belong to all three. Yet the Task system is, in many ways, at odds with the Identity and Governance systems, and vice versa.

THE TASK SYSTEM

In industry the Task system is called "management". In health care it's called "administration". I use the generic term Task system to mean either one.

Health care professionals do one or more of four tasks requiring coordination: (1) Patient Care; (2) Education; (3) Research; (4) Administration. Each task is independently valuable to a reasonably complete health care system. These tasks constitute the work of medical centers, hospitals, clinics, and health maintenance organizations.

Patient care, education, and research superficially resemble business functions like production, marketing, or research and development. These superficial similarities encourage the use of industry-based technologies, like program planning and budgeting, management by objectives, and organizational development.

These create an illusion of rationality that disappears quickly when scrutinized, for there are radical discrepancies between industrial and medical Task systems. They lack commonality *exactly* on the four features that make industry such a fertile laboratory for OD.

In industry, management attempts to obtain organizational support for a common definition of interdependence, authority, goals, and measures, while avoiding financial loss. But as Figure 15-1 shows, in complex medical centers goals tend to be abstract, authority diffuse, interdependence low, measures few and controversial. Since there are three systems, not one, it is extremely hard to achieve organizational support, and even harder to avoid financial loss. Let us discuss each of the four features in turn.

TASK INTERDEPENDENCE

Industrial managers each do one task at a time in an enterprise of any size. A person works in production, marketing, sales, or finance, for example, and while a manager might build a sequential career in various functions, none

FIGURE 15-1

DIFFERENCES BETWEEN INDUSTRIAL AND
HEALTH CARE SYSTEMS

INDUSTRY (one system)

Task/(Management)

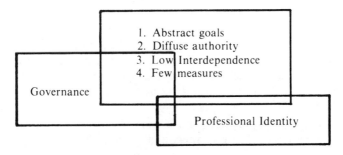

1. Concrete goals
2. Formal authority
3. Task interdependence
4. Performance measures

HEALTH CARE (three systems)

TASK/(Administration)

1. Abstract goals
2. Diffuse authority
3. Low Interdependence
4. Few measures

Governance

Professional Identity

Overlapping Identity and Governance systems function to
thwart the application of goals, authority, interdependence, and
measures in the Task System.

would conceive of trying to perform these tasks all at once. Nevertheless, the
functions are interdependent. The organization requires all to be performed
well if it is to be successful. This mixing requirement—called "task interdependency"—rests on two concepts: the differentiation of function, and the
integration of functions towards specific goals.

Lawrence and Lorsch demonstrated empirically how these two concepts
complement each other in high-performing business.[6] They showed that
people need different social/emotional orientations for different tasks.
Differences that make a difference include time horizon—how fast the

feedback?; interpersonal relations—how important?; goals—how precise?, and so on. Such matters seem to vary with environmental complexity and rate of change. Successful managers recognize this.

Of course these differences, however necessary, create conflict because different groups in the organization have necessarily different goals. The more productive managers were found not only to differentiate skillfully, but also to integrate or manage effectively conflict between diverse functions. Examples of integrative mechanisms, as opposed to people, include information, cost control, budgeting, and planning systems.

Now, consider problems of differentiation and integration in health centers. First, health centers are differentiated primarily by specialty. Each specialty runs its own little "business" called a service. Within each service, several tasks may go on simultaneously: patient care administration, teaching and research. Moreover, these tasks are *all* performed by people wearing multiple hats. Few health center professionals do only one of the major tasks, for to do a single task seriously hampers status and mobility in the other two systems. The most complex example is a one-person entity called a "department chairman" in a medical school whose title masks the fact he is often not only doing all four major tasks, but managing many other people who also do two, three, or four things at once.

To make sense out of this reality, Lawrence, Charns, and I found we had to turn Lawrence-Lorsch theory upside down.[7] Imagine the organizational confusion when task differences exist not only between functions, but also wi.hin each individual. As Figure 15-2 demonstrates, coordination is often left to the whim of the individual.

How can one manage such a system? With difficulty. The reason it runs at all is because individuals are so adept at differentiating and integrating what they do. Health professionals identify much more task conflict "in general" than they do "in my own work."[8]

To me this means multiple hats are not so much a personal problem as an *organizational* one. Task system managers do not know what to do if they can not predict how much of each task is being performed on a given day, the strategic goals this work supports, how much it will cost, and who will pay for it.

This fact accounts for much conflict between administrators and professionals. The one tries to coordinate towards institutional goals, and the other sees this effort, given their personal goals, as bureaucratic constraint which hinders, not helps, their performance and reduces their autonomy.

CONCRETE GOALS

Setting priorities, upon which rational resource management depends, is central to industry. "Only if targets are defined," writes Peter Drucker, "can

FIGURE 15-2

TWO DIFFERENT TASK ORGANIZATION PROBLEMS

INDUSTRIAL FIRM

Sales	Production	Research

3 People, 3 Hats

Problem: Integration. What's the strategic goal?

MEDICAL CENTER

Patient Care	Teaching
Research	Administration

One Person, Many Hats

Problem: Differentiation. Who's Doing What?

Are the goals compatible?

resources be allocated to their attainment, priorities and deadlines set, and somebody held accountable for results."[9]

Health priorities are hard to set, for everything seems equally urgent. Hospital managers consider patient care central, medical deans education, clinicians their own specialty. For many teachers research matters most, because academic advancement, peer recognition, and personal satisfaction are wrapped up in it.[10]

THREE-LEGGED STOOL

The famous "three-legged stool"—equal commitment to service, research, teaching—permits each person to defend whatever he does as high primacy of one or another task at any point in time. Besieged on all sides to accommodate every social and political need, a service institution, writes Drucker, "cannot concentrate; it must try to placate everyone." Thus, the critical question for medical centers is: Can we pay for it? The organizational question is: Does it make sense for us to do it?

One way out of this intolerable goal dilemma is to specify which services or customers come first. Narrowing goals makes coordination with existing technologies more feasible. This strategy has made limited-service private hospitals a successful growth industry while local medical school affiliates are going broke.

It is much easier to run a "businesslike" operation when profit is predicated on treating selected diseases, while limiting or eliminating teaching and research entirely. At the same time, there is a professional cost in this. Physicians attracted to academic medical centers wish to choose for themselves which mix of tasks they need to do to remain at the cutting edge in their fields. They resist the implication they could learn, grow, create, and contribute if limited to working on one task at a time.

This obstacle, however, is not insurmountable. Task differences are subject to rational analyis, even without forcing people to take off some hats. For example, it is possible to write separate contracts for each hat a person wears, instead of lumping tasks into one undifferentiated person labeled "Professor and Chairman."

PERFORMANCE MEASURES

In industry, accountability hinges on managing to a set of numbers. Having goals, dividing up and coordinating work, seem pointless unless you can track progress and make course corrections. Business firms use three major indices: Costs, productivity, and profitability.

Customers are the judges who enforce accountability. Their behavior affects the numbers by which managers manage. Customers can go elsewhere, lobby Congress, write Ralph Nader, picket, boycott, in short make life as miserable for a firm as its faulty products do for them. Health care customers—patients, students—have fewer options. They can do the above, but they are fighting three systems, two of which have cultural/international roots, rather than a single entity with offices somewhere.

The health care Task system uses three major indices, each measuring quite different dimensions: (1) size of budget; (2) space; (3) salaried "full-time equivalents." More of each is held to constitute good performance, and less equals bad, because, as Drucker says, "No institution likes to abandon anything it does."

Quality control, while an issue for administrators, is very difficult for them to manage; for quality standards come not from customer to manager to organization, but from the Governance system to the manager to the customer. Given the nature of medicine, public expectation, and physician training, it is physicians who set and enforce quality standards.

Until recently this has been an extremely individual, rather than organizational, act. "Such evaluation," writes the Joint Commission on Accreditation of Hospitals, "isn't done systematically. . .in a way that reflects the bulk of care given in a hospital." Therefore, the "onus is on the reviewer rather than the system," making it hard for the institution to learn and perform differently.[11]

Thus, while most physicians have and practice high standards, there are few organizational procedures for connecting standards, good or bad, to dollars, space, and staffing decisions. The JCAH's new focus on outcome audits (how well did the patient do?) is a step in the direction of better organization—if such data can be linked to Task system decisions, and not just to physician competence. But so long as the two sets of standards are managed independently of each other, health costs will continue to spiral.

FORMAL AUTHORITY

To enforce and link Governance with Task system measures requires not only a cognitive act but decisiveness. Industrial managers are acknowledged to have the right to decide, even when people question their good sense. The marketplace, in the long run, determines whether they are right or wrong.

In industry, it requires formal authority to sanction "teambuilding," a democratizing process which spreads influence to those who have had too little. In addition, the formal boss-subordinate relationship provides a setting that permits the scrutiny of dynamics important for task accomplishment: anxiety; group collusion to maintain problems; unrealistic expectations for the boss, and vice versa; intolerance of mistakes; reluctance to speak candidly; and the impact of interpersonal feedback on working together.

Health administrators are not exempt from these dynamics. Many have legal responsibility for the consequences. Their formal authority, though, extends in practice only to nurses, aides, technicians, service employees, and other administrators. It excludes physicians and scientists. In this situation business tools and training have limited utility. Health administrators find themselves more often playing the political game of engineering consent rather than the managerial game of implementing decisions.

Lawrence, Charns and I have asked hundreds of medical school faculty to whom they were responsible when wearing each of their medical task hats. From 20+ percent for undergraduate education, to 55 percent in patient care, to 70 percent on research have said "no one," or left the item blank, or named a person or group outside their medical center. While accountability is a much discussed and much valued concept, when applied to others, a great many medical faculty cannot imagine Task system accountability at all. For them, it is purely a Governance matter, based on setting standards for the identity system.[12]

The Identity System

It is the salience to the doctor of the physician Identity system that is key to understanding why health care is so hard to organize. There is a complex interplay of forces: The medical personality, how doctors are socialized, what society expects of physicians. All of these forces reinforce a physician self-concept based largely on the technical expertise needed to diagnose and treat disease, and the mental toughness to make life-and-death decisions alone. This symbolic system exists inside each physician. It is based on public recognition of professional credentials which confer status and a sense of self-worth. Four binds result from this emphasis.

The Self-Concept Bind

The scientific definition of knowledge relevant to disease is extremely limited. All data outside a medical model of life are difficult for many doctors to internalize, let alone act upon. This in no way denies the impressive achievements of modern medicine. It does result in doctors paying a high price, internally, to maintain identity. Most consider task-related feelings, for example, as irrelevant. Some grow quite emotional at the suggestion emotions constitute "scientific" data worthy of study, codification, understanding, and integration with whatever specialty they practice. Many share, in the extreme, a common cultural belief that to show feelings is an unprofessoinal retreat from reason and a sign of weakness.

They tend to see no middle ground of choice between uncontrolled, hysterical catharsis and extreme self-control. Yet few people do work that continually stirs up so much anger, fear, and helplessness. Thus, physicians have few ways of using their emotions constructively toward the solution of problems, in the same way they use their expertise. This seriously limits the degree to which they can invest in joint work with others, and in the utility of their contributions when they do.

This bind extends to positive feelings too. To a great extent trust, in such a disorderly system as health care, is a valuable commodity. Often one's good feelings about another provide a reliable indicator of relevant expertise; many physicians use personal relationships and intuitive trust as important variables in their professional judgments.

Medical theories cannot easily accommodate this fact. Unless your conceptual frame includes (a) a sense-making view of the interplay among feelings, behavior, and relationships, and (b) the impact of these on medical practice, you cannot utilize such data systematically. In fact, a high percentage of important medical decisions are made from such a framework—which constitutes, by formal standards, an extremely unscientific view of medicine.

THE ACCOUNTABILITY BIND

Doctors do not judge each other's work publicly. However valued the concept, it is difficult to practice it. This makes sense where identity is so closely linked to narrow expertise. Only those with equivalent specialized knowledge are presumed to be able to judge one's work. Moreover, at least until recently, such judgments—even when made formally, as part of a hospital audit—were based on "How I would have handled this case," rather than the result for the patient and the impact on the hospital.[13]

Paradoxically, each physician has strong opinions about health system goals, and what roles *all others* (non-physicians) should play in achieving them. They "often regard themselves as expert in medicine at large," writes a public health school dean, which "includes all parts of the hospital . . . and, beyond that, the community, since so many aspects are 'health related.'"[14]

"CATCH-22" OF MEDICINE

Accountability is the Catch-22 of medicine. The demonstration of expertise in one specialty, which is critical to self-esteem, is taken as admission of incompetence in all other areas. Thus, physicians accept medical administrator claims to management expertise—so long as no clinical matters are involved.

The trouble is that in hospitals nearly everything is health-related. Yet accountability—for the system as a whole—is extremely fragmented. Though most physicians care very much about quality, they have few procedures for linking this concern to institutional management.

THE KNOWLEDGE BIND

Identity hinges on state-of-the-art skills and knowledge. Yet nobody can keep up any more. "If I did nothing but read journals all day," one doctor told me, "I'd just fall behind at a slower rate." To maintain status, doctors must maintain an illusion of keeping up. Knowing the impossibility of doing this, they do the next best thing. They narrow their focus and become sub-specialists.

This has a curious organizational consequence. It cannot be predicted when a new technique, piece of equipment, or care concept will be developed. It *can* be predicted at what point in time physicians will pressure their medical facility to acquire an innovation: at once. From an Identity system perspective this makes sense. Whether it makes sense from a patient care or teaching or institutional management standpoint varies considerably from place to place.

To put it another way, knowledge is piling up at a rate beyond the ability of anybody to assimilate it—and it is easier for physicians to blame bureaucracy for their inability to keep up than to accept their own human limitations.

THE TASK INTERDEPENDENCE BIND

The only reason to be organized is that the problems you are trying to solve require it. Certainly this is true of complex health facilities. At the same time, organizations, for optimal performance, require some cooperation—which implies give and take. Physicians, caught in their other binds, feel compelled to direct, control, decide and be responsible for every patient and patient decision within their purview. It is hard for doctors to share life-and-death risks with anybody, even the patients themselves. What is more, this bind is growing tighter. A growing number of malpractice suits seem based on the premise that infallibility, rather than best effort, should be the minimum standard.

Physician identity has serious consequences for medical organizations. It is the department, rather than an institution, which undergirds Identity. Medicine is organized by specialty to a greater degree than generic tasks like service, teaching, research. Specialty is so pervasive that without the label it is difficult to achieve status in a medical center. Budgets tend to flow through departments. Programmatic activity—integration of knowledge around patient problems—often suffers.

Except for science-based R&D, there is nothing in industry remotely comparable to the medical Identity system. To a remarkable degree industrial managers measure self-esteem and organizational achievement together. They feel good about themselves when the numbers improve, and badly when they do not. The needs of Task and Identity systems work hand in glove. Enhancing one will also enhance the other. It is this chance that makes organization development valuable and welcome.

THE GOVERNANCE SYSTEM

The Governance system sets and maintains health and medical practice standards. It is the "appreciative" mechanism, in Vickers' phrase, which performs the valuing function that makes the Identity system so potent.[15]

Governance exists both in and outside institutions. Inside, it includes trustees, hospital and medical boards, audit committees, and—in medical schools—faculty senates, executive faculty (chairmen), task forces, and committees on everything from admissions to curriculum and grading. Outside are professional societies, specialty boards, accrediting groups, granting agencies, and government. These influence admission to the field, ethical practice, funding, and educational, clinical, and research criteria.

Governance, in its own terms, is the best organized of the three systems. From the standpoint of health care systems, however, Governance mechanisms tend to have three flaws.

LICENSURE BY A GOVERNANCE GROUP, NOT AN EMPLOYMENT CONTRACT, UNDERGIRDS IDENTITY

It is not necessary to demonstrate competence in working with others, nor an understanding of organizational complexity, to achieve status in medicine. Moreover, it is not necessary to demonstrate achievement in a particular Task system. Once technical competence is certified, all else is assumed.

GOVERNANCE SYSTEMS TEND TO BE MORE CLOSED THAN THE TASK SYSTEM, WHICH REQUIRES DAILY INTERACTION WITH PATIENTS, STUDENTS AND THE PUBLIC

There have been few pipelines into health policy which lay people can use, although this is changing.

In addition, links between Governance and Task systems are spotty, rather than well institutionalized. In most hospitals, for instance, utilization review, under cost pressure from third party payers, is an important Task problem. Meanwhile, hospitals are also under pressure to phase-in outcome audits, as a means of insuring uniform, high quality care. The latter is a Governance function. As hospitals are presently structured, whether physicians will have an opportunity to analyze with managers the relationship between both sets of data and their impact on goals and costs is questionable. Another result of this is that administrators are called upon to implement standards which they are not considered competent to judge. This exacerbates still more the inherent conflict between physicians and managers.

GOVERNANCE SYSTEMS WORK AGAINST INTERDEPENDENCY

Internal committee meetings, by far the most frequent type in medical centers, tend to be long, frustrating, and often non-productive. Departmental loyalties are more intense than loyalty to the whole which Governance represents. Without concrete institutional goals, it is hard to favor anything except what will be least restrictive of one's own freedom of action.

The High Costs of Poor Linkage

Throughout, I have tried to show the significance of the lack of links between Task, Identity, and Governance systems, and to demonstrate how this works against rational management and incurs costs.

This lack of links among the three systems requires more Task system administrators. This drives up fixed costs, which are then squeezed from professional budgets as a sort of "coordination tax." Despite this, integration remains elusive. It takes place in a vacuum. Toward what ends is the system being integrated? If ever there was a cat chasing its tail, it is the addition of administrative systems in the absence of goals that professionals share.

Second, is cost in alienation. An anomaly of medical centers is the degree to which the Task system so slavishly imitates industry's least appropriate bureaucratic mode. Functional specialization defines status in health, despite a crying need for programs integrated on behalf of whole people—patients, students, communities, the professionals themselves.

To cite one example, consider a connection between deteriorating doctor-nurse relationships and rising hospital costs. There are in the main three things hospital patients need: Clinical care, personal attention, and help in getting a complex system to focus on their own case. Doctors provide the first service. Increasingly, aides do the "hands-on" care, clerks the paperwork, allied technicians the clinical tests, and ombudsmen the patient advocacy. Nurses, who might provide a link between clinical and administrative tasks, are being squeezed out. RNs often don't want the narrow jobs, for they are trained to greater responsibility.

They cannot use their knowledge well in the present setup, despite the fact they spend more time with patients, and often understand better than anyone the complex relationship among physical, emotional, social, and administrative problems.[16] With clinical and administrative training, they might make excellent hospital integrators—much better, in fact, than doctors or administrators. Instead, they are opting for the Identity game—seeking to become nurse practitioners—because nobody, themselves included, can visualize a more appropriate use for their training.

Why OD Hasn't Worked—So Far

Since face-to-face interdependence is so important for solving medical center problems, it seems plausible that applied behavioral scientists, with OD skills, would have some useful procedures. Alas, we have our binds too.

First, our knowledge is inadequate. Though we have some ideas about how to coordinate the major tasks, industrial theories shed no light at all on how to link the three systems in ways so that both individuals *and* organization are enhanced. They do not, in particular, account for the consequences of a highly competitive Identity system, based entirely on individual achievement.

Second, our structure-reducing, interdependence-enhancing technologies do not work where there is no organizational payoff for interdependent behavior. To practice structure reduction in such a competitive environment is to raise professional anxieties even higher, for these technologies seek to improve a set of conditions physicians do not value to begin with.

The OD repertoire needs structure-*creating* interventions, consistent with our humanistic values. Yet we share with health professionals a profound mistrust of mindless bureaucracies.[17] To the extent we can find no middle ground between free-flowing "organic" relationships and industrial constraints, we may resist the persistent—not intermittent or temporary— commitment that the invention of innovative structures calls for.

The Health Manager's Bind

The risk for all of us is falling prey to what Maslow called "the dangers of unrealistic perfectionism."[18] It is this syndrome which probably accounts in part for the short half-life of deans, chiefs, chairmen and administrators. Knowing the scene firsthand, many go into management believing they, unlike their predecessors, will avoid the big mistakes.

They see the pitfall—there is little evidence to the contrary—as personalities, not systems, and soon discover they cannot easily change others. Instead, they seek to change themselves, in the same mode that made them competent physicians or scientists—by acquiring new skills and knowledge. They study MBO, PPBS, and the more adventurous OD, as if these were anatomy courses through which the system, once understood, can be manipulated. However, the courses are based on industrial practice and deal with a very different anatomy.

Where their industrial counterparts use technology strategically, they use it ad hoc, to patch up this situation, to damp down that one. They find themselves constantly saying No to people they like, rejecting ideas they value, holding the creativity of others at bay, unappreciated for the good things they have done, attacked for the numberless things others think they *should* have done. Only a few redefine the problem as something beyond technology: how to discover/translate/invent wholly new modes.

How can this be done? The paradox is profound. Though the Identity system names the game, and the Governance system makes the rules, the Task system is the playing field. Those who play by technical expertise alone win only at the expense of many others, jeopardizing an already fragile system. A critical variable is cognition of the missing linkages, for managerial changes which lack Governance sanctions or threaten Identity are not likely to be stable.

Paradoxically, to introduce a new management practice sensitive to all three systems requires, in the absence of relevant organization theory, innate political and interpersonal skills. These skills, though in short supply, are not lacking entirely. Some administrators with whom I have been privileged to work over the years are doing things worth studying:

- Budgeting both by department *and* program to encourage integrative activity
- Clarifying the center's institutional and departmental goals
- Involving professionals in managerial tasks
- Planning resource management more deliberately

FIGURE 15-3

SYSTEMS LINK-UP NEEDED IN MEDICAL CENTERS

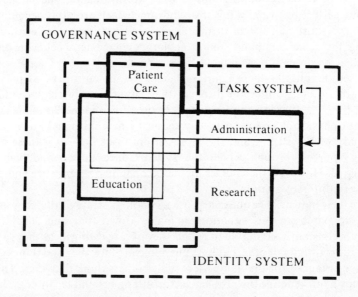

1. TASK SYSTEM itself requires coordination of major tasks—the target of management technologies.

2. In addition, links are needed with GOVERNANCE and IDENTITY systems. Theory is inadequate to this.

- Bringing physicians and scientists into institutional budget discussions
- Educating others to the complexity of these tasks.

Judging the efficacy of these efforts by "all-or-nothing" medical standards seems inappropriate, for no one knows what "all" looks like, and "nothing" is unacceptable in a system strangling for lack of organizational innovations equal to those of medicine.

A sensible goal for health managers, it seems to me, is to try to make small improvements, say 10 percent, in the congruity of goals, interdependence, authority, and measures. Small rationalizations, sanctioned by Governance, mindful of Identity, contribute importantly to more human medical centers.

Figure 15-3 charts the complex interdependencies I think must be taken into account in any new theory of individual/organization fit in medical centers. Present technologies seek to rationalize the Task system (solid lines). Whether they also can be used to link the three systems is one test of their practicality. Those unwilling to experiment with new structural relationships cannot facilitate change, for the changes called for may be the very ones they resist. If that is an exaggeration, the changes called for are certainly structures of a different sort than any of us know much about. They are structures that encourage, support, and utilize creative, individualistic, and idiosyncratic behavior for socially desirable ends.

If we can own up to our ignorance, and to our values in such matters, then I believe we are ready to have the "right" problem: how to create, in health-care-specific situations, a better fit between people and work.

REFERENCES

1. Georgopoulos, Basil S. (Editor), *Organization Research On Health Care Institutions*. Institute For Social Research, The University of Michigan, Ann Arbor, Michigan, 1972.
2. Friedlander, Frank, "OD Reaches Adolescence: An Exploration of Its Underlying Values." *The Journal of Applied Behavioral Science*, Vol. 12, No. 1, 1976.
3. Freidson, Eliot, *Professional Dominance: The Social Structure Of Medical Care*. Aldine Publishing Co., Chicago, Illinois, 1970.
4. Maslow, A. H., "Synergy in the Society and in the Individual," Chapter 14, *The Farther Reaches of Human Nature*. The Viking Press, New York, 1972, pp. 199–211.
5. French, Wendell L., and Cecil H. Bell, Jr., "A History of Organization Development," *Organization Development*. Prentice-Hall, Inc., Englewood Cliffs, New Jersey, Chapter 21, pp. 21–29, 1973.
6. Lawrence, Paul R., and J. W. Lorsch, *Organization and Environment*. Homewood, Illinois: Richard D. Irwin, Inc., 1969.
7. Lawrence, Paul R., Marvin R. Weisbord, Martin P. Charns, "The Organization and Management of Academic Medical Centers: A Summary of Findings."

Unpublished Report to Four Medical Schools, Organization Research & Development, 1974.

8. Lawrence, Weisbord, Charns, op. cit., page 7.
9. Drucker, Peter F., "Why Service Institutions Do Not Perform," *Management—Tasks—Responsibilities—Practices.* Harper & Row, 1974, Chapter 12, pp. 137–147.
10. Lawrence, Paul R., Marvin R. Weisbord, and Martin P. Charns, *Academic Medical Center Self-Study Guide,* Report to Physicians' Assistance Branch, Bureau of Health Manpower Education, National Institutes of Health, 1973.
11. Jacobs, Charles M., J. D., *Procedure for Retrospective Patient Care Audit in Hospitals,* Joint Commission on Accreditation of Hospitals, Third Edition, 1973.
12. Lawrence, Weisbord, Charns, op. cit., page 6.
13. Jacobs, op. cit.
14. Lynton, Rolf P., "Boundaries in Health Care Systems" (Backfeed Section), *Journal of Applied Behavioral Science,* Volume 11, No. 2, 1975, page 250.
15. Vickers, Sir Geoffrey, *The Art of Judgment,* Basic Books, New York, New York, 1965.
16. Charns, Martin P., "Breaking the Tradition Barrier: Managing Integration in Health Care Facilities," *Health Care Management Review,* Winter, 1976.
17. For a sensible, humane statement see, Culbert, Samuel A., *The Organization Trap and How to Get Out of It.* Basic Books, Inc., New York, 1974.
18. Maslow, A. H., op. cit., p. 217.

16 | Working with the Primary Care Team: The First Intervention

Ronald E. Fry
Bernard A. Lech
Irwin Rubin

Two bodies of knowledge—organizational psychology and organizational development—were used in the design and implementation of the strategies, interventions, and activities that comprised the M[assachusetts] I[nstitute of] T[echnology] pilot program for team improvement at the Dr. Martin Luther King Jr. Health Center in the South Bronx.

Put briefly, organizational psychology provided us with a theoretical framework for dealing with groups and individuals within the organizational setting.[1] Organizational development (OD), which is the application side of organizational psychology, provided us with a set of educational strategies and methods, emphasizing experiential learning.[2]

In this chapter we describe our experiences with two of MLK's eight health care teams, each of which we worked with for some fifteen hours over a period of five weeks. As a first step, it was necessary for us to examine or diagnose the environment in which the health teams operated. To do this, we needed a framework within which to proceed.

AUTOTHERAPEUTIC MODEL

The conceptual framework we used to help guide us in our work with the health teams consisted of an autotherapeutic or self-renewing model, which is

Portions of this chapter were abridged from an unpublished Master's Thesis at the MIT Sloan School of Management, R. E. Fry and B. A. Lech, June 1971. Reprinted with permission from *Making Health Teams Work*, copyright 1974, Ballinger Publishing Company.

shown in Figure 16-1. The basic assumption underlying this framework is that the environment in which the teams operate inevitably produces uncertainty, anxiety, and frustration. Unless team members can effectively manage these negatives, they will be caught in a downward spiral, which will lead to more anxiety and poorer performance on the job. If, however, they are able to manage the situation effectively, the result will be less anxiety and improved health care delivery.

We call the environment in which a team operates its "life space," which is shown in Figure 16-2. Many aspects of this life space are slow, difficult, or impossible for the health teams to change. For example, nothing the teams can do is likely to have much effect on the city bureaucracy or the ghetto neighborhood within which the teams must operate.

We might say that the team's job is to manage its interface with this life space. "Manage" as used here means that the team must be able to handle conflict; work out relationships between doctors, nurses, family health workers, etc.; socialize new members; and make decisions so as to effectively cope with and solve the social-medical problems presented by the life space.

Our thesis is that if the teams communicate, support their members, problem solve, etc., the result will be autotherapeutic or self-renewing, like recharging the "team battery" (the upper loop in Figure 16-1). But if team members fail to communicate, support, etc., we believe they will experience more anxiety, which will drain team energy and spirit; in other words, they will be caught in the negative spiral or lower loop in our diagram.[3]

Now let us briefly step through the model. The environment—slow and difficult to change as it is—generates the frustratingly heavy workloads and uncertainty about work priorities. Team members may ask any of the following questions:

- Doctor: "Can I get enough valid information from the family health worker about this family's situation to be sure my medical prescription will help?"
- Public Health Nurse: "Can I really function as a nurse-practitioner when my training has taught me to follow doctors' orders and ask no questions?"
- Family Health Worker: "Do I really know enough to be able to give the doctors and nurses the information they need?"

The anxiety, uncertainty, and frustration reflected in such questions must be dealt with *by the team.* If members do not support the nurse in her new role, if communication is so poor that the family health worker cannot provide doctors and nurses with the feedback they need, if the family health worker does not feel she is trusted or respected, then the lower loop of Figure 16-1 will operate to increase the anxiety. On the other hand, if communication among team members is sufficiently good, and trust is high, the team will then operate on the upper, autotherapeutic loop of Figure 16-1.

FIGURE 16-1

THE HEALTH TEAM AS AN AUTOTHERAPEUTIC ORGANISM

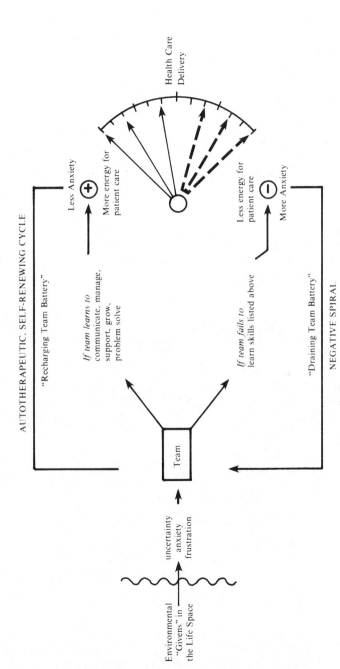

FIGURE 16–2

THE LIFE SPACE OF A HEALTH TEAM

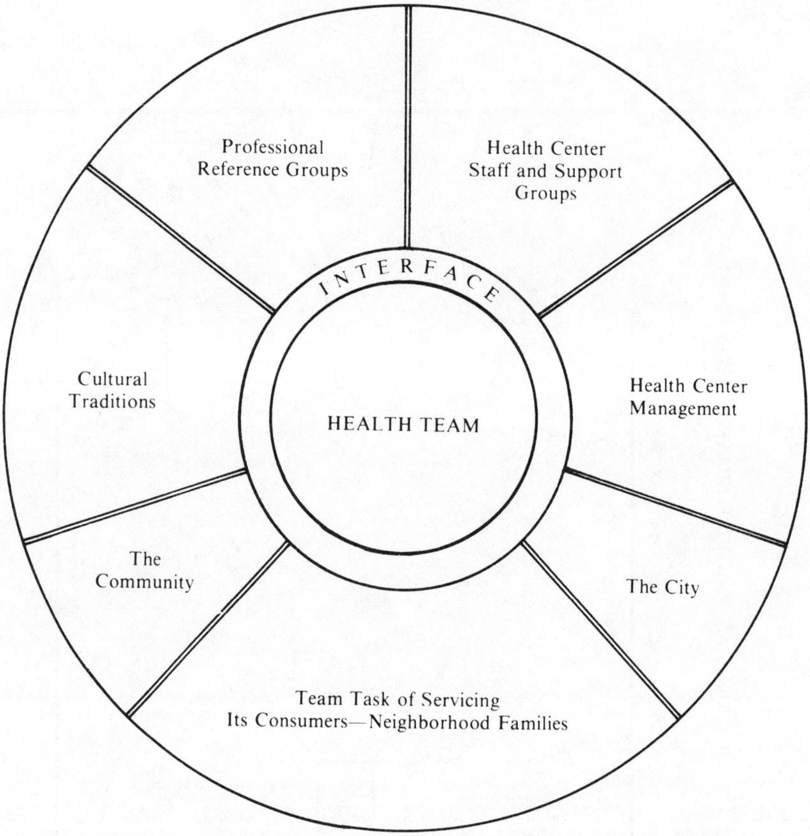

ENVIRONMENTAL FACTORS

Keeping this model in mind, we will now look at the environmental factors that impinge on the health teams, briefly indicating how they are likely to affect team members in the performance of their jobs.

THE TEAM'S TASK

The primary task of the health care team is to deliver comprehensive, family-centered health care to the residents of the community it serves.[4] Any task stated in such global terms is likely to produce some anxiety. For instance, what does "comprehensive health care" really mean? And how can care be family-centered when most patients are seen as individuals? Even when this is not the case, how is a family defined? If the small children live with an aunt or other relative during the week while their parents work and only come "home" on weekends, who comprises the family?

The team's task is also made more difficult by the lack of clearly defined and measurable goals. While the complex and frustrating environment makes this unavoidable, the ambiguity the team faces tends to dilute any successes that do occur, causing uncertainty and often depression.

Chronic problems with no easy or clear medical solutions are also a specific source of anxiety for health team members. They not only yield few successes but they afford little if any positive feedback or reinforcement from the patients. A family health worker remarked that what made her happiest was "when Mrs. Y stopped by our office to thank us. But people just never seem to do that very much."

Then there is the problem of patient demands. Beyond being asked to respond to the normal health needs of a patient, some patients also "ask the impossible of me," as one family health worker put it. These "impossibles" range from resolving marital problems to doing the grocery shopping. Even if not actually impossible, such tasks at least create many conflicts around what a team member expects his role to be.

Difficulties also arise around team members' expectations of each other. A family health worker, for instance, who has been trained in practical nursing and community development, may be seen as an "errand girl" or "messenger," and hence treated as such by other team members. This can only cause additional frustration and uncertainty about what her job really is.

Often team members are forced to work in relatively new or unknown areas such as a doctor getting involved in social welfare problems, family health workers in psychiatric problems, or a nurse in the supervision of paraprofessionals. Such behavior is generally at odds with the expectations created by prior training and experience. Adjusting to such roles takes time. And worrying about one's qualifications makes it that much more difficult to act confidently.

All these factors contribute to the complexity of the health teams' task of providing comprehensive patient care.

GHETTO COMMUNITY

The following are elements of the community which, inherently, create anxieties for the health teams:

1. Inadequate law enforcement threatens the safety of everyone in the neighborhood, including team members.

2. Low level of education and lack of understanding of or appreciation for preventive medicine add to the health teams' task of educating the community in health care, family planning, nutrition, drug rehabilitation, sanitation, etc.
3. Cultural and economic differences often create communication problems. For example, a doctor's prescription which reads, "To be taken three times per day after meals" reflects a white, middle-class perspective. Poor people often do not have the luxury of three meals a day.

Seemingly obvious, straightforward solutions like getting the walls painted, getting children in day care centers, or getting a homemaker into a household are generally only partial solutions. And even then, implementation of any such social prescription is no simple task. Total success is nearly impossible and clear-cut success is infrequent. Against such odds, team members cannot help but react in frustrating, depressive, critical manners which create anxieties among themselves and in their patients. One family health worker summed it up: "I'm told not to worry about social problems that I can't handle, but then I have to tell the family I can't help them. And that makes me feel lousy."

THE URBAN MONSTER MEGALOPOLIS

The bureaucracy, politics, and staggering demographic enormities of the city engulfing this health center easily conjure up the image of an unwieldy, thick-skinned creature. Insensitive and unresponsive, the creature moves slowly, uncontrollably, down paths that seem to many, including the "little" health team, to lead nowhere. To the health team serving the community's needs, dealing with both city and large private agencies providing welfare, housing, hospitalization, transportation, and law enforcement services is often a time-consuming, frustrating experience.

For example, a family health worker who arranges her schedule so that she can accompany one of her patients to a hospital for treatment not provided by the health center may find herself with the following dilemma: Should she leave the frightened, Spanish-speaking woman in a waiting room with little hope of adequate communication with doctors (the sick woman may flee) so as to see other needy patients or to attend an important team meeting? Or should she scuttle the remainder of her schedule to stay with the woman? The dilemma increases her uncertainty and, hence, her anxiety.

CULTURAL MIX OF TEAM MEMBERS

Health care teams are composed of members ranging widely in nationality, color, religion, and social background. Caucasian, Afro-Americans, Europeans, Asians, Puerto Ricans, Americans, Jews, Catholics, Protestants, residents of poor, middle, and upper class urban and suburban neighbor-hoods, unmarried, married, with children, without children, separated, divorced—all are represented on the teams. While it might be helpful for teams to have nonwhite doctors, nothing the team can do is going to greatly affect the number of Black or Puerto Rican medical students graduating in the next few years.

Formal education of team members ranges from the M.D. degree to less than a high school diploma. And this directly affects the status of team members. Doctors are at the top, nurses are subordinate to doctors, and family health workers, without recognized professional job roles, are still lower. These vast differences produce gaps in communication, understanding, and expectations that may only be closed through long hours of special effort. Yet the pace of the work tends to preclude any such effort being made.

While the differences in skills and experiences are necessary, the anxiety caused by them needs to be managed. It should be a task of the team to find methods to reduce the uncertainties and frustrations that naturally occur from this cultural mix. Ignoring and suppressing this anxiety will only worsen the situation. For example, a family health worker, intimidated by a doctor's higher status and by her own background of subordination, finds it impossible to ask the doctor about terminology she is not familiar with. This inevitably affects her self-confidence when she communicates with her families and tries to implement a plan of action the team has decided upon. And in the end it is the family who suffers.

TUG–OF–WAR: COMMUNITY AND TEAM

The family health worker is supposed to cultivate the skills of questioning, probing, and collecting information that she needs to perform her job effectively. The community, in many instances, is withdrawn, suspicious, and silent. Since she is also a member of that community, she is certain to experience some uncertainty and frustration centered around violation of community norms and her own sense of survival. Sharing information and feelings openly with other team members may be just too threatening—based on her past experiences in the community. For example, should she communicate private, confidential information about a friend of hers who is also a team patient and the subject of a team conference meeting? Should she reveal that the husband is not living with the family so that his wife and children can enjoy the relative comfort of an apartment in a new housing project which is made possible by Aid for Dependent Children welfare payments? Such a disclosure, she knows, could result in the family's eviction. Unless the resulting anxiety, in addition to the specific problem, is dealt with, the situation can only worsen.

The team approach to health care may require that the long-standing tradition of privacy between doctor and patient be expanded to a team-patient relationship. However, for most team members the tendency is to revert to the established medical model: labeling, diagnosing, and prescribing "in one's head" with only the result shared.

MLK MANAGEMENT

Finally, the health center's management is an important aspect of the health teams' life space. It affects the teams in many ways. Our observations suggested that the interaction between health teams and management did not, on the whole, improve the delivery of patient care. Sometimes quite the reverse.

Briefly, the center's organization structure was patterned along traditional hospital lines, with a top-down chain of command. This meant the health delivery teams fell at the bottom of the structure and were, more often than not, the passive recipients of decisions made at the top of the hierarchy, with the latter often lacking the information required to be really responsive to the needs of the teams.

The reporting system also tended to work against facilitating a team operation. As in hospitals, pediatricians reported to a chief of pediatrics, internists to a chief of internal medicine, nurses to a chief of nursing, etc. This had the effect of drawing people outside the team and lessening the cohesive factors. What we encountered in many instances was a group of individuals each doing his or her own tasks independently of other so-called team members. It was a team in name only.

These then were the major factors making up the environment or life space of the health teams over which members had relatively little control. We now will look at the area of greatest potential control—the team's management of itself. It is here that we, as consultants, planned to focus our efforts to help the teams help themselves.

THE PROCESS FACTORS

To understand how any group manages itself, it is necessary to look at the group's processes—that is, how it goes about doing its work. For instance, how are decisions made? Do people listen to each other? Do most members participate in discussions or do a few consistently dominate? These and other process factors tell us how the group operates, how it goes about doing its tasks.[5]

To evaluate the health teams' managerial effectiveness, we looked at six key process variables, which are critical in all groups: (a) goals or mission, (b) role expectations, (c) decision making, (d) communication/leadership, (e) norms, and (f) conflict management.

It is important to note that all these factors are amenable to change. While the elements of the life space of the teams are slow to change, how a team *manages* its life space is assumed to be subject to change through learning. The key, then, in striving for the autotherapeutic ideal is that the team learn to manage its life space effectively. We will now look at how the teams dealt with each of the process factors listed above.

GOALS OR MISSION

Any team or group has a purpose. A reason or reasons exist for the formation of the group in the first place. Questions relating to goals are (a) Who sets the goals and how clearly are they defined? (b) How much agreement is there among members concerning the goals? How much commitment? (c) How clearly measurable is goal achievement? (d) How do group goals relate to broader organizational goals? To personal goals?

As we have already seen, members of the MLK health teams experienced considerable uncertainty over their global mission of attempting to provide comprehensive, family-centered health care. Anxiety was also generated because teams did not really know when and if they were succeeding. Questions of priorities and time allocations were also complicated; how does one decide between competing activities in the absence of clearly defined goals? These were some of the unresolved problems relating to goals that the teams needed to work on.

ROLE EXPECTATIONS

Multiple role expectations is another critical factor affecting members of most groups. Each person, in effect, has a set of expectations of how each of the other members should behave as the group works to achieve its goals. In any group, therefore, there are questions about: (a) the extent to which such expectations are clearly defined and communicated (role ambiguity); (b) the extent to which such expectations are compatible or in conflict (role conflict); (c) the extent to which any individual is capable of meeting these multiple expectations (role overload).

In the two teams we worked with there was little discussion as to what one's job responsibilities really were. Even where a role was clear, it was often not accepted by all team members or not utilized properly. A nurse remarked, "I'm supposed to supervise but I don't have any power to do anything if I find something is wrong." A doctor remarked that he "wished nurses could do more nursing, but they have too many other things to do." Family health workers, perhaps more than any other team members, were not used adequately and their roles were not clear. While they were told they were the team "experts" on the community, more often than not their opinions were not solicited.

Such frustrations and uncertainties result from and reinforce unclear goals and priorities for the total team: "The patient is No. 1." "Medical problems are No. 1." "Social problems are my main concern." "We have to change the community before we can provide comprehensive health care." These differences were rarely discussed; rather, for the most part they were ignored.

A team member's failure to communicate his feelings about what he thinks others expect of him, about what he'd like to do, and about what he feels he has to do results in uncertainty for both himself and the rest of the team. Conflicts and dilemmas that could be dealt with if they were allowed to surface are instead submerged; only the frustration surfaces. The level of concern now becomes "how to cover up what I really feel in order to avoid a fight or argument that I will probably lose." The assumption is that by avoiding such interactions, the team will have more time to perform its task in the community.

Actually, the opposite is true. Energy that might have been expended on the task instead goes into these elaborate cover-ups of feelings. And since any discussion of such problems is avoided, nothing gets resolved.

A nurse remarks that she feels like a "juggler with too many balls." Another says, "I can't keep my head above water." Instead of being in a position to deal with the unavoidable anxieties caused by the environment, the team adds to its frustration, depression and uncertainty by ineffective management of its own processes. By not spending the time required to achieve common goals and clear roles, the resulting anxiety actually interferes with the team's providing effective health care.

DECISION MAKING

A group is a problem-solving, decision-making mechanism. By this we do not mean to imply that an entire group must make all the decisions as a group. The issue is one of relevance and appropriateness: Who has the relevant information and who will have to implement the decision? A group can choose from a range of decision-making mechanisms, including decision by default (lack of response), unilateral decision (authority rule), majority vote, consensus, or unanimity.[6]

Any of these forms may be appropriate under certain conditions. And each will have different consequences both in terms of the amount of information available for use in making the decision and the subsequent commitment of members to implement it.

Probably the most obvious requirement in attempting to deal effectively with the South Bronx community and its patients is the need for many different inputs into the decision-making process. While some purely medical problems can be resolved unilaterally by the physician, more often the nature of the task dictates that many skills and resources will be needed to diagnose and treat complex social-medical problems. Furthermore, all team members must be commmited to team decisions if those decisions are to be effectively implemented. But such commitment, we know, is rarely forthcoming unless all members have participated in the decision-making process.

The decision making we observed most frequently on the teams could be characterized as being made by a minority, with most team members noncommittal. Decisions by majority vote and unanimity were not seen at all. Consensus was often solicited, but usually had to be assumed from silence. This kind of decision making is best understood as the "plop effect." At first glance, this hardly seems a method at all, but its invisibility belies its power. When a team member suggests an idea, the result is no response at all, and then another member suggests a new idea. The first member's suggestion has "plopped" without as much as a single response concerning its merits or disadvantages.

Another member, seeing his first "plop," may think, "if that is what happens to his ideas, I won't stick my neck out." The effect spreads until only the most outspoken members offer their ideas. They become the minority making the decisions. While they may sense some uncertainty as to the degree they are supported by others or as to their authority, in the face of an environment that demands action they forge ahead, often railroading a decision through. Such decisions not only limit participation but, even more detrimental, severely reduce commitment to the decisions.

Majority vote and true consensus seem most appropriate in terms of sharing ideas and feedback among all those who should be involved. This puts great emphasis on effective communication: Necessary information and feelings *must* be shared if the team is to manage the anxiety and frustration caused by the environment. The less sharing of such information, the more anxiety is created.

What we observed was little sharing and much anxiety.

COMMUNICATION PATTERNS/ LEADERSHIP

If, indeed, a group is a problem-solving, decision-making mechanism, then the effective flow of information is central to its functioning. Anything that acts to inhibit the flow of information will detract from the group's effectiveness.

A range of factors affects information flow. At a very simple level there are architectural and geographical issues. Meeting space can be designed to facilitate or hinder the flow of communication. Geographically separated facilities may be a barrier to rapid information exchange.

Numerous more subtle factors also exist. Participation—frequency, order, and content—may follow formal lines of authority or status. High status members may speak first, most often, and most convincingly on all issues. The best sources of information needed to solve a problem will, however, vary with the problem. Patterns of communication based exclusively on formal lines of status will not meet many of the group's information needs. The degree to which people feel free to participate, to challenge, to express opinions also significantly affects information flow.

Very much related to the processes of decision making and communication is the area of leadership. To function effectively a group needs many acts of leaderhip rather than one leader. People often misinterpret such a statement to mean "good groups are leaderless." But this is not what we mean. Rather, depending on the situation and the problem to be solved, different people can and should assume leadership. For instance, the formal leader of a group may defend the organization's official position on a particular issue. Another member may express sharp disagreement and a third may provide help in clarifying the disagreement. This would be an example of some useful acts of leadership. We repeat: It is highly unlikely that in any group there will be one person capable of meeting all of a group's leadership needs.

The communication patterns and leadership we observed on the MLK health teams in general relied on the model team members knew best—in this case, *"follow the doctor."* Acts of leadership by other team members were seldom attempted; and when they were, we saw very little support forthcoming from other members. Several family health workers stated to us (in interviews, not publicly) that since they were closest to the families, they ought to have more of a say in what gets done and how it gets done. These few forceful family health workers either eventually influenced a team decision or "went down swinging," saying ". . . that just won't work with that family!" But they were in the minority, and had little support from the others.

The effect of this traditional model of leadership was decision making by expert medical power, with lack of commitment and support from quiet team members.

Norm Structure

Norms are the unwritten rules that govern any group. Whether they are understood as such or just "felt," they are powerful determinants of how members will behave. They define what is good or bad, acceptable or unacceptable if one is to be a functioning member of this group. They often take on the quality of laws: "It's the way we do things around here." Their existence is most clear-cut when they are violated—quiet uneasiness, shifting in one's chair, joking reminders are all observable. Repeated violation of norms often leads to psychological or even physical expulsion.

Norms take on particular potency because they influence all of the other areas we have discussed. For instance, the MLK teams we studied exhibited the following powerful norms:

1. In making a decision, "silence means consent."
2. Doctors are more important than other team members—we don't disagree with them; we wait for them to lead.
3. Conflict is dangerous, both task conflicts and interpersonal disagreements—"it's best to let sleeping dogs lie."
4. Positive feelings, praise, support are not shared—"we're all professionals here to do a job" (as if professionals were not people).
5. The difficulties inherent in our task preclude the possibility of our being flexible in respect to our own internal group processes.

The effect of these norms, and others like them, is to guarantee that a team gets caught in a negative spiral. The task demands flexibility; the teams are inflexible. The task underscores the need for some place to recharge one's emotional battery; the team does not provide this opportunity. The task demands maximum flow of information and frequent decisions by consensus; but team members are reluctant to share ideas and feelings; decisions most often are made by a minority, with other members noncommittal.

The cost of failing to develop norms of flexibility, support, and openness of communication is high indeed. For in addition to precluding these norms, it also precludes the development of a set of higher order or meta norms, which involve developing the capacity to become self-renewing or autotherapeutic. For this to take place, controlled experimentation must be sanctioned, along with risk taking, failure, and evaluation of outcomes. In the absence of norms that support and reinforce these kinds of behaviors, a team will end up fighting two enemies—its task and itself.

CONFLICT MANAGEMENT

Conflict management, although overlapping considerably with other process factors discussed, is important as a separate process factor because it determines whether team members will be able to work together successfully despite their many differences. When we use the term "conflict management," we mean both solving a problem involving disagreeing parties and getting adversary parties to accept and live with their differences without compromising the overall team functioning.

Openness is often the key to successful conflict resolution, regardless of environmental givens. Lawrence and Lorsch lend support here by saying, "In organizations existing in quite different environments, we have found that effective conflict management occurs when individuals deal openly with conflict and work the problem until they reach a resolution which is best in terms of organizational goals."[7]

In the health center we observed few members who allowed conflict to surface as it developed. There appeared to be an implicit norm for smoothing over conflicts, as if to preserve the myth of the perfect team. Several members said, "I keep quiet about what bothers me so it doesn't interfere with daily activities." And although three members of one team each spoke to us in private about the same issue, not one of them permitted the conflict to surface in the team meeting, where it might have been resolved.

While we never observed the direct effects of such buried and smoothed-over conflicts, we were told that such conflicts produced an intolerable buildup of anxiety which eventually resulted in a blowup or personnel turnover. At the very least these conditions must result in a loss of motivation and commitment, with communication seriously impaired within the team. For instance, during our sessions we noted some members consistently avoided others when voluntary subgroups were formed. This behavior, we suspect, was the effect of unexpressed feelings about some past conflict which had not been effectively managed.

But perhaps the most important result of this failure to deal with conflicts is the link between team processes and team members' ability to work with the families they serve, particularly family health workers, who are supposed to constructively intervene into family conflicts. Unwillingness to risk surfacing such conflicts within the team and deal with them is likely to be reflected in sidestepping family conflicts. Such avoidance also deprives team members of the opportunity to practice and develop intervention skills. While the immediate result of sidestepping is relatively painless, ultimately the price is increased anxiety and ineffectiveness in helping the patient-families.

Family-centered comprehensive care requires a team to operate much as a family *that deals with or manages its own problems*. When it has achieved this goal it will be in a far better position to serve neighborhood families.

Before moving to a description of the specific consultant interventions designed to help teams learn to manage their processes more effectively, we will examine the overall consulting model we relied upon in our work.

THE CONSULTING MODEL

Models give the consultant an organized way of thinking. Instead of responding only on the basis of what "feels good" or "seemed right at the time," conceptual models can help the consultant begin to make thought processes explicit that previously were implicit or uncertain to both consultant and client.

If a consultant finds himself without some reference point—some way of explaining "where he's at"—his uncertainty leads to anxiety, which can be sensed by even the most naive client. This is likely to lead to an increase in the client's anxiety, which then means that the consultant has made life tougher in terms of readiness for change. One only has to be stopped unexpectedly in a hallway during his first visit to the client system and asked, "What are you going to do on the teams? And have you done this before?" by a person who has only one minute to listen, in order to realize the importance of some consistent model, framework, or guidelines. The use of a model—in this case the Kolb-Frohman model for planned change—to which we could relate our perceptions, behavior, and activities proved invaluable to us in the program.

Following is a brief look at the seven phases of the Kolb-Frohman model (see Figure 16-3) and how we made use of them, with emphasis on a few key learning points we felt were particularly important. This seven-phase Kolb-Frohman model is an elaboration of the basic action research approach, which involves four phases: (1) data collection, (2) summarization and feedback, (3) action planning, and (4) evaluation.

SCOUTING, PHASE ONE

Since the entire health center was our first "client system," a way had to be found to enter the total system in order to determine which of the eight health teams wanted to consider working with us. Some of the questions we had to answer were: Can we let the administration choose the teams? Should we work through the formal power structure? What about the inevitable rumors—how will we deal with them?

In a highly interdependent organization with a diffuse power base, we were most concerned with soliciting and sending valid information. This meant dealing directly with the teams as much as possible rather than through the administration. We avoided the assumption that all information from the top of the organization was valid, particularly when it concerned the teams at the lower end of the system. In many cases the right hand really did not know what the left hand was doing. All this led to our scheduling a mass meeting with the eight teams.

ENTRY, PHASE TWO

The meeting provided a formal introduction to the potential clients. It was also the beginning of contract setting—a process in which perceptions, expectations, and clarification of the roles of both client and consultant are

FIGURE 16–3

THE KOLB-FROHMAN MODEL FOR PLANNED CHANGE

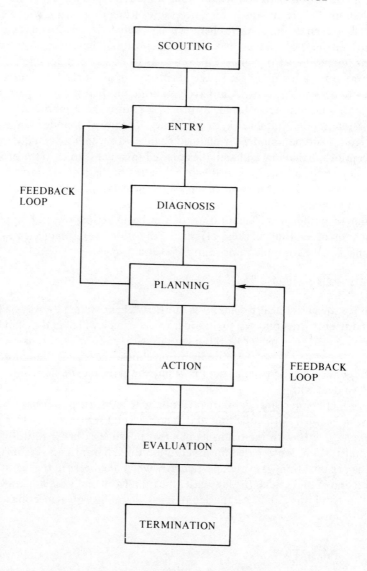

Source: D. Kolb and A. Frohman, "An Organization Development Approach to Consulting," *Sloan Management Review* 12:1 (Fall 1970).

shared, to the end that working agreement is reached. Since we were very much outsiders, we had to make clear our background, expectations, and goals. And since it was important to be legitimized, we asked the head of the center to introduce us, sharing his overall needs and goals with the health teams and how he thought that we, as consultants, might help them. However, legitimacy can be other things too. "Who is paying you?" was a question asked. The statement behind that question of course was, "If your pay comes from operating funds, we'll take a very skeptical look at the whole activity." While this was not an issue, since our work with the teams was funded by a special grant from the Carnegie Foundation, if the question had not been raised and clarified, it could have interfered with our work without our being aware of what the problem really was.

DIAGNOSIS, PHASE THREE

To reinforce free choice and encourage internal commitment, we used a shared decision process (explained at the mass meeting) to select the two teams. Then we began the formal diagnosis. This consisted of individually interviewing each member of the team and collecting data on the various process issues discussed in the previous section. Although diagnosis occurs throughout the consulting process, the interviews provide a way to get client needs and resources out in the open and match them with consultant needs and resources. It is a negotiable continuation of contract setting. While our interviews clearly focused on team issues, we were committed to feeding back all the data. An open, trusting relationship was enhanced by our commitment to collaborate on action planning with the team. The more the team became involved, the more valid the information and the more team members were committed to taking action.

In working with the teams to diagnose their data and define their priorities, silence or reluctant or vague responses told us that we needed to rethink our previous stage in the overall consulting process. Remarks like, "I don't know what this meeting was supposed to do for us" indicated that we had not effectively dealt with the contract issues, which meant we needed to go back over our expectations with the teams. In a sense, the contract was really renegotiated at each weekly session by discussing where we had been and where we were going. This also led to a basic change in our overall goals: we moved away from attempting attitude change and decided to try for early successes through structural and behavioral changes. We had misread the teams' level of readiness and were about to push too fast. This also had implications for the future: some quick successes might "unfreeze" team members sufficiently to make them willing to take more risks later on.

PLANNING, PHASE FOUR

The decision to push for some early success experiences affected our planning. It required our using expert power as opposed to trust-based power, which has its own element of risk. However, by (1) sharing our diagnosis of the data with the teams, (2) sharing our design for quick success experiences around improving team conferences, and (3) selecting an activity that all team members recognized as an important and legitimate task, we tried to build a trusting climate. In this way it became less risky to assert our "expertise" and be more directive in planning specific interventions.

But we also had to recognize that increased reliance on us as experts rather than facilitators resulted in increased dependency, which then had to be reduced in the termination stage of the consulting process. Although we tried to design specific actions to make team members aware of their own resources and capabilities, our participation at times overshadowed this objective. Using a consulting model to assist in anticipating such problems helped us. With 20–20 hindsight, it is clear we could have used it more.

ACTION, PHASE FIVE

Whatever actions are taken, whether they result in outright failures or just unanticipated consequences, they only become dysfunctional when the consultant loses sight of his framework, strategy, and contract with the client. When either success or failure—or anything in between—is related back to the diagnosis and to the overall learning goal, it can be helpful to both consultant and client. While dealing with resistance is crucial (sufficiently so to be discussed separately below), we will only emphasize here that client resistance to change at the stage of implementing actions can and should play an expected and helpful role in innovation.[8]

EVALUATION, PHASE SIX

The importance of clear, verbalized, shared criteria for evaluation cannot be overemphasized. The team's recognition of a need to develop flexibility led to selecting activities requiring experimentation. Experiments, to be useful, require descriptive evaluation from which team members can learn and grow, not win or lose.

It was important to emphasize personal team ownership of action plans and results. If the teams decided to try something new at a team meeting, we suggested that they take the following actions to insure building the base for internal commitment: decide who was going to carry out an individual task, who was to observe the new behavior or procedure for later evaluation, and when the experiment would be discussed. In this way, team members were more likely to experience a sense of controlling their own processes as opposed to being controlled by the consultants.

In our "where we've been" introduction to each session we evaluated the learning and progress to date. We ended every session with a sharing of observations and evaluations aimed at improving the following week's session. We also began a transfer to the two teams of more and more ownership of planning, evaluating, and follow-up in anticipation of our termination.

TERMINATION, PHASE SEVEN

Anticipating and planning for termination of the client-consultant activities is a consulting necessity. While a consultant may be attaining great objectives while pushing a team and using his "expert" power, his sudden, casually planned exit can create such anxieties on the team as to negate all his previous efforts. Use of a consulting framework such as the Kolb-Frohman model can help to avoid this and aid in proper planning.

We attempted to consider termination issues such as client dependency throughout our work with the teams. Some of our interventions emphasized the team's ownership of the data. As we have pointed out, we hoped in this way the teams would realize they had the responsibility and the capability to carry on at their own initiative rather than at the consultant's. However, again with hindsight, this was not sufficient. We should have placed greater emphasis on termination beginning with the entry phase and proceeding throughout the entire consulting process.

DEALING WITH CLIENT RESISTANCE

How the consultant reads the signals of client resistance is crucial to effective diagnosis. Behavior such as refusal, criticism, silence, etc., should be interpreted as valid information for checking and possibly altering the diagnosis. For example, resistance in the form of apprehension, reluctance or refusal at the implementation phase of the program may indicate the consultant misread the team's readiness in an earlier phase in the consulting process such as contract setting or action planning. Should the consultant react defensively, seem overwhelmed, or be overly saddened, he may increase the very anxiety he is trying to help the team control. He may be implicitly signaling that he cannot handle his client: that the client is in worse shape than either had imagined, or that the consultant's perceived competence is less than the client had anticipated.

If the consultant is to use the client's resistance productively, he must assume that this behavior is the client's way of sending another message as to "where he is at" and thus his readiness for change. By sensing the resistance, determining the underlying message and supporting the feedback, the consultant is also reinforcing one form of effective diagnosis and problem solving: feedback, evaluation, and reduction of anxiety associated with the risk of resisting.

SUMMARY

Planned change is enhanced whenever a process can be explicitly described, which is what we have attempted to do here.

It should be emphasized that the seven phases of this model overlap, and that looking back and ahead are appropriate processes in any consulting phase. For instance, data collection and diagnosis is not merely a formal one-shot process; it occurs throughout the client-consultant relationship. Hearing over the public address system the names of doctors, nurses, and family health workers being called to the mass meeting instead of teams being asked to assemble represented informal data gathering which we used to diagnose the state of this complex social system.

The more we understand why we did something that "felt good" at the time, the more we can teach and transfer the skills of planned change to others, thereby improving the health of the group, organization, system, or society within which we are working. Had we to do it over again, we would put even greater emphasis on learning about the consulting process throughout the program. The results are helpful to both client and consultant, both immediately and in the longer run.

We will now describe some of the interventions we used in helping the teams unfreeze.

CONSULTANT INTERVENTIONS

Intervention has been defined as a direct attempt to influence the ongoing behavior of organizations by coming between or among persons, groups, or subsystems. In the broad sense, everything the consultant does (or does not do), *including* the establishment of the relationship between consultant and client, is an intervention. And *what* he does may range from observing a group of people at work and commenting on their process to asking them to perform specific tasks, the goal of which is experiential learning.

Our initial activity with the teams, as we have already stated, was to interview each member individually, using both open-ended questions, as shown in Table 16-1, and a team interaction form, which is shown in Table 16-2. We explained at the beginning of the interview that many of the team

TABLE 16–1
INTERVIEW AGENDA

Name _____

Team _____

A. Contract setting issues
   1. note taking
   2. confidentiality—data will be fed back anonymously
   3. check back at end of interview on what has been written down

B. Perception of own role/job
   1. what, how, with whom

C. What could other team members do to make you more productive/satisfied?

D. What do other team members do which makes your job more difficult and less satisfying?

E. Team's major strengths and weaknesses

F. Weekly staff meetings—how useful/what could make them better?

G. Kinds of decisions team does/should make as a team
   1. what constitutes a "crisis" for this team?

H. Fill out team interaction form

members' remarks would be anonymously fed back to the entire team. As might be expected, the data from the interviews showed many problem areas. There were concerns about team goals, individual roles, relations with the rest of the agency, interpersonal conflicts, and so on. After we had categorized and summarized all this material, we fed back the data at our first meeting with the team as a whole. (See Table 16–3 for data summary.)

Team members' reactions to the data presented during the feedback session were varied. For some, the result was one of surprise—"I didn't realize people felt that way about this team!" Others had been unaware that many of their own concerns were widely shared by other members of the team. Before the feedback session, many people believed that they were the only ones experiencing certain difficulties. The most frequent reaction could be

TABLE 16–2
TEAM INTERACTION FORM

A. *Communication*

I often feel as if no one really listens to anyone else	1 2 3 4 5 6 7	People really listen to one another's ideas and points of view
I often feel hesitant to speak up in team meetings	1 2 3 4 5 6 7	I feel free to speak up in team meetings

B. *Teamwork*

Around here it's everyone for himself— we really operate as separate individuals	1 2 3 4 5 6 7	Everyone pulls together— we really support and help one another

C. *Team Management*

A few individuals really make most of the decisions on this team	1 2 3 4 5 6 7	We all contribute to the decisions made by this team
Disagreements are ignored or avoided on this team	1 2 3 4 5 6 7	We deal directly and openly with disagreements on this team
I often feel I have more to contribute to this team than others seem to recognize	1 2 3 4 5 6 7	I really feel as if others recognize the many contributions I can make on this team
I often feel as if I have no power/influence over what happens on this team	1 2 3 4 5 6 7	I really feel as if I can influence what happens on this team

TABLE 16–3
SUMMARY FEEDBACK OF INTERVIEW RESULTS

The following suggests one way of feeding back a large conglomeration of remarks so as to help a team begin to set priorities for issues it feels are relevant. The examples here were collected from both teams, with names omitted to perserve anonymity.

A. *How Work Gets Done*
  1. Team goals; examples:
     (a) we react to crises rather than planning
     (b) we never have decided on what team should be doing: we *should*
     (c) differing priorities; teaching, medical, social, build agency
     (d) very little time for joint planning with nurse for patient/family

  2. Individual roles/responsibilities; examples:
     (a) FHWs not adequately utilized, roles not clear; should feel it is her patient
     (b) nurses should do more medical and delegate more to FHWs
     (c) team coordinator should be more of an administrator and not concerned primarily with medical care
     (d) follow-up weak
     (e) our roles should be better defined
     (f) you can't ask someone for something if it's not their job

  3. Decision making; examples:
     (a) we should never decide what a family should do without them involved, except for absolute medical problems
     (b) we should spend some time assessing how the team is doing
     (c) decisions should be made only by people involved
     (d) FHWs are closest to patients and *ought* to have more to say about what gets done, how, etc.

  4. Relations with other groups/rest of agency; examples:
     (a) I'm worried about this place, no managers and no goals
     (b) arbitrary decisions handed down from top don't help
     (c) no real autonomy as a team, no control over budget; many of us are responsible to bosses outside the team
     (d) no ability to choose our own staff

TABLE 16–3, *continued*

B. *What It Feels Like to Work Around Here*
   1. Praise, support, feedback; examples:
      (a) more praise, support would help us cope with crises/mundane tasks
      (b) we should appreciate each other's pressures
      (c) little credit/respect given for a job well done
      (d) you can really trust some people to do a job—this is very satisfying

   2. Individual worth and contribution; examples:
      (a) FHWs used to speak up; now we won't buck the nurse or Dr.; we've been put down and have given up fighting back
      (b) lots of roles dumped on nurses; FHWs may feel at "end of the line"
      (c) often made to feel untrusted/inadequate in my job
      (d) my opinion not as valued as the "authority"
      (e) people always checking up

   3. Pace and sense of accomplishment; examples:
      (a) around here everything pulls you down, there is nothing pulling you up
      (b) this job is an ongoing crisis
      (c) the work day never seems to end
      (d) environment problems seem to have no solutions

C. *Interpersonal*
   1. Communication style; examples:
      (a) some doctors should try to check with nurse more
      (b) I feel bad when someone else deals with my patient and we haven't arranged to swap patients

   2. Communication frequency; examples:
      (a) some people talk too much, others talk too little
      (b) one team member not keen on lab report put on desk by another without instructions
      (c) one team member makes me feel stupid so I don't ask questions anymore.

TABLE 16–3, *continued*

3. Interpersonal conflicts; examples:
   (a) personality frictions have to be resolved; we should cultivate individual strengths instead of ignoring personal conflicts
   (b) one team member is sometimes too harsh in judgment when a task isn't done—sometimes people just plain forget or make mistakes

D. *Issues Outside the Team*
   1. There are too many problems we have no control over, that seem to have no solutions (lead paint, lousy police protection, rats, drugs, welfare, psychological problems in families, alcoholism)
   2. Lab, X-ray work, and getting records often slow
   3. We have no ability to choose our own staff
   4. We are just too crowded together
   5. We have no real autonomy as a team, no control over budget
   6. Lots of research but no implementation and no benefit to us
   7. Arbitrary decisions at the top are based on whims, not reason
   8. I can't get any satisfaction bucking welfare and having to tell family I can't help them
   9. You can't expect to have an efficient team in a sloppy organization

E. *Team Conference Issues*
   1. Mechanism:
      (a) minutes help, rotating chairmanship is good
      (b) conferences are only good when we present a problem, work on a solution, try the solution and then review the results
      (c) always FHW who presents a family case; doctors and nurses should too; "implies" doctors and nurses are not concerned about families
      (d) they are sometimes all talk and no action
      (e) time-keeping and agenda are important
      (f) rotating leader not good

   2. Objectives:
      (a) should be a place to learn from each other
      (b) should be able to develop plans of action but there is little goal setting or agenda setting

TABLE 16-3, *continued*

   (c) we need to focus on common, solvable problems; we waste too much time on impossible social problems

   (d) it is useful to get together as a total team to talk together, develop consensus of all members, get some people to say more, and others to say less

   (e) for the team, they seem to range from great to poor; they are great when something is solved; they are poor when you don't stick to the task; for instance, meeting spent analyzing FHW's role was a poor meeting

3. Participation:
   (a) if everyone gets interested, we can really get at it
   (b) professionals can be overpowering
   (c) conference is not useful for me—I'm in the outer ring
   (d) communication flows well; everyone attends
   (e) push people to do more of their own case summaries
   (f) quiet FHWs have a lot to contribute

characterized as: "These problems have been around—*under the surface*—for a long time. Now they have been collected, summarized, and are out on the table for all of us to see."

In other words, the teams were provided with an image or picture of their present state based on information collected from the most valid sources available—the team members themselves. As a result of the interview-feedback process, teams owned the information and shared the image of their present state. This shared ownership helped to create a heightened desire and commitment on the part of team members to solve their own problems. Now we could go on to help them set priorities for the multiple issues reflected in their data; generate alternative solutions to the problems identified; and develop a clear and shared set of change objectives or goals—an image of what a more ideal or improved state would be.

This data collection-action planning approach that we used in our work with the MLK teams helped us in a number of ways:

1. It enhanced our knowledge of the environment and the team in a short period of time.
2. Through interviewing we began to establish an open, trusting rapport with the team members.
3. Allowing the team to decide what it wanted to work on from the data it

generated counteracted the fear that everyone (administration, patients, researchers) only wanted to take from the team and that no one was really interested in helping. By sharing control of the issues to be worked on, we reinforced our goal of helping team members help themselves instead of coming to them with predetermined or hidden agendas.

4. Finally, this approach provided a basic problem-solving model where those who are part of the problem are involved in the solution; where information is solicited from the most valid sources—team members themselves; and where alternatives are generated in terms of specific actions, which are then evaluated and either continued, modified, or stopped.

The tasks we asked the teams to work on all related directly to the problems that were apparent in their data. They ranged from the relatively safe task of planning an agenda to a collage exercise, the purpose of which was to get 'feelings expressed and recognized as a legitimate part of the real work situation. Our role as consultants became more facilitative and somewhat less directive as our relationship continued, although we did exercise leadership and control in specific exercises. In all the assigned tasks our goal was to provide our clients with the opportunity to learn from experiencing directly rather than read about or hear a lecture on a subject, although we also made use of these as helpful reinforcers or backups.

Focus on Team Meetings

Since we had decided that the teams needed a quick success experience to increase their confidence in what was for them essentially a new approach to learning, and since team members themselves saw this as valid, it was agreed that the initial focus should be on a relatively easy task—improving team meetings.

To achieve this objective, the teams undertook the task of analyzing the data from the interviews that related to team conferences (see section E of Table 16-3 for a summary of team conference issues). They then selected one or two "behavioral prescriptions" to implement at their next conference. The goal was to make that next meeting the "best meeting ever."

Formal "observer" roles were given to volunteers who would evaluate changes in the team conference; on one team formal "helper" roles were also given to volunteers to assist the team conference leader if he or she requested help.

A formal planning procedure was introduced. Each week several team members met a few days prior to the team conference to evaluate feedback from the last meeting and plan an agenda for the next meeting. The resulting "behavioral prescriptions" were structural or procedural: use of a checklist for the conference chairman, giving each person an opportunity to speak, rotating the chairman, passing in evaluation cards or hearing from formal observers at the end of meetings, and trying different types of presentations.

The structural changes provided an opportunity for new inputs from quiet team members. For the first time, in most cases, family health workers became involved in planning; and medical assistants were, for the first time, invited to attend the meetings. Various team members took on new roles (chairman, planner, observer, helper) before the entire team.

Quick improvements—such as a reduction in uncertainty about what the meeting was supposed to be about and the opportunity to become involved with planning a case presentation—generated noticeable interest and eagerness to attend. The team began to observe, evaluate, modify, and reinforce some of is processes.

Some members, however, were reluctant to try the new formal helper and observer roles for fear that their lack of skill and practice would show. They expressed the need for more direction as to what to observe. Therefore, in our sessions with the teams we began devoting time to sharing our observations for the purpose of helping them develop their own observational skills. Also the growing acceptance of a formal observer role gradually lessened the risk for other team members to share ideas and feelings even when they were directed at a particular person. This kind of participation began to be appreciated as helpful to the team since it generated useful and valid information. Anxiety also seemed to be reduced as team members expressed willingness to help and be helped.

COMMUNICATION-FEEDBACK EXERCISE

To emphasize the importance of open communication and feedback, we devised a communication-feedback exercise that made use of the doctors' power base, since physicians were clearly the most powerful team members. Our goals were to emphasize the usefulness of helpful feedback; reinforce the new norm of experimentation by encouraging individuals to try new styles of behavior; and underscore the importance of sharing valid information. Working together (without consultants present), the doctors devised individual behavioral prescriptions for "improving my communications style."

Some prescriptions were:

"I will not be the first one to fill silences."

"I'll listen more and won't clarify or restate unless asked to do so."

"I won't run on over two minutes."

"I'll check when I bring up something new to see if it is relevant."

Each doctor decided to evaluate each other doctor, share their prescriptions with the entire team, invite others to give feedback and to meet briefly after each team conference to check on their progress.

Particularly significant for our team-building efforts was the effect on the nurses and family health workers at seeing doctors experiment with communication and feedback. If the physicians on the team were willing to take risks, to try out new behavioral styles, and to share these experiences with other team members, it must mean that the doctors trusted their teammates and were concerned with overall team functioning. Nondoctors too, they reasoned, could now start to experiment behaviorally and offer feedback to others—tentatively at first but then with growing confidence. Thus the sense of team became enhanced.

Working with the doctors as a group was an example of effective consultant use of an "environmental given," i.e., a professionally and culturally defined subgroup of the team. Using their roles as "image setters" and "givers of power," the doctors began to build the team instead of just controlling it.

ROLE NEGOTIATION PROCESS

To decrease dependence on the consultants and to teach new facilitative skills to team members, one of our interventions involved a role negotiation exercise.[9] The design called for the development of the "third-party facilitator" role on the team to help other team members solve a problem.[10]

As homework, each team member was asked to fill out and sign individual worksheets for all other team members. The signer was asked to briefly state at least one good example of what "you think the team member named at the top of the sheet could do:

1. *more* or *better* in order to help you work more effectively
2. the *same* which is now helping you
3. *less* of in order to help you["]

These sheets were given to the person whose name appeared at the top prior to the negotiation session.

When the team met with the consultants, two volunteers were asked to negotiate a conflict, using the consultant as the facilitator, with other team members observing. (Such a setup is often called a fishbowl exercise where the "inside" group is doing something while encircled by an "outer" group that is observing the inside group's behavior.) After the demonstration, our plan had been that the other members would pair off with a facilitator and do their own negotiations. However, they were not ready to take the plunge—they needed to ease into this new activity and manage it at their own pace. Some balked at the rigid structure; others said there was not sufficient time, which may have been a way of avoiding what they saw as a risky situation. During the discussion that ensued a team member remarked, "I can't see why we need this procedure to get at problems between us. Wait—I do so. It's because we just don't do it otherwise!"

While we did not push the teams to focus on feelings (in order to minimize the initial risk associated with the new exercise), feelings did come out, and prompted some healthy discussion. Examples of issues were: family health worker to internist: "I felt bad when you said what you did . . . ."; doctor to FHW: "It would help me more if you tried to describe with facts, rather than label with opinions and judgments, the situations you relate to me."

Their sense of ownership of the information on the sheets prompted some team members to say that they would see to it that negotiations took place in the future—at a more convenient time and place. One doctor remarked, "These sheets fascinate me! I'm certainly going to try to see some people about them in the next few weeks."

COLLAGE EXERCISE

As we neared the end of our pilot work with the two health teams, we sensed that team members were now ready to deal more explicitly with feelings—if they could be provided with a reasonably safe vehicle for this. We also felt it important to encourage the sharing of feelings about the team and the individual's relationship to the team.

The vehicle we selected to try and get at such feelings was a collage exercise. The homework for this session was to express, on a large sheet of paper, "what it feels like to work on this team," using sketches, words, magazine cutouts, or any combination of these the team member wished. The sheets were not to be signed.

When we met, the papers were posted around the room and members eagerly viewed the artistic expressions of their fellows. The discussion started with team members volunteering what they thought the picture said or what they thought the person who made the collage was feeling when he or she did it. Before the session ended all members had given their interpretations of the collages. For example, one collage pictured the team as a battery to which members could "hook up and get charged." There was general agreement that to be effective (autotherapeutic) the team needs to recharge the emotional batteries of its members which get drained by the anxiety-producing environment.

An exciting outcome of this exercise was that some team members said they now could see that their difficulty in expressing feelings of frustration, isolation, or inadequacy was really a fear of being seen as weak or unable to cope with the job; but it was *good* to get these feelings out if the person expressing them received help and support in an atmosphere of trust and openness.

Theory Memos

While our learning strategy obviously stressed the experiential approach, we also used theory inputs at times. The memos we selected we hoped would reinforce, in our absence, the concepts or methods the team had already worked with. This we felt would reduce dependence upon our presence, yet at the same time legitimize us as a source of useful knowledge.

Two short papers on "Group Process" and "Chairmanship" were distributed following our session on behavioral prescriptions for improving team meetings. A subgroup of a team received a "Force-Field" memo to use as a diagnostic tool for a problem they were going to work on. And at the request of some members, an "Observation-Feedback" memo was distributed to the teams after the evaluation session, which concluded our main activities with the teams.

Although it is hard to judge the effectiveness of these memos, we expect that the best read and most used was the one requested by some team members. Here we were responding to a felt need on their part—not an implied or presumed need on our part.

We do know that reactions varied in terms of professional training. Doctors expressed interest in reading the memos. A group of nurses said they could not use the "Force-Field" memo because it was too abstract and academic. Family health workers gave no indication of having read the memos.

Synergism

Synergism is a process by which individual pieces summed together produce an outcome which exceeds the sum of the individual parts. In this case, while each of the interventions we have described produced specific results, taken together these activities achieved an outcome over and above the sum of all the interventions. As one team member put it, "We have *experienced* the meaning of team. It is no longer an abstract concept." This higher order phenomenon, or "meta-learning," is the experience of the autotherapeutic process. It is demonstrated by the following outcomes:

1. The teams gained a new sense of self-control and efficacy. Many of the members began to sense a real team identity. One team could confront the administration as a team in support of one of its nurses. Another team could stand firmly by its rules regarding visitors to team meetings, even when faced with the risk of an administrative decision forcing them to act against their will. The awareness and ownership of their own rules, norms, feelings, successes, and failures gave the teams a greater sense of legitimacy.
2. The teams began to sense the growth of a climate in which all members

could express ideas and feelings. The risk of doing this and being hurt, ridiculed, ignored, or taken for granted was now manageable. They began to experience ways to reduce the risk (and the anxiety it created) through support, feedback, trust, and openness.

CONCLUSIONS

Our pilot work with the two teams was quickly followed by similar efforts with four other teams. This meant that by the end of the summer of 1971, six of the eight health care teams at the center had had some fifteen hours of training to help them start dealing more effectively with their own team processes.

What was the outcome? What could be accomplished in such a limited time frame? To begin with, results were somewhat uneven. Not all the teams reacted as positively as the two pilot groups. Like individuals, teams vary in their responsiveness to a training program that is new and different. If a doctor on the team was unenthusiastic or negative (which did happen), other members tended to follow his lead. And team members often found it hard to relate their training experience to their everyday work. Generally, however, the reaction to the training was positive.

But our limited time frame had other consequences. For one thing it meant that our intervention objectives of necessity had to be modest. While we observed increased clarity of role expectations, greater flexibility in decision making, and more widely shared influence and participation, the question of permanence and the relationship of these internal changes to the more ultimate measures of improved delivery of health care remain unanswered.

Actually much of the new behavior exhibited by the teams could best be described as being in the "awkward stage," which is to be expected since team members were trying to do something new and difficult for the first time. The danger here is that without some reinforcement or follow-up activities to help reduce the awkwardness, the chances of reverting to the older anxiety-driven behavior are great. If attitudes are to be changed and the new learning internalized, continuing OD support is essential. While fifteen hours is enough to initiate change and to unfreeze the teams, no team can be "OD'd" in a one-shot program and expect to be "healed" forever. OD is a process more resembling health care than a health cure.

Two things do seem clear at this point:

First, it is naive to bring together a highly diverse group of people and to expect that, by calling them a team, they will in fact behave as a team. It is ironic indeed to realize that a football team spends 40 hours per week practicing teamwork for those two hours on Sunday afternoon when their teamwork really counts. Teams in organizations seldom spend two hours per year practicing when their ability to function as a team counts 40 hours per week!

Second, behavioral science knowledge and techniques, developed in a variety of nonmedical settings, are relevant and appear to be transferable to organizations involved in the delivery of health care.

We turn now to some broader issues and generalizations:

Whenever a team is formed to perform a task, certain predictable issues will arise which, if not effectively managed, will operate to impair the team's ability to function.

A unique connection exists between what a team does (its task) and how it goes about doing it (its internal group processes). At a very simple level, the health care analogy would be: If a team is to treat a family as an integrated unit (its task), the team itself must in many ways operate as a highly integrated family unit (its internal group processes). When a team's internal processes are inappropriate, it is likely to be no more than a collection of single entities treating subparts of single patients.

The action research model we have discussed (in this case the Kolb-Frohman model) represents a methodology and set of values that will help a team become a self-renewing or autotherapeutic organism. In some ways it demands of a team that it treat itself as a patient—periodically diagnosing its own state of health, prescribing its own medication, and subjecting itself to regular checkups to insure that the prescription is working. Although this process may require the assistance of an outsider initially, the "patient" team can learn to do many of the things itself.

The internal process issues we have discussed will occur in any group. They cannot be wished away or ignored for long without cost. Nor are they the result—as is frequently assumed—of basic personality problems. More often team members have difficulty functioning together because of ambiguous goals, unclear role expectations, dysfunctional decision-making procedures, and other such process issues. These issues should be anticipated and effectively managed when they occur.

But it is not enough for the teams alone to handle their internal processes effectively. The administration supporting the teams must also be willing to experiment with flexible modes of decision making, open communication, and problem solving. One compelling reason for this is that the processes of decision making, communication, and problem solving developed at the top of an organization set norms and reinforce behavior throughout the organization. *What happens within the administration is reflected and magnified at the team and support levels.* For example, a vague decision-making process by the administration seemed reflected in the MLK teams' difficulty in decision making.

The interdependencies of most modern organizations, particularly this health center, suggest that successful organization development efforts be organization-wide and managed from the top.[11] Since we know that in traditional pyramidal bureaucracies, orders are communicated from top to bottom (the first line supervisor tends to mirror the overall organization style unless he is extremely strong willed or independently wealthy), the top must set the right example. Therefore, we would like to see this health center's administration develop an image as an environmental resource available to facilitate the team delivery of health care as against, say, a collection of medical people running the place. And this is not impossible, since the administration constitutes a part of the team's life space that is capable of responding to team needs.

Undertaking such an effort would mean that rather than a traditional pyramidal organization in which the bottom supports the top, the center would become a large team, sharing needs, setting priorities, and combining resources so as to most effectively support the primary delivery system of the organization—the health teams. In this way, not only would the right hand of the center know what the left hand is doing, but the right hand would also be able to help.

NOTES

1. Edgar Schein, *Organizational Psychology*, Englewood Cliffs, N.J.: Prentice-Hall, 1965.
2. For a broad look at the current practice of organization development see Addison-Wesley Series on OD, 1969, edited by Warren Bennis, Richard Beckhard, and Edgar Schein.
3. Conceptual support for our framework is drawn from two sources: Edgar Schein, *Organizational Psychology*, p. 70; and R. W. Revans, London, *Standards for Morale: Cause and Effect in Hospitals*, Oxford University Press, 1964, Ch. 9. Schein identifies the dual function of any group as meeting the organizational task needs and its own social needs. Revans identifies the outstanding social need of the hospital organization as the effective management of anxiety. Our assumption in the health team setting is that a certain level of "teamness" is needed to manage this anxiety, uncertainty, and frustration.
4. Harold Wise, *Fourth Annual Report of the Dr. Martin Luther King, Jr. Health Center*, 1970, p. 8.
5. For a detailed discussion of "process factors" in teams, see Edgar Schein, *Process Consultation*, Reading, Mass.: Addison-Wesley, 1969; and I. Rubin and R. Beckhard, "Factors Influencing the Effectiveness of Health Teams," *Milbank Quarterly*, July 1972, Part I. Vol. 50, pp. 317–335.
6. Edgar Schein has identified six methods by which groups come to decisions: [1] decision by lack of response (silence equals consent); [2] decision by authority (informal or formal leader makes final decision); [3] decision by minority (a few "railroad" the decision); [4] decision by majority (vote or poll taken); [5] decision by consensus (majority concur; dissenting minority is willing to go along); [6]

decision by unanimous consent (all agree) E. Schein, *Process Consultation,* Reading, Mass.: Addison-Wesley, 1969, p. 58.
7. P. Lawrence and J. Lorsch, *Developing Organizations: Diagnosis and Action,* Reading, Mass.: Addison-Wesley, 1969, p. 14.
8. D. Klein, "The Defender Role," in *The Planning of Change,* W. Bennis, K. Benne, and R. Chin (eds.), New York: Holt, Rhinehart & Winston, 1969, p. 498.
9. R. Harrison, "*Role Negotiation: A Tough Minded Approach To Team Development,*" Development Research Associates, unpublished.
10. For a detailed analysis this role and its uses in conflict management, see R. Walton, *Third Party Consultation,* Reading, Mass.: Addison-Wesley, 1969.
11. R. Beckhard, *Strategies of OD,* Reading, Mass.: Addison-Wesley, 1969, p.9.

Appendix

Portrait of a Heath Care Team*
Thomas F. Plaut

I have worked as a pediatrician on several health teams, both in New York and Kentucky. I'd like to describe the team on which I have worked for the past three years at the Dr. Martin Luther King, Jr. Health Center in the South Bronx. I will point out some strengths and weaknesses of a team and describe a few important events in the life of our team, especially the work we did with the MIT consultants.

Background and Goals

The catchment area of the MLK Center is made up of forty-five blocks containing approximately 45,000 residents. Compared to the rest of the Bronx, this area has a high rate of venereal disease, tuberculosis, out-of-wedlock pregnancies, and families on welfare. Residents of our area accounted for half the clinic visits to Morrisania City Hospital, though they comprise only one-sixth of its population.

Forty-seven percent of the residents are Black and an equal number are Puerto Rican. The majority of these people live in four- to six-flight walkup tenements, with 17,000 living in a large housing project and a few in private homes.

The health center was founded in 1966 by Dr. Harold Wise. The center's operations are sponsored by Montefiore Hospital and funded by OEO.

Its goals were and are:
• To provide comprehensive family-centered medical care for a low income neighborhood.

*Based on a paper presented before the Maternal Child Health Seminar, Johns Hopkins School of Hygiene and Public Health, Baltimore, Maryland, December 1971.

- To develop training programs for nonprofessionals.
- To employ community residents.
- To involve community residents in policy making.
- To determine if this system is effective enough to be replicable.

Our doors were opened to patients in June 1967 in what was to become a satellite center. When the main center was opened in September 1968, MLK had between 300 and 400 employees, with eight health care teams, each responsible for a specific geographic area.

STRUCTURE

Team E, of which I am a member, consists of thirteen full-time people: six family health workers, two public health nurses, two internists, a pediatrician, a secretary, and a dentist. We are responsible for the health care of 1,576 families living in eleven buildings of a large city housing project. At present more than 70 percent of these families are registered for care.

Population	No. of Individuals
Black	1,827
Latin	2,414
Other	153
Total	4,394

All our patients live within three blocks of the health center.

The family health workers are community residents, each of whom joined the team after six months of training for the job. They handle housing, welfare, family, court and school problems, and provide some home health care. All six family health workers on our team are married women with from three to six children. None had worked in the health field before. Their roles and tasks are still in the process of definition.

The family health workers have been trained for a new job for which there was a theoretical need but little practical understanding. They obtain medical histories, which are often ignored; they are used as messengers by physicians and nurses. They have been unable to increase their own social and health knowledge to the degree necessary to make their work more helpful to the patient and more meaningful and satisfying to them. They have been termed "the neglected people" of the health team and health center.

A total of four nurses has filled the team's two nursing positions. Their average tenure is eighteen months, age at employment is thirty, and they had an average of seven years of nursing experience at the time they joined us. None of the nurses is a community resident. Two are Black.

The nurse is a practitioner who cares for well children and prenatal patients and provides family planning services during four half-day clinic sessions. She is the coordinator of team activities. It is her job to set priorities and see that problems relating to families and the team itself are taken care of rather than ignored. Until November 1971, she was responsible for supervising the family health workers—making daily plans with them and reviewing their patient charts.

The jobs of the team internists and pediatrician are easy to describe. They see patients in their office eight half-days per week, care for some chronically ill patients at home, and visit hospitalized patients in rotation with their colleagues.

The following tabulation presents data on Team E members as of September 1971.

	Current Staff	Left Team	Avg. Tenure	Age When Hired	Job Clearly Defined	Minority Race (%)	Have Children (%)
FHW	6	3	26 mo.	40	Poor	100	100
PHN	2	2	18 mo.	30	Fair	50	50
MD	3	1	21 mo.	33	Good	0	25

INTRATEAM RELATIONSHIPS

Some family health workers resented the nurse supervising their activities. Often they had worked at the health center longer than the nurses. They felt more knowledgeable about the problems of the community since they lived there and the nurses did not. Some felt more experienced by virtue of being older and having raised more children. Differences in background and race also led to misunderstanding and discord. Hostility was at times real and at other times imagined.

In order to give the family health workers more responsibility and to provide them with an opportunity for growth, they were removed from the supervision of the public health nurses in November 1971. They may still call on the nurses and physicians freely for help; but they answer only to the medical care evaluation committee and the team as a whole for their performance.

When the team was formed three years ago, the two nurses resisted the efforts of the pediatrician to help in the supervision of the family health workers. Although they wanted to develop their own competence as practitioners before concerning themselves too much with this aspect of the job, at the same time they wanted the supervisory role to be open to them when they became ready for it.

The pediatrician was responsible for teaching the nurses well child care and provided consultation when requested. This worked out well. However, it took six months before the nurses and pediatrician could work together on team matters (as distinguished from pediatric matters) without friction. At that time, they began planning weekly team meetings together and working out plans for family care.

While the internists on the team have always been competent and conscientious in caring for their patients, they never took any initiative in working to improve the function of the team until after MIT consultants were brought into the center in February 1971 (which I will discuss later). Since that time an understanding of team membership has developed on their part and they have begun to hold informal teaching sessions for family health workers, which are well received.

The team meets as a body once a week for one and a half hours to discuss families with difficult problems or problems from which we can learn. We also exchange information of common interest. Since the MIT intervention I have been meeting weekly with the nurses. These meetings deal with common pediatric problems and enable the nurses to take over more clinical duties. I also meet weekly with the family health workers to discuss specific patients as well as general problems affecting patients.

By spending more time with the family health workers and nurses, the physicians are now demonstrating their respect for them. This demonstration of respect has been followed by a decrease in friction between physicians and other team members.

An example of genuine teamwork occurred in August 1971. At that time, the health center found that a new census was urgently needed for planning and billing purposes. The physicians decided to share this tedious but necessary job with their teammates. Every member of Team E participated in the census—several on evenings and weekends. This happened in no other team.

EXTRATEAM RELATIONSHIPS

Many outside demands are made on team members. The physicians and nurses have conflicting loyalties. The nurse, for instance, is involved with the nursing group, the pediatric nurse practitioner program, the obstetric program, covering other nurses, and outside organizations. Physicians are involved with weekly pediatric or internal medicine meetings, emergency room coverage, covering other physicians, hospitalized patients, the intern-residency program, and health center committees. The family health workers, in constrast, generally owe their allegiance to and get their primary support from the team.

IMPORTANT EVENTS IN THE LIFE OF TEAM E

September 1968:	Formation.
	Continuous staff changes.
December 1968:	Successfully confronted the health center administration: limited visitors to team meetings.
February 1971:	MIT consultation: Improved communication, growing awareness that our satisfaction is important in contributing to teamwork.
April 1971:	Fired psychiatric consultant.
July 1971:	Health center administration changed.
August 1971:	Unit management system begins: includes team's involvement in hiring.
November 1971:	Family health workers removed from supervision by nurses.

There has recently been a change in the way team members relate to the administration. Before August 1971, they related to and brought problems to the health center administration through their respective peer groups: nurses, pediatricians, internists, family health workers. There was no system of team advocacy. The team often had no say and was merely informed of a change in its life—e.g., you will get two interns February 1; Professor A will visit your team conference as an observer; Dr. B will become your second internist; you will care for the following new families, etc. Starting in August of 1971, the team became responsible for hiring its own staff, approving leaves of absence and controlling intake of new registrants. Our team had asserted some autonomy previously by restricting visitors and firing a psychiatrist. In each case, facing a common "enemy" brought a feeling of unity and togetherness.

THE MIT INTERVENTION

I have already referred to the MIT consultation. Now I'd like to describe their goals, methods, materials and effect on the team. Professor Irwin Rubin and his student Ron Fry came to us under the auspices of the Carnegie Foundation, which is interested in the operation of health care teams. We first met them at a general medical staff meeting in January 1971, at which they described the consultation process. They stated that their goal was to help the team help itself function more effectively. They asked that the teams interested in working with them list the pros and cons of consultation as they saw them. From a group of six interested teams, the MIT people chose two, mainly on the basis of understanding of the consultation process and the unanimity of the decision.

Rubin and Beckhard have described their method as consisting of four parts: data collection, summary and feedback, action planning, and evaluation. This is exactly how Rubin and Fry worked with Team E. Each team member was interviewed for an hour and a half on such process related factors as team goals, priority setting, role definition, decision making, support and feedback among team members, and whether the team member experienced a sense of accomplishment in his work. These data were summarized and fed back to the team at its first meeting with the consultants.

Team members were surprised to see that they were not alone in their judgments and feelings about the team. Rubin and Fry discussed the material with us and suggested that we take as our initial task the improvement of our weekly team meeting, since these meetings involved all team members and we all agreed they needed improving. To this end, we took the following actions: used a planning committee to develop an agenda for the meetings, rotated chairmanship among all team members, and started on time. A written evaluation occupied the last ten minutes of each meeting. The comments were later used by the planning committee in preparing for the next meeting.

The same format of data collection, feedback, planning and evaluation was used in small groups also. The three physicians met and each wrote a recommendation for each of the other two to follow at the next meeting. The recommendations for one physician were:

1. Do not repeat yourself until others have responded. You may have been understood perfectly the first time.
2. Be more concise.
3. Do not be the first one to always fill quiet spaces.
4. Improve listening skills.

Adherence to these recommendations was discussed by the physicians at the end of the next meeting and the improvement in behavior was supported. Our consultants also supplied us with tracts discussing feedback, chairing a meeting, and role negotiation.

We met with our consultants for a total of sixteen hours over a two-month period. In all our dealings with them they emphasized the importance of openness and support among team members. I believe they were successful in what they tried to do. Last week, eight months after the intervention, I polled my teammates. In the words of one family health worker: "I feel more important. The importance of everyone's job has been explained, and I am more efficient. As for other team members, they are more considerate, more willing to give. The new teaching program is a good example of this."

EFFECTIVENESS OF THE TEAM

What gives a team strength? A feeling of accomplishment which brings satisfaction; a feeling of working together for a common goal. The feeling of accomplishment can come only if one has a clear-cut goal which is attainable in a reasonable period of time. Crash immunization programs are a beautiful example of this: everybody feels great when the measurable accomplishments are read off at the end of a single day.

The members of Team E at the Dr. Martin Luther King, Jr. Health Center have an unending job. The goal set out for us to bring to an optimal state of health all 6,200 individuals living in our area can never be attained with our resources. We haven't even agreed upon the components of the goal. In short, although we are the best team at the best health center in the country, there is plenty of room for improvement.

GROWTH STAGES REQUIRED FOR
TEAMWORK AT MLK

Each individual must go through the following stages before he can function as part of a team. The time spent at each stage varies with the personality, previous experience, competence, job category, stage of fellow workers, and other responsibilities. Advancement may occur in several areas at the same time.

1. *Groping.* Everyone starts here. No one knows his or her role or tasks. Evidenced by purposeless movement or by inaction.
2. *Orientation to tasks and roles.* Easy for physician—because trained for majority of his tasks. Hard for nurse because of quadruple role and previous training in only one area. Impossible for most family health workers until the rest of the team gets itself together to support her.
3. *Development of individual competence.* Once this has been achieved, a helping role becomes possible.
4. *Reorientation.* Necessary for MD with regard to relationship to teammates and also to new tasks—for example, community orientation.
5. *Setting priorities.* When several people are oriented and competent they can join together to set priorities and work together, bringing their teammates along.

17 | Survey Feedback

George F. Wieland
Robert A. Ullrich

THE SURVEY FEEDBACK TECHNIQUE

SURVEYS IN GENERAL

Surveys consisting of interviews or questionnaires have enjoyed widespread use in organizations as sources of information on internal functioning. It is a rare employee who has not responded to at least one survey of his or her morale, feelings, attitudes, beliefs, or opinions. The rationale for conducting organizational surveys—whether they are conducted by outside consultants or in-house staff such as personnel specialists—is to assemble information that will aid management in diagnosing problems and selecting remedies for them.

Be that as it may, problems with survey procedures frequently limit their usefulness to management. As Katz and Kahn (1966) indicate, top management occasionally feels that it has done the right thing just by authorizing a survey. It is assumed that workers will feel much better after having blown off steam and gotten the impression that management was interested in them. In cases such as this, findings are likely to be filed away in the personnel office and forgotten. In other cases, top management routes findings to subordinates unaccompanied by directives for their use. If the survey results are read by the subordinates (which is problematic in some cases), selective inattention possibly will distort their meaning. All of us have a tendency to select information that is congruent with our current views and beliefs and to disregard findings that are contrary and indicate a need for change. When this happens, the usefulness of the survey is diminished.

When survey results are not utilized, the organization may suffer harm

Adapted from George F. Wieland and Robert A. Ullrich, *Organizations: Behavior, Design, and Change* (Homewood, Ill.: Richard D. Irwin, Inc., 1976) pp. 497–513. © 1976 Richard D. Irwin, Inc.

above and beyond the waste of time. A survey's immediate effect may be somewhat positive; respondents sometimes experience mild catharsis in expressing their attitudes and feelings. But in responding, employees may be led to expect that survey information, including their own statements, will be used to rectify the problems and unpleasant situations they describe. These employees may become cynical, if not angry, about management's motives in instigating the survey. One can make a strong case that it is better to "let sleeping dogs lie" and not conduct a survey than it is to raise expectations inadvertently and leave them unfulfilled.

SURVEYS AND OVERLAPPING GROUPS

Mann (1957) developed a procedure for group discussion of survey results which atttempts to put the information to good use. Survey data provide the basis for discussion and analysis in appropriate *organizational* families throughout the organization under survey. Organizational family refers to a supervisor and all employees reporting to him directly. Many employees belong to two families: those in which they are superior to subordinates and those in which they are subordinate to their bosses. Hence, the organizational structure comprises overlapping family groups.

Mann takes advantage of the hierarchical character of organizations by starting the feedback process with the top organizational family: namely, the presidents and vice presidents. In this initial meeting, the consultant helps the group discuss and interpret survey data. Following this, a series of feedback discussions are held at the next organizational level. In these meetings, each vice president meets with the department heads who normally report to him. This is followed by a third set of meetings between department heads and their subordinates, and so on, down to the organization families comprising foremen and shop floor workers.

Reliance on organizational families attempts to produce cohesive work groups. In addition, the technique draws on a phenomenon noted by Lewin (1952) in a now famous experiment. This experiment suggested that individuals taking part in a decision were more likely to execute the agreed course of action than were those who were not involved directly in the decision-making process. This phenomenon is incorporated in the survey feedback technique; for example, the vice presidents participate with the president in discussing the survey results in the initial feedback meeting. In addition to discussing the nature of the findings, the group plans the kind of feedback to be used at the next level down. Because the vice presidents participate in a comparable discussion with peers and chiefs, they are exposed to a model for conducting the discussion in which they, as superiors, meet with their own subordinates. According to the logic of the argument, having participated in planning the feedback session for subordinates, the vice president will be committed to its execution, even in the event that the survey team is unavailable for help and support.

Tailoring Data to Hierarchical Levels

The nature of survey data presented for discussion will vary depending on the group's status in the organizational hierarchy. Data must be of direct relevance to the group in which it is studied; for example, a branch chief meeting with his or her department heads will be given company-wide totals for employee attitudes and breakdowns for the various branches including his or her own. In addition, data pertinent to the branch in question will be broken down further according to the specific departments represented at the meeting. Thus, each participant will be provided sufficient information to compare: (1) branch performance with overall company performance, (2) branch performance with that of other branches according to the dimensions measured by the survey, and (3) relative standings of departments within the branch. Similar procedures will be followed throughout the organization. For instance, the individual department head will next meet with supervisors under him or her to discuss department standing vis-à-vis other departments in the branch as well as each supervisor's standing vis-à-vis his peers.

Comparison and discussion of the data for this hypothetical meeting may indicate that members of one department are more dissatisfied with their jobs (and with supervision in particular) than are members of other departments. The objective data upon which discussion is based may confirm vague feelings that previously existed in the absence of objective evidence. Alternatively, the data may indicate that job satisfaction is high and, in so doing, lay to rest contrary rumors. Either outcome is potentially beneficial to the organization, insofar as the survey findings are valid.

In either event, members of the group are likely to contribute their own observations as they attempt to understand the objective data. In so doing, they may reveal further areas in need of attention. By defining the data according to its own experience, the group will define the problem in terms to which it can respond. The next step for the group is to plan a program of change that will modify dissatisfying situations.

According to Mann, one important aspect of the survey feedback technique is the objective atmosphere it creates. Use of survey data (facts and figures), together with emphasis on task orientation, lends a degree of rationality to issues that are usually clouded by emotionalism.

The use of organizational families for these rational, task-oriented discussions is important because members possess not only relevant information to supplement the data but also solutions to problems brought to light by the survey.

The technique attempts to solve problems at their locus in the organization. Top levels of management lack detailed information for solving complex problems at lower levels in the organization. By the same token, lower level personnel cannot be expected to cope adequately with the problems of top management. The disaggregation of survey data allows pertinent information to be routed to the parts of the organization that can understand and respond to it. The technique involves the "right" people in both diagnosing and solving the problem. Individuals who have participated in planning a solution usually are committed to implementing the course of action on which they have decided.

PREREQUISITES TO SURVEY FEEDBACK

Mann suggests that certain conditions must be met if the survey feedback method is to operate effectively. As mentioned above, an objective, task-oriented climate must be maintained. Second, each organizational family must be allowed discretion to consider the implications of findings for its own organizational level. While each group plans the feedback for the next lower group, planning must allow leeway for the lower group to add its own observations to the data. Similarly, each group must be given prerogatives to implement changes at its level, as these are suggested by analysis of the data. The latter point is a delicate one, for changes made by a group at one organizational level cannot be so pervasive that they preclude discretionary action at lower levels. Rather, groups are advised to work at one level as broadly as possible, leaving specific details that affect subordinates to their discretion.[1]

Meeting these prerequisites enhances the likelihood that members of organizational families at each level will perceive genuine opportunities to participate in decision making and become involved in and committed to the process. In the absence of discretion, discussion of survey results will be perfunctory. Employees will view the feedback and discussion process as a mere sham.

An account by Hall (1966) of an application of the survey feedback technique in a university setting illustrates the points made above. The individuals conducting a survey of the university's staff were researchers, not consultants, and apparently lacked the power to establish the proper prerequisites. Specifically, the researchers failed to secure top management's commitment to provide feedback and to allow discretion for change to lower organizational levels. Instead, top managers resisted delegation and sought to act on the findings themselves.

Hall was successful in pressing for divisionwide meetings, but these were overly large and inadequate to the task of problem solving. Hall's recommendation that organizational family meetings be held was generally ignored.

Middle managers did not seem to perceive themselves as members of overlapping groups; since they were not involved in planning the meetings they were to lead (by virture of the absence of former meetings in which they were subordinates), they generally were unprepared and uninvolved in the process. Furthermore, these managers seemed somewhat anxious about the survey in the first place. The combined result was that meetings were not held. Needless to say, organizational changes did not eventuate from survey findings.

TWO-WAY REPORTING

An early experiment by Mann (1957) demonstrates the technique's superiority to simple surveys in producing organizational change. A branch of a large electrical utility used survey findings; four departments were involved in survey feedback while two others received survey data in the absence of feedback and discussion sessions. A follow-up survey conducted a year and a half later indicated considerable changes and improvements had accrued in the four departments using the technique. Comparable progress was not indicated by surveys of the two departments that merely received survey data.

Generally speaking, these findings indicate that survey feedback is effective in resolving problems brought to light by survey results. In addition, the experiment suggests that the feedback process may improve interpersonal functioning within the organization—specifically, communication and understanding among managers, their peers, and subordinates. Further analysis of findings from the four experimental departments led Mann to conclude that departments that had achieved the greatest change were those that held the most meetings and involved the most employees in these meetings.

In addition to highlighting the importance of participation, Mann's study illustrates the importance of reporting the results of feedback sessions to higher levels of management. For example, when a department had found satisfactory answers to some of its problems and was ready to make specific recommendations, the department head reported back up the line, presenting the findings at a subsequent meeting of peers and the superior. In this meeting, the department head was able to report on matters to be resolved within the department and also on problems that seemed to stem from conditions over which the branch, or perhaps top management, exercised some authority. Similar meetings followed in which branch managers met with their superior for the same purposes.

This two-way reporting is useful in several ways. First of all, it establishes the accountability of organizational family groups to other, higher level groups. Results of the survey cannot be ignored or "buried," but must be acted upon and these actions reported to groups of higher level managers. In some cases the report back will consist merely of additional questions raised by the survey data and, perhaps, requests for additional information. Even in this event, the outcome can lend direction to the change activities of higher level managers by indicating that existing problems or alternative solutions are inadequately defined.

In addition, the managers who know that they will eventually report back to a group comprising their peers and superiors will be moved to "touch all of the bases"—to involve, rather than bypass, significant employees in the problem-solving and change processes. This can be quite important, given the propensity of some managers to act unilaterally rather than to take time to seek the cooperation and opinions of others.

THE SURVEY FEEDBACK PROCESS

THE CONSULTANT'S ROLE IN SURVEY FEEDBACK

Mann and Likert (1960) argue that if survey results are to be used effectively, managers must *understand* the results and their implications *and incorporate this information with existing attitudes and behavior.* In order to be effective in producing change, survey results must produce more than cognitive learning. In order to make use of new cognitive experiences people must alter their attitudes and feelings. Problem solving, especially in ambiguous situations, necessitates a psychological structuring of reality and, to some extent, psychological closure. Hence, altering people's information base will not necessarily alter their perception of reality, attendant feelings and attitudes, or consequent behavior. This problem is overcome to some extent by involvement in data feedback and problem-solving sessions. Participation fosters emotional involvement with the problem, the data that describe it, and other members of the problem-solving group. Emotional involvement is instrumental in changing perceptions, attitudes, and motivations. By participating in feedback sessions, the members can translate survey data into terms that are meaningful to them. Furthermore, the ideas of the group, to which they have contributed, are more likely to be transcribed into practice than are the suggestions of outside experts.

Mann and Likert contend that participation must start at the outset of a survey project. Consultation with top executives provides their views of major organizational problems and the kinds of data they desire of the study. This information, in turn, serves as a basis for the survey design. Other members throughout the organizational hierarchy must also be given the opportunity to learn the purposes of the survey and to suggest problems and data to be investigated.

At the conclusion of the survey, participation continues via the feedback and discussion activities of organizational families. In fact, Mann and Likert make it a rule that no report containing recommendations based solely on their own analysis of data will be given to the client. Instead, they present data in preliminary form and involve members of the client organization in interpreting the data and deciding on specific courses of action.

By disaggregating the data according to its relevance to managers at different levels in the hierarchy, functional areas, and geographic locations, the consultants match their input to the interests of the groups with which they work. The more relevant the survey results, the more likely they are to elicit the interest and motivation of management. Also note that the consultant serves as a model when he or she participates in interpreting and acting on survey findings. Hopefully, managers will engage in similar behavior as they work with organizational families at the next lower hierarchical level.

When conducted effectively, the survey feedback technique improves the "fit" between the formal and informal aspects of the organization. Small group dynamics can be aligned with formal organization authority. The survey process begins at the top of the organization and, thus, carries with it the authority of top management. Each organizational family includes what Likert (1971) has termed a "linking pin"—a member of management from the next higher level in the chain of command, who can lend legitimacy and authority to the decisions and activities of subordinates. Involvement of line management in the process is essential. Line managers, rather than staff, generally have the authority to implement changes. Finally, the linking pins that bridge the membership of contiguous organizational families facilitate complementary decisions. They serve to relate the decisions taken by one group of managers to those at successively lower levels.

Use of organizational families brings a number of favorable attributes to the problem-solving process. Individual group members are able to contribute a wide range of experience to the definition and solution of problems. Furthermore, since these groups contain overlapping membership, matters of authority and higher level responsibility can be incorporated into the group's actions. Problems emerging from survey activities become public and, therefore, amenable to the contributions of numerous other individuals in the organization. This contrasts notably to the normal modus operandi wherein problems are handled in confidence by one, or a few, individuals who may be ignorant of potential support available from others. Finally, as we have seen, a group decision based on general, public commitment has a potent effect on the behavior of the individual, whether or not he or she is a member of the group in question.

Several other points guide the consultant's role in the survey feedback process. Feedback on performance can be motivating and cause the individual to raise his or her aspirations for future performance. Similarly, knowledge of results is essential to the learning process. A program of repeated surveys and feedback sessions can foster organizational learning that leads to productive change, increased motivation, and more effective organizational behavior in general.

Mann and Likert caution the consultant against the temptation of playing expert. Faced with difficult problems, clients naturally seek expert advice. However, the consultant's job is to help clients develop their own solutions, for their participation and consequent learning, not the consultant's advice, set the stage for productive change.

Timing and pacing are also important. In some situations survey results turn out to be disconfirming, quite dissimilar to the client's expectations. Caution is essential when this occurs, as clients must be allowed to establish the tempo. As Harrison suggests (see Chapter 14), management must be allowed to limit the rate and depth of organizational change to levels where they can work comfortably and effectively. However, it is the discrepancy, or mildly disconfirming nature of the information compared to what was expected, that is the source of motivation for change (Bowers and Franklin, 1972).

The consultant's presentation of survey findings should be made within a positive group setting. Favorable results should be emphasized as well as those that indicate problems. Furthermore, when dealing with negative findings, emphasis should be on means for improving these shortcomings, rather than on the shortcomings themselves.

Surveys are not easily designed. Although a wealth of literature has been written on the subject, the design of questionnaires and interviews that produce valid, reliable data is a demanding task—the success of which cannot be guaranteed a priori. Even carefully designed surveys contain misleading questions and omit important data. Clients frequently question the accuracy of data and the validity of procedures. These questions should be handled objectively. Examination of other relevant information such as organizational records is useful in cases such as this. However, rigid defense of the survey's accuracy can only serve to arouse client resistance.[2]

A MODEL FOR DIAGNOSIS WITH SURVEYS

Likert (1967) remarks that surveys often are no more informative than fever charts and are of limited value in improving an organization. We shall explore this analogy in some detail, since it provides some major implications about the ways in which surveys ought to be designed and conducted.

Physicians need two kinds of information to diagnose illness. They need general information about health and pathology, stemming from research on bodily conditions and relationships between symptoms and diseases. The second kind of information they need is obtained from appropriate measurements taken from the patient at a particular point in time.

Managers face an analogous problem when attempting to diagnose organizational problems. First of all, they need to understand the fundamental nature of the system: the ways in which the parts function (e.g., make adaptive responses to the environment). Second, they need diagnostic measures of the organization's internal state and functioning at a particular point in time. The problem is that many survey efforts focus on the measurement of *end-result* variables such as absenteeism and turnover rather than on causal variables.

End-result variables provide after-the-fact kinds of information. They are similar to the patient's fever which may result from a variety of conditions (e.g., any one of a number of bacteria causing infection). What the physician needs to learn is the cause of the fever; namely, the type of bacteria causing the infection and, thus, the fever. To attempt to reduce the fever without knowing the infection's source is an ineffectual approach to medicine. Similarly, treating organizational symptoms often fails to cure the source of the problem.

Likert recommends measurement of *causal* and *intervening* variables that provide information on the internal state of the organization and the causes of problems (as evidenced by end-result variables). For example, he suggests that participative decision making, a causal variable, improves communications, reciprocal influence, confidence, and trust. These intervening variables in turn lead to end-result variables, such as reduced absenteeism and turnover and increased productivity. To measure only absenteeism and productivity would be futile. What management needs to know is the relationships among intervening and causal variables and end states. Ignorance of these relationships renders effective organizational change problematic at best. However, even when such relationships are known, attention limited to end-result variables (e.g., horses running out of the barn) is likely to tell us that a problem has occurred (e.g., someone left the barn door open). Measurement of causal and intervening variables will more likely call management's attention to potential problems and the need for preventive action.

WHY SURVEY FEEDBACK WORKS

Most of our tentative conclusions about the way survey feedback works are based on Bowers' (1973) research cited in Chapter 14. A more detailed review of his work will shed additional light on the subject. Please recall that Bowers studied the effectiveness of various OD techniques in 23 organizations. His findings indicate survey feedback to be more effective in producing organizational change than the other techniques studied.

The OD techniques examined in Bowers' study can be arrayed according to a number of dimensions; for example, they differ according to what Harrison (1972) terms depth of intervention (Chapter 14). At the extremes, both "deep" (T-group) and "shallow" (data handback) strategies were employed. Survey feedback appears to lie somewhere between these extremes, which may account for its effectiveness.

Bowers also directs our attention to the temporal dimensions of the change processes studied. Laboratory training focuses participants' attention on experienced behavior that occurs in the "here and now." Interpersonal and task process consultation are somewhat similar in this regard. In contrast, survey feedback deals with "then and there" data as well as immediate perceptions (Bowers and Franklin 1972). Thus, a variety of organizational characteristics such as roles, regulations, policies, and technologies as well as immediate interpersonal reactions are explored and evaluated.

Three other dimensions can be used to differentiate survey feedback from other techniques studied. Bowers identifies these as: (1) extensiveness of coverage, (2) extent of "unfreezing," and (3) relevance. Regarding extensiveness of coverage, it is apparent that survey feedback is the only technique in which change activities "fan out" into the organization. Survey data are disseminated throughout the organization and problem-solving activities are assigned to various appropriate levels in the organization. Moreover, the feedback format employed by the technique produces information about the organization which most members are anxious to see and act on.

As we indicated in Chapter 14, various parts of a system must be loosened up (unfrozen) before they can be modified or rearranged. One way to unfreeze an organization is to present members with data that disconfirm existing perceptions of the organization. Sensitivity training may have powerful unfreezing effects in a small group. However, survey feedback tabulations are more likely to contain disconfirming information about the organization per se. Furthermore, such tabulations may be more persuasive than feedback within sensitivity training or other small groups. The former comprise aggregated perceptions of fairly large numbers of people, and are permanent records that can be considered from time to time, whereas the latter usually are verbalized observations of a single individual. In short, survey tabulations may be harder to disregard than interpersonal communications and, thus, more effective in preparing an *organization* for change.

The final dimension to be discussed, relevance, refers to the degree of "fit" between the OD technique employed and the manner in which the organization normally functions. Analyses of day-to-day problems usually are based on data obtained from the organization's information system (e.g., production statistics, grievance rates, sales records, and the like). Thus, as Bowers observes:

> Against this background, it perhaps seems quite natural to launch a problem-solving discussion of "people" issues from a base of tabulated, quantitative data whose accuracy is attested by an outside expert (just as the other data with which they work come from the comptroller, the quality control department, or the production control office). Alternative treatments, of a process consultation or laboratory training variety, may seem, on the other hand, to be a bit peculiar. They are asked to accept the observations of an outsider who, they may feel, knows neither them, their business, nor their problems, and to accept them in off-the-top-of-the-head format, rather than in the more customary form of tabulated data.
>
> Thus a credibility gap may ensue. It may also be enlarged by some of the change agent's more confronting interventions. It may be, for example, that a change agent who spends most of his work time in a confrontation mode becomes somewhat jaded, such that what, to client group members, is terribly confronting—just barely within tolerable limits—is to him a "cop-out," whereas what to him is confronting is to them an outrageous assault upon propriety. (Bowers 1971, p. 34)

CLIENT PERCEPTIONS OF OD TECHNIQUES

Bowers' observation that organizational members did not view the various OD techniques as particularly important elements of the change process is particularly interesting. Where survey feedback was used, individuals acknowledged the occurrence of change and viewed survey tabulations as useful. However, credit for the resulting change often was given to organizational members themselves—not the technique employed. Similar observations are reported for the other OD techniques. Bowers' interpretations of these observations are reproduced below:

> In fact, some anecdotal evidence would suggest that client reactions were connected more to the personality and style of the change agent than to what he accomplished. In certain instances, the change agent played, as Interpersonal Process Consultant, a lower key, more ambiguous role; despite the fact that, in those sites, one could usually point to significant improvements in leadership behavior in the organization as a whole, the months toward the close of the project, and those immediately following its termination, often resulted in blame-fixing upon him as one reason for what was perceived to have been a non-success. In other instances, the change agent responsible for the intervention strategy was, in personal style, more active and charismatic. Despite an overall pattern of little change, anecdotal evidence suggests that he is highly regarded, that he is seen as having been responsible for much constructive change. In still other instances, especially those focusing around Laboratory Training, enthusiasm waxed greatly at the moment, but rapidly waned to indifference or disillusionment shortly afterward.
>
> Although far from constituting convincing evidence, these bits of anecdotal

information certainly suggest the possibility that client system affect is whimsical and no reliable measure of what has really changed. Client system affection may be both useful and necessary for continuation of projects and contracts, just as disaffection is a rather reliable precursor of their cancellation, but they may bear little or no relationship to real accomplishment. (Bowers 1971, pp. 31–32)

This anecdotal evidence suggests a source of much of the present-day confusion about the relative effectiveness of different OD techniques. In the absence of rigorous, experimental evidence, managers and OD practitioners have used client attitudes as surrogate measures of contributions toward organizational improvement—attitudes which may be unrelated to the actual effectiveness of the technique employed.

REFERENCES

Bass, Bernard M. When planning for others. *Journal of Applied Behavioral Science*, 1970, *6*, 151–71.
Bowers, David G. Development techniques and organizational change: an overview of results from the Michigan Inter-Company Longitudinal Study. Technical Report, Office of Naval Research, 1971.
Bowers, David G. OD techniques and their results in 23 organizations: the Michigan ICL Study. *Journal of Applied Behavioral Science*, 1973, *9*, 21–43.
Bowers, David G., and Franklin, Jerome L. Survey-guided development: using human resources measurement in organizational change. *Journal of Contemporary Business*, 1972, *1*, 3 (Summer), 43–55.
Hall, Richard H. The applied sociologist and organizational sociology. In A.B. Shostak (Ed.), *Sociology in action: case studies in social problems and directed social change*. Homewood, Ill.: Dorsey, 1966, Pp. 33–38.
Harrison, Roger. Role negotiation: a tough minded approach to team development. In W. W. Burke and H. A. Hornstein (Eds.), *The social technology of organization development*. Washington, D.C.: NTL Learning Resources Corp., 1972, Pp. 84–96.
Katz, Daniel, and Kahn, Robert L. *The social psychology of organizations*. New York: Wiley, 1966.
Lewin, Kurt. Group decision and social change. In G. E. Swanson, T. M. Newcomb, and E. L. Hartley (Eds.), *Readings in social psychology*. New York: Holt, 1952, Pp. 459–73.
Likert, Rensis. *The human organization: its management and value*. New York: McGraw-Hill, 1967.
Mann, Floyd C. Studying and creating change: a means to understanding social organization. In C. M. Arensberg et al. (Eds.), *Research in industrial human relations*. New York: Harper, 1957, Pp. 146–67.
Mann, Floyd, and Likert, Rensis. The need for research on the communication of research results. In R. N. Adams and J. J. Preiss (Eds.), *Human organization research: field relations and techniques*. Homewood, Ill.: Dorsey, 1960, Pp. 57–66.
Wieland, George F. Evaluation report. In G. F. Wieland and H. Leigh (Eds.), *Changing hospitals*. London: Tavistock, 1971, Pp. 211–401.

NOTES

1. See also Bass (1970).
2. Something can be said for using ambiguous, although valid, data. Wieland (1971) found unclear survey data to be more effective in creating attitude changes among hospital managers than unambiguous data. If the data were clear, managers tended to look at survey results and conclude: "Right! Here is the answer!" Provided more ambiguous data, managers tended to discuss them with others, puzzling over the findings with consultants and colleagues. In the course of these discussions, the managers learned about one another and, with the help of the consultant, formed cooperative working groups. These changes led to changes in the attitudes some managers had about one another and other members of the organization. In some cases, the process beginning with ambiguous data led to new patterns of work and cooperation.

18 | Managing Change in Health Care Organizations

Newton Margulies

There has been a good deal of attention over the last decade to the current attitudes and capabilities of organizations to respond to rapid sociological and technological changes in our society. While all organizations, some more than others, experience the pressures to change, there is little doubt that changes in both societal values and technology have created stresses and strains in health care and health care delivery organizations unequaled in other areas.

Demands of the society for improved health care, for consumer involvement in health care planning, for personal involvement and participation in the health diagnosis and the treatment process itself, provide one set of forces which create pressure to change. Increased involvement of governmental agencies and of legislative regulation have provided still another source of pressure to change, and organizational innovations such as interdisciplinary health teams and the use of organizational matrix designs provide still another source. The internal and external environments of health care organizations seem to be in a turmoil and the need for ways to add some rationality to the turbulence and to assist in the management of these changing environments is clearly before us.

This paper describes a promising process and technology which is in part a response to the need for ways to manage rapid change. While the process itself is not new, the growing list of methods associated with it is new and is providing some relief as a "field" which administrators can call upon to cope with problems and dilemmas of managing change. A specific application of this process is also described herein and some things we have learned from it are discussed.

Reprinted with permission from *Medical Care*, Vol. 15, pp. 693–704, Copyright 1977.

THE NATURE OF ORGANIZATIONAL DEVELOPMENT

As implied, there is a new and emerging field, derived in part from the applied behavioral sciences; Organizational Development, as it is called, is a response to a much-felt need on the part of administrators in all types of organizations to better prepare themselves and their organizations for the rapid social and technological changes which seem to be enveloping the society as a whole. While management philosophers and theoreticians have talked about the need for the development of techniques to manage change and the need for organizations to become more responsive to the environments in which they are embedded, Organizational Development (OD) is an attempt at translating the conceptual groundings of the behavioral sciences into concrete technologies to facilitate the planning and implementation of organizational change.

As with any emerging field, there are a variety of definitions of organizational development, just as there are differences in approaching the problems of change. Most writers agree, however, that OD is a long-range effort,[1] involving the total organization (at some time or another)[2] in planned interventions which are aimed at increasing the organization's effectiveness. OD is an activity reflecting the application of behavioral science concepts and knowledge about human beings in organizations in order to make the organizational environment *both* a productive and satisfying one. To be sure, organizational development is a value-based process and technology[5] since the methods, techniques, and strategies imply the kinds of organizational processes that should be utilized for the mutual achievement of the productive-satisfaction goals.

Organizational Development is intended, by its nature, to "strike" at the culture of the organization—those characteristically dysfunctional patterns and processes which in fact are more hindering than helpful in the achievement or organizational goals. Many of these patterns and processes are products of the bureaucratic form of organization so prevalent in our society. Other patterns are products of a time when such ways of doing things were probably appropriate; but new times and new technologies make these characteristics outdated and obsolete. Many organizations, when given the opportunity, find that their current behavioral patterns (the way in which they make decisions, the way in which they proceed to solve problems, the way in which they deal with rewards and punishments, the way in which they deal with evaluation, the way in which they deal with discipline, etc.) are in fact no longer useful in terms of present and future goals of that organization. Moreover, these traditional aspects of the organization's processes are like ghosts without real substance in terms of the current societal milieu and present-day requirements.

Organizational development has emerged as a problem-solving process and a technology which an organization can use to facilitate assessment of where and how to make useful changes, how to implement these changes, and how to evaluate the outcomes. One important aspect of this "culture change" orientation is that the organization learns to *continually* assess its organizational patterns, assess its current functioning, and diagnose and introduce those changes which are most meaningful in terms of the goals it wishes to achieve. This process of *natural* change and *ongoing* change is incorporated into the organization's life pattern along with other necessary functions.

In summary, the process of organizational development can be described in the following way: *First,* it involves the generation and exploration of pertinent information regarding the organization's functioning. *Second,* it involves an evaluation of that information and a diagnosis of current functioning with specific emphasis on those aspects of organizational behavior which are dysfunctional. And, *finally,* it involves the formulation of an interventional strategy, based on that diagnosis, which can bring about changes so that more of the organization's behavior is functional in terms of its goals.

As for "OD technology," very specific methods and techniques have been developed for helping organizations perform the above three steps most effectively.[5] In addition, there tends to be more and more experimentation with ways in which the generation of data, the processes of organizational diagnosis, and ways of developing interventional strategies can be achieved. These techniques and methods which constitute the OD technology are increasing both in number and in the quality of their effectiveness.

The Nature of Action Research

For many practitioners and theoreticians who link themselves to this field, there is strong sentiment that early pioneering work in organizational development had as its basis the action research model. Using the research skills of the social scientist was a basis for proceeding with organizational change programs. In addition, action research represented a core philosophy which is central in the development and implementation of change. This philosophy incorporates the use of relevant "scientific" information with practical application to real and experienced social problems. The approach was able to bring together the orientations of social science and the action orientations of problem solvers in a variety of settings.

One of the strongest proponents and contributors to the action research concept was Kurt Lewin. Lewin's work and conceptualization of the process of action research is particularly relevant since he also pioneered the concept and theory of planned change. Lewin was especially interested in social change and felt that the processes and techniques of research could play an important role in the generation, direction, and implementation of change efforts. Action research, as it is currently viewed, involves a process of analysis, information gathering, action planning, action, and evaluation. The cycle is then repeated. This perhaps simplified description is a way of incorporating ongoing change strategies into social problem solving. Although Lewin and his colleagues were particularly interested in using action research as a way of influencing the attitudes and values of groups and the subsequent human relationships, the concept obviously has a much wider range of application.

Most definitions and models of action research follow the basic Lewinian concept. The process described in one way or another treats action research as a way of developing sound information and knowledge which can be applied directly to practical problems with the intention of bringing about social change. The model, including the basic steps in the process, is summarized in Figure 18-1.

Action research, then, incorporates five different but related aspects, all very significant in the process of change and development. Action research 1) is a *methodology for generating knowledge* about the processes of an organization, 2) is a *mechanism or strategy for disseminating that knowledge* and for generalizing the knowledge to other similar situations, 3) provides a *logical sequence for organizational and individual problem solving*, 4) may be thought of as a *powerful interventional strategy* in the process of organizational change, and 5) represents a *philosophical view* which strongly encompasses the need and desire for ongoing organizational review.

ACTION RESEARCH AS A CHANGE STRATEGY

Action research is closely analogous to the process of organizational development as previously described. In combining action processes (planning, execution, and evaluation) with research processes (problem identification, hypothesis formation, and testing) the result is a sequence of steps and activities which identify the relevant things that have to happen in the initiation and implementation of change. It is clearly a process of change which is built upon the premise that rationality provides a solid and sound springboard for determining change goals and the subsequent action designed for achieving those goals.

As an interventional approach to organizational change, action research is appealing to practicing managers who place high value on the importance of

FIGURE 18-1

THE ACTION RESEARCH PROCESS

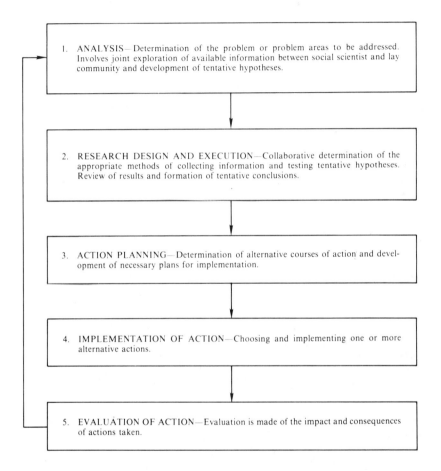

1. ANALYSIS—Determination of the problem or problem areas to be addressed. Involves joint exploration of available information between social scientist and lay community and development of tentative hypotheses.

2. RESEARCH DESIGN AND EXECUTION—Collaborative determination of the appropriate methods of collecting information and testing tentative hypotheses. Review of results and formation of tentative conclusions.

3. ACTION PLANNING—Determination of alternative courses of action and development of necessary plans for implementation.

4. IMPLEMENTATION OF ACTION—Choosing and implementing one or more alternative actions.

5. EVALUATION OF ACTION—Evaluation is made of the impact and consequences of actions taken.

knowledge and research as a basis for managerial decisions.[4] It is also compatible with the values of our culture that hold science and technology in high esteem. Action research has the additional advantage of appealing to reason and logic as a basis for action and, therefore, can be used not only as a basis for change decisions, but also as a way of reducing resistance to change. It is difficult to argue with the facts, especially when those concerned have participated in the generation of those facts. In this regard, action research is a strategy for bringing about the acceptance of change as well as a process to be followed by those interested in creating and managing change.

A final word about action research as an interventional strategy in organizational change may be in order. "Intervention" is the term generally used to describe the technology used by managers and/or change agents to bring about specific organizational changes. Action research can be used as an approach to organizational change by focusing on specific organizational problems and by involving organizational members as participants in the research process as well as in the planning and implementation phases of the change effort. In this light action research can be viewed as an overall strategy for changing an organization. This, then, was the strategy employed in the following case example. The *research* and *data feedback* processes were the core of this change program.

A word of caution! I believe that any theory or model of change must be evaluated in terms of its utility. Action research makes logical sense; I have no clear empirical foundation to support the value of this approach although clearly the process provides an opportunity for enlightened self-assessment not currently practiced in medical oriented organizations.

Basically then, what faces health care organizations today and in the future, is the problem of analyzing and responding to the different and complex demands of the "patient system." Patients are individuals with a variety of physical, emotional, and social problems, all of which interact with the health care delivery system. The health problems of the patient system tend to be interdependent as well as complex and therefore require capabilities in many areas which lead to proper diagnosis and treatment. The issues for the health care organization are:

What is the appropriate structure which will facilitate the most effective accomplishment of tasks?

What configurations of health care teams make the most sense in our situation?

What distribution of authority will help make decisions in the most timely and expeditious manner?

What kind of communication and information system will provide us with the best available information when we need it?

How do we maintain a patient-oriented delivery system as well as a well-motivated staff of different disciplines whose members will work together?

The action research model presented here is one way for health care organizations to start looking at these organizational issues in a systematic and programmatic fashion.

THE KAISER PROJECT

In January, 1973, a large organization involved in a medical care program in Southern California decided to administer its first attitude survey and feedback project for administrative and staff support employees. The project was initially intended to explore and measure employee perceptions of the working climate within the program and to relate those climate dimensions to both organizational effectiveness and experienced organizational problems. At a later point in time, the goals of the project shifted toward more careful identification of issues of concern to both exempt employees and key physician leaders and to the development or processes to bring about local and region-wide improvements.

This project was by no means a simple or easy task. First of all, the organization itself is a complex structure of roles and responsibilities and intricate relationships. Secondly, the process described herein was certain to initiate a process of organizational change that the organization needed to absorb and see through to some conclusion. The size of the project was in itself a gargantuan undertaking. It involved approximately 25 suborganizations (medical centers, regional support groups and departments, etc.) and about 800 key people, region-wide, who were asked to become involved with the data, feedback and eventual diagnosis and organization improvement processes. As the project grew, about 25 new temporary working groups in the form of task forces and representative groups emerged and required some form of management. Clearly the amount of time and energy committed to the project was not insignificant.

RESEARCH PHASE

The early research activities focused on tailoring an organizational climate instrument developed by researchers at Texas Christian University* to the Kaiser Permanente work setting. This involved selection of appropriate climate dimensions and modifying the language of specific questionnaire items to fit the people and the organization. Twenty organizational dimensions were chosen and included such aspects as organizational communication, interdepartmental cooperation, decision-making decisiveness, leadership effectiveness, roll clarity and job pressure; the survey included approximately 100 questions about the organization and its effectiveness.

The questionnaire was then pretested with a group of Kaiser Permanente

*This instrument has been developed by Dr. Lawrence R. James and his associates at the Institute of Behavioral Research, Texas Christian University.

employees to identify any difficulties with concepts and formats and final modifications were made. The key research questions which were of interest and provided the primary focus were:

1. Are we (top management) aware of the problems faced by our administrators and supervisors?
2. What are the strengths and weaknesses of our organization?
3. Are we using our people resources appropriately?
4. Are our key people motivated and committed to improving medical care?

The final form of the organizational climate questionnaire was then administered to all the management and supervisory people in the region. While each individual's anonymity was maintained, the information was organized according to organizational unit; for example, questionnaires from each medical center and even for units within a medical center were used to develop a profile for that particular organizational entity. On an organizational unit basis then, a computer program developed statistical information (means, standard deviations, and percentages) for each of the approximately 100 items in the survey. In addition, pictorial profiles using the 20 organizational climate dimensions were developed so that areas for further exploration and discussion could be examined at a glance.

ACTION PHASE

During the rest of 1974, top administrators at five of the medical centers designed and carried on elaborate follow-up programs aimed at turning the survey data into concrete operational improvements. Although each center developed different approaches according to their own needs and requirements, the following characteristics were present in all situations:

Each center had the opportunity to review its own organizational climate data in detail and test its accuracy with others in small group meetings (with or without the boss).

Each center spent additional time in group meetings to do further "sensing" of "soft spots" and strengths in the medical center operation.

Each center identified five to ten priority improvement areas that could increase their evaluation of the organization's effectiveness.

Each center elected representatives to serve on hospital and clinic-wide action planning committees. These committees represented a diagonal slice of the medical center management team (top management usually participated in committee meetings).

GENERAL PROJECT DESIGN

The general format for the project consisted of five phases represented in Figure 18-2 and described as follows:

Phase 1: Action-planning meetings with top local administrators. With the help of an organizational consultant, the top administrative team at each location studied the survey results, discussed the general project design, and decided on how they would proceed in their Medical Center. Typically,

FIGURE 18–2

ORGANIZATIONAL CLIMATE IMPROVEMENT PROJECT

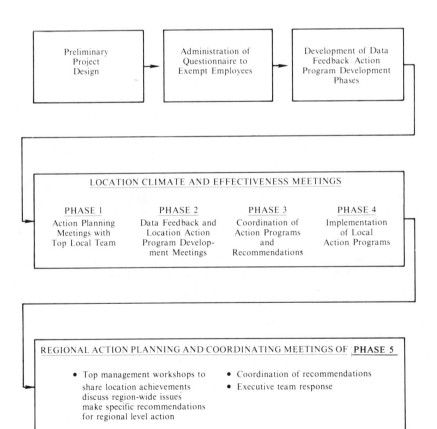

hospital and clinic components designed separate plans for feedback and action planning. These plans usually provided for joint action planning meetings at advanced stages of the local design.

Phase 2: Data feedback and action program development. In all situations, people had the opportunity to review their own climate data in detail and test its accuracy with others in small group meetings (without the boss). The consultants helped the groups further identify organizational climate and effectiveness issues. Additionally, each group began the process of relating climate results to organizational effectiveness and to identify the issues and areas for further consideration by representative task forces.

Phase 3: Coordination of action programs and recommendations. Task forces were elected from the feedback groups to follow up on identified issues. These committees represented a diagonal slice of the medical center management team (top management usually participated in committee meetings). The task forces pulled together ideas and suggestions from the earlier meetings, developed recommendations and timetables, and drafted final reports. In many cases, top local administrators (physicians and non-physicians) participated in the complete series of task force meetings.

Phase 4: Local implementation. A great variety of implementation activities occurred locally. In most cases, the local task force reports and wrap-up meetings led to changes with direct response from management. Some improvements were scheduled into the 1975 Objectives Program efforts. Other issues were further reviewed and resolved through the work of ad hoc committees.

Phase 5: Regional action planning and coordination. The local meetings surfaced some issues which were thought to need regional review. Top management groups in each suborganization entity met to review local progress and to further identify regional issues.

The Regional Phase 5 meetings were conducted by entity, with some divisions within entity. For example, Nursing Directors met separately from Hospital Administrators in the early stages of Phase 5. During those meetings, at least three levels of concern were typically addressed. First, the participants discussed locally identified "regional issues," however stated. Second, the groups addressed climate and effectiveness issues within their own groups (for example, how well clinic administrators are working together as a team). Finally, the groups addressed issues of relationships with upper management groups in other entities and to the next level of management.

Given this mix of interests, clear definitions of "regional issues" are difficult to state. There did seem to be, however, the need for region policy formulation and change to facilitate the changes identified at local levels.

USING THE ACTION RESEARCH MODEL

In a general sense, an action research process was followed throughout the project. Data about the organization and its effectiveness were collected from people, tabulated, and fed back for verification and the planning of further actions. At each phase, the design was reviewed and modified to reflect experience.

The questionnaire findings served as a springboard for discussion and as an organizing framework. Typically, five to ten new statements of concern were created, based on the findings and discussions. The new statements of concern were placed in priority of importance, typed up and returned to original participants for further review. This iterative process was carried upward in the organization, and participants decided at each stage precisely which issues should be communicated upward and the mode in which issues could be addressed.

The dynamic nature of each of the above processes is worth clarification. At each step, key managers participated in the review of the feedback/follow-up experience, and helped identify and select next steps. This led to joint ownership of the overall process between consultants, managers, and to some extent all participants. Second, participants retained ownership of the products (or content issues) that were to be communicated upward to the next level of management.

Throughout the program, administrators and consultants creatively modified the activities of each phase to mesh with the environment. Through this process, the local and regional projects kept pace with current issues and stimulated improvements on a broad scale.

ISSUES IDENTIFIED

The climate survey itself identified some general areas of concern to employees that were widely shared in the Southern California region. Among these concerns were the quality of leadership and supervision received (specifically, help from immediate supervisors with job-related problems, and planning and coordination of work requirements), feedback to employees on job performance, management awareness of employee needs and problems, decision-making decisiveness, opportunities for growth and advancement, and fairness and objectivity of rewards. These themes were partly validated in feedback meetings, but there were important departures by location and organizational component.

During local small group feedback meetings, people had the opportunity to review their own data and redefine issues in their own terms. In the process, people reviewed both the *quality of work life* and the *effectiveness of their organizations*. The lists of priority concerns that fell out of this process reflected local experiences and were clearly related to the effectiveness of the organization. The following is a partial list of priority concerns that seemed to emerge from discussions at the medical centers:

1. *Communication.* A pervasive problem. The major focus is on the amount and quality of information flowing downward from management and problems with interdepartmental communication. Upward communication is also an issue. Information upward is scant, distorted, or sometimes non-existent. In addition, supervisors should be able to communicate freely to solve common problems.

2. *Hospital-clinic relations.* Differences in the hospital and clinic cultures were identified as the basis for some interorganizational conflict. There was also a good deal of concern about the quality of support services provided by "the other side." Organization policy and procedures often impede the establishment of effective working relations between the two organization segments.

3. *Relations with physicians.* Managerial employees at some locations felt that physicians lacked a "Program" orientation, were unaware of the pressures they place on employees and support departments.

4. *Interdepartmental cooperation.* Some support department/line department conflicts exist over quality of resources provided and joint responsibility to ensure that projects and improvements are completed. Decisions made in one department often affect other departments and yet are made without this consideration.

5. *Clarity on responsibilities and authority.* This is of particular concern in parts of the organization which face dual supervision. Unclear and uneven division of responsibility between physician and nonphysician leaders. Decision-making changes unclear or complicated. Some defunctions are contradictory.

6. *Opportunities for growth and advancement.* Widespread concerns exist that the organization lacks program for development and advancement of

employees. Information on job opportunities is difficult to get and is not disseminated effectively. Need for new practice theory.

7. *Concern for members and patient care.* There was a widespread concern for more patient-centered improvement programs. A belief that many residual benefits (fewer complaints, less work pressure, etc.) to physicians and staff could accrue through real concern for members. Patient education should be developed and conducted by both hospital and clinic personnel.

SOME EARLY RESULTS

Outside organization development consultants worked with the medical center administrative teams at all phases of the project, including the development of action plans. Some of the plans and activities are listed below:

Clearer roles and improved relationships. One clinic's task force (which includes the medical director and representatives from all levels of clinics administration) designed and has begun to carry out an elaborate program for clarifying roles and improving relationships among supervisors, administrators, and chiefs of service.

Improved patient care. Counterpart departments (e.g., Hospital/Clinic, Pediatrics) at one location arranged for temporary exchanges of staff, joint meetings, and other programs aimed at improving continuity of care for patients. Other locations are working on improved feedback to Health Plan members on complaints and problems.

Increased interdepartmental cooperation. At several medical centers, specific conflicts between nursing departments and interdependent support departments (e.g., Laboratory, Pharmacy, Housekeeping) were identified and ad hoc groups of key managers were created to resolve them. Combined Medical Center meetings of peer-level people were initiated for purposes of problem solving. Programs of orientation to acquaint departments with the role and functions of other departments were designed and implemented.

Improved relationships with physicians. At some locations orientation programs to better acquaint physicians with Medical Center and Department procedures were initiated. Programs were aimed at familiarizing physicians with lines of communication, responsibility delegations, and determination of areas of problems which should be resolved by administration or jointly by administration and physicians.

Increased involvement in medical center directions. Some medical centers revised their goal-setting and planning processes to provide more input from personnel at all levels. In addition, better coordination between medical center goals and region-wide goals was reported within a relatively short time period.

New organizational norms. In some ways, the questionnaire and feedback process itself can be considered as an elaborate listening device aimed at encouraging more participation and involvement. Increasingly, people report that more openness of expression exists, and "it's becoming okay to question the system."

SOME CONCLUSIONS

To reiterate earlier observations, while action research is not the "cure all" method for administrative ills, the use of action research as a change strategy and as a specific intervention in organizational development has several advantages but should be applied with several cautions. The following is a sample of the potential advantages this method has as a way of beginning organizational assessment and change.

Level of involvement. The survey method described herein provides a system-wide involvement of organization members in the process of generating data about the organization's functioning. It also provides by its nature a high level of enthusiasm in the problem-solving process as well. Surveys are generally a quick and economical way of generating such organizational information. Because of its concentration on data, action research is often seen as a legitimate method for exploring the various dimensions of the organization's operations in a way that moves easily from data/diagnosis to action problem solving.

Multiple strategy. The example presented in the case illustrates the way in which the action research process can be used simultaneously at a number of different organizational levels. In this instance the data were used at the "local" level, the medical centers, as well as at the regional level. The medical centers, and even suborganizational units within the medical center, can make use of the data which is pertinent to that organizational unit. Data which has wider ramifications can be dealt with at appropriate higher levels. This method, then, has the distinct advantage of being able to address issues which require action solutions at different levels in the organization. Because this process occurs simultaneously, the actions taken at lower levels do not necessarily have to wait for policy decisions at the high levels; the process occurs in tandem.

Data collection as a beginning. The action research process provides a significant input into the data and diagnosis phases. Importantly, the survey data provide a reasonable and meaningful springboard to examining other issues not necessarily covered by the survey per se. The other obvious advantage is that this method provides an easy transition from data collection to organizational diagnosis. The feedback process additionally permits logical movement to the problem-solving phase. It is also possible to simply diagnose organizational problems and then plan for appropriate problem-solving sessions which might include others more closely associated with a particular issue but not present at the feedback session. The most important aspect of the action research process described herein is that it initiates and legitimizes discussions of organizational issues and analysis of the effectiveness of the organization. In this light, careful planning of the research process is essential. While validity of data collection methods is critical in establishing credibility of the information, highly sophisticated research methods may serve only to complicate the process and detract from the primary purpose of action research.

Consultant role. Very often the use of a consultant can be quite facilitative in moving an organization through the data collection and feedback process. The consultant can provide a sense of optimism and a sense of reality which very often get obscured when organization members become emotionally involved with the data. Some aspects of the role of the facilitator are to:

1. *Assist with the interpretation of the data.* If there are statistical analyses presented people are often interested in what the statistics mean, what this kind of analysis says about the organization. Someone experienced in this kind of interpretation can be valuable in examining and exploring data and getting the most from survey information.

2. *Facilitate discussion of material.* The consultant also acts as a discussion leader and monitor, pointing to the communication and information sharing process.

3. *Encourage additions to the data.* There often is an exploration of other pertinent information, perceptions, or feelings that can be added to get a more complete picture of the organization's functioning.

4. *Helping with transitional steps.* The consultant can provide ways of moving from one phase to another. The feedback sessions may need some structure so that shifting emphasis from data examination to organizational diagnosis to problem solutions can be accomplished with minimum difficulty.

Impact on attitudes. Feedback sessions were primarily focused on the data collected in the survey and were intended as data discussion—diagnosis meetings. Information sharing, both of an organizational nature and of a more personalized nature (feelings, perceptions, etc.) in and of itself has a profound effect on the relationships among participants in the meeting and on attitudes toward change and improvement. This does seem to correlate with other experiences with action research as an approach to organizational change.[3] Willingness to engage in change activities as well as a sense of potency in the change process seems to be related to information sharing, the establishment of congenial and supportive relationships, and involvement in some level of diagnosis. In addition to generating specific problem areas as targets of change, an added benefit of the action research strategy is the formation of more positive attitudes toward change and toward the organization.

The case described in this paper is perhaps like other such examples of the use of action research. There are several general cautions learned from this experience which seem important in the conduct of action research as an intervention in the service of facilitating organizational change.

Follow-up. The action research method will not work without carefully planned follow-up and explicit attention to problem solving. No doubt the feedback sessions are in fact useful in and of themselves; they allow people to discuss issues sometimes never verbalized before and to express feelings and perceptions of the organization which impede the performance of the job. If, however, the feedback sessions remain at the level of catharsis, no real change and improvement will occur. Action solutions mean that explicit necessary steps must be taken to ensure that solutions to issues identified are implemented and evaluated.

Use of internal resources. The development of active and involved internal people who are trained in this methodology can be a valuable organizational asset. The knowledge of the organization, its setting, its client population, etc., are important in data exploration; an empathy for the issues and problems related to the health care was an important ingredient in the success of the process setting. External consultants can be used selectively: in the training of internal resources, in the planning of the survey, and in the design of feedback meetings. Real ownership on the part of trained, involved internal people can make a vast difference in the degree of follow-up and in the availability of ongoing consulting help to the project.

Overresponse to data. The data once again are merely a starting point. Too much time can be spent on the "nitty-gritty" details of how the data collection was constructed and conducted, what the statistical analysis means, and why questions were worded in one way rather than in another way. While some attention should be paid to these questions as a means of placing the data in a realistic and valid context, an overabundance of time spent on these details detracts from the real mission and goal of the action research process; i.e., to explore issues and problems in the organization that when resolved would lead to greater overall performances and satisfaction of organization members.

Training of organization members. For many people in organizations, the use of data, of the sort generated through action research, is a foreign experience and generally the level of acquaintance and experience with this process is rather limited. Some training in the intent and goals of action research, in utilizing the kind of data which is generated, and in the interpretation of this data can be a very useful starting point. First of all, the level of anxiety about the process can be reduced considerably, and secondly, the feedback meetings themselves will move efficient and productive rates if people understand the process and have some facility with the data/diagnosis steps.

SUMMARY

A successful action research project requires an organizational commitment of time, energy and resources to design, conduct, and follow-up with necessary implementation of problem solutions. Probably, more than anything else, success depends on the organization's "staying power," the ability to struggle through with patience in order to reap future advantages. Clearly, aborted projects occur when administrators are short sighted, have unrealistic expectations of results, and require immediate success. While action research is not an immediate panacea nor a substitute for good management practice, it can provide a logical and systematic strategy for organizational change and improvement which can be used as an important tool in the management of health care organizations.

NOTES

1. Beckhard, R.: Organizational Development: Strategies and Models. Reading, Mass., Addison-Wesley, 1969.
2. Bennis, W. G.: Organization Development, Its Nature, Origin, and Prospects. Reading, Mass., Addison-Wesley, 1969.
3. Brown, L. D.: Research action: Organizational feedback, understanding and change. J. Appl. Behav. Sci. 8:697, 1972.
4. Jenks, R. S.: An action research approach to organizational change. J. Appl. Behav. Sci. 6:131, 1970.
5. Margulies, N., and Raia, A. P.: Organizational development: Values, process and technology, New York, McGraw-Hill, 1972.

19 | Management by Objectives

Jeanne Palmer

When you know what you are trying to do you are more likely to succeed in doing it. This, very simply, is the basic idea behind the more complex process of management by objectives. In essence, management by objectives works this way: subordinates at various levels of an organization, in conjunction with their superiors, set specific goals for themselves; they then measure their performances in relation to these goals.

Management by objectives focuses attention on, and provides a logical framework for, achievement. It provides for leadership and motivation and is a basis for review and control. It is a system whereby objectives become directional guides for all activity.

Management is not an end in itself but an integral part of an organizational enterprise—an enterprise which consists of individuals. One requirement in a management position is that the individual's vision be directed toward the attainment of these goals.

In brief, management by objectives is a process whereby superior and subordinate managers jointly identify common organizational goals or objectives, define each individual's major areas of responsibility in terms of results expected, use those objectives as operational guidelines, and assess each person's contribution on the basis of objectives achieved or not achieved.

According to George S. Odiorne, "management by objectives goes beyond being a set of rules, a series of procedures, or even a set method of managing . . . it is a particular way of thinking about management." He places the system of management by objectives in its conceptual framework: a primary assumption is that an organization has as its basic structure an organizational form often referred to as a hierarchical structure, which can be shown by a vertical organizational chart. That structure is made to work by means of a system of management by objectives, making the action of the people within it personal and vital.

A secondary provision of management by objectives guides the orderly growth and the maintenance of the organization by stating the expectations for each of the individuals concerned, and provisions for measuring the achievement of those expectations. The responsible leaders must be assigned risks, and the results produced by them should determine their progress, and even tenure. Their achievement and ability will be stressed and personalities minimized in importance.

A system of management by objectives is particularly useful when applied to managerial and professional workers, and can even be applied to first-line supervisors as well as many staff (advisory) and technical positions. The concept of management by objectives helps in meeting many of the common problems arising in the management of professionals and other managers by allowing for measurement of the real contribution of these personnel and by giving definition to the shared goals of the organization and its people. Without giving up the aspect of personal risk taking, defining goals stimulates coordination and teamwork.

Management by objectives also helps solve the problem of assigning major areas of responsibility for each person in the group, including responsibilities shared by more than one individual. Moreover, it puts emphasis on the achievement of objectives, rather than on personality characteristics. Other benefits from this system include a clear definition of each manager's area of control, an accurate and fair means of allocating pay increases when payment is awarded for results, and indicates channels for advancement of promotable personnel.[1]

The system of management by objectives is a cycle, as shown in Figure 19-1. The feature in the cycle which is often most time-consuming is the joint establishment of subordinate goals.

The way in which the manager spends his time is an important aspect of management by objectives. This is a system of managing and not an addition to the manager's time. The one who adopts management by objectives as his system of management should plan to drop some of his more time-consuming activities. That is, he must delegate certain activities which he personally controls or oversees in too much detail which could just as effectively and efficiently be done by someone else. By delegating these activities, he now has more time for teaching the subordinate his duties and to perform more independently. The system of management by objectives thus entails a behavior change on the part of both the superior and subordinate. The subordinate, because he knows what his goals are, becomes more result-oriented. The superior exemplifies the behavior and provides the instruction and help that will aid the subordinate to succeed.

FIGURE 19-1

THE CYCLE OF MANAGEMENT BY OBJECTIVES

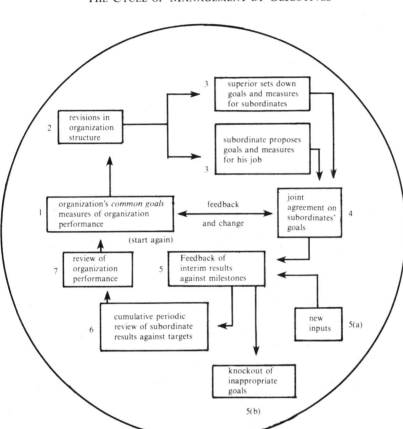

From MANAGEMENT BY OBJECTIVES by George S. Odiorne. Copyright © 1965 by Pitman Publishing Corporation. Reprinted by permission of Fearon Pitman Publishers Inc., Belmont, CA 94002.

SETTING OBJECTIVES

Forming the real basis for planning or for other day-to-day activity is the establishment and identification of the objectives toward which the activity is directed. Objectives should be formulated for every area where performance and results directly and vitally affect the survival and purpose of the organization. Among other things, objectives should enable one to predict behavior, appraise the soundness of decisions while they are being made, and analyze one's own experience and, as a result, improve one's performance.

Ideally, the objective-setting program should start with the chief executive officer, such as the hospital administrator, with the assistance and concurrence of the board of directors. It is at this top management level that the broad overall organizational objectives are set and from which subordinate levels of management will build their objectives. Without these broad organizational objectives, the objectives of subordinate levels of management may be at odds with each other and with the direction of the organization as a whole. Without central organizational objectives, subordinate levels of management may be misdirected, their efforts wasted, and instead of teamwork there is apt to be friction, frustration, and conflict.

Typically, the overall objectives include a plan for the ensuing five years—probably built on a year-by-year basis. Using the hospital as an example, once the administrator has established objectives, the objectives must be translated or communicated to all levels of management. Usually this involves an in-depth briefing of the organization's officers, such as the assistant administrators, by the administrator at which time he discusses the overall objectives for the target period. Each assistant administrator must leave the briefing with an understanding of the objectives and an appreciation of the responsibilities which they place on him and his particular area of responsibility.

Once each assistant administrator understands the overall organizational objectives, he must then think through, plan, and formulate the specific objectives he plans to accomplish within a target period. Naturally, these objectives will be narrower in scope than the overall objectives of which they are a part and will be concerned with the assistant administrator's own area of responsibility. Once the assistant administrator has formulated his objectives, he then takes them to the administrator for review. Once his objectives are approved, they become his guide to required action and a standard against which he will be measured or evaluated.

Because each assistant administrator understands the overall organizational objectives and those he has set for his area of responsibility, he must not assume that his managers and personnel understand them. Thus, because the assistant administrator for nursing service, that is, the director of nursing service, understands the hospital's overall objectives and those she has accordingly set for her department, she must not assume that her supervisors, head nurses and other personnel understand them equally as well. It, therefore, becomes her responsibility to define and interpret these.

When the assistant administrator has set the goals for his area of responsibility and interpreted them to his personnel, he is ready to assist those reporting directly to him in setting their objectives for a target period—again usually for a year. Thus, the assistant administrator for nursing service is ready to help her assistant directors of nursing service, or whatever might be the title of those reporting directly to her, in setting their objectives for the next target period.

In setting objectives for the next year, Odiorne suggests that a supervisor set a date for discussing his subordinate's objectives, which the subordinate brings in written form to the meeting. The supervisor should also list objectives he would like to have the subordinate include—noting especially any innovations and improvements required of the subordinate's function. After reviewing the subordinate's objectives, the supervisor should offer his suggestions. When final agreement is reached, two copies of the objectives should be typed with the superior and subordinate each retaining a copy. At this time, also, the superior should ask the subordinate what he can do to help him reach his objectives—this should be noted on the superior's copy of the subordinate's objectives.

During the year, Odiorne continues, the superior should check each subordinate's objectives as expected goals are accomplished. Thus, it should be asked: is he meeting his targets as they are measured by time, cost, quantity, quality, and service? Would it now be appropriate to change his targets? It must be noted that one should not hesitate to get rid of inappropriate goals, or to add new ones if the opportunity presents itself. Are you, as supervisor, carrying out your part of the agreement to help the subordinate accomplish his goals? A list of objectives, mutually agreed upon by the supervisor and subordinate, should be used as a tool for encouraging and developing each subordinate's performance. Calling attention to success reinforces good performance. A subordinate should be allowed to make mistakes without being hounded and his errors should be a platform from which to coach him on to better results.[3]

The objective-setting process is a key aspect of this total system. If an organization is only beginning to use management by objectives, goals should be set for periods of only three or six months rather than for the usual year, providing more practice at goal setting and faster feedback for appraisal of the objectives. As personnel become more skilled at setting objectives, the time periods may be lengthened.

Objectives, if the management by objectives approach is to be effective, must be structured along certain lines, thus: First and most important, objectives must be made specific in terms of what must be done and when it must be finished. As far as possible, the objectives must be qualified, as for example:

Poor: Reduce medication errors.

Better: Reduce medication errors by 50 percent in the next 12 months.

Objectives should be set so as to be realistic and attainable. But if they are too easily reached, they may be destructive because the group will not have earned or received the value due it during the period. Additionally, the manager's development is hampered because he is without sufficient incentive to improve his performance. Unattainable objectives, on the other hand, cause loss of confidence on the part of managers in this kind of management, and they will lack the feeling of achievement that one derives from attaining goals.

Objectives should be formulated to suit the manager's experience and capability. He must be either trained for the job or removed from it, if he cannot achieve the necessary action and consequences. Obviously a newly appointed manager should not be expected to perform as a veteran manager might, although more would be expected of him as he gains experience and skill.

The objectives of a manager must be in line with the constituted authority of his position. It is defeating to give him the freedom to set a goal which he does not have sufficient authority to carry out, and may lead to dissension as well as defeat.

In order to allow for changing organizational goals and also to keep appropriate priorities, it is likely that the objectives for most managers ought to be changed during subsequent target periods. To formulate a general rule: the same *what* and *when* should not ordinarily be repeated unless there is an unusually good reason to do so. Care should be taken that it is not simply a way of carrying on the same familiar routines.

Objectives should be carefully stated to have the same meaning and clarity for both the subordinate and the superior. Often management effectiveness is lost when terms are not interpreted in the same way by everybody involved.

Finally, two questions should be applied to all objectives under consideration: (1) Is the work necessary? and (2) Does it fit in with the other goals for the same time span? The activities of greatest importance should be emphasized in the objectives; lesser objectives may either be assimilated into the more important goals or postponed until the important ones have been fulfilled.[4]

Once a subordinate has prepared his objectives, they must be reviewed and evaluated by the superior in the light that these are the goals toward which the subordinate proposes to work and against which he will be measured. This the superior does by asking himself the following questions, as conceived by McConkey, about each recommended objective:

1) Is it enough of a task to be worthy of the manager, during the measuring period?
2) Can it actually be accomplished, and is it practical?
3) Is it plainly expressed regarding the task, the time allowed, and the means of measurement?

4) Does it fit in well with the organization's other plans and goals for the period?[5]

Only after the superior has answered these questions is he in a position to pass judgment on an objective.

Following are but a few of the many possible errors which may be committed by superiors in setting objectives: common objectives are not clarified for the whole area for which the superior is responsible; objectives are set too low to challenge subordinates; objectives are inappropriate or impossible to achieve; objectives of subordinates are always approved without consideration given to a plan for successful achievement; intermediate target dates are not set by which to measure progress; there is rigidity in pursuing previously agreed-upon objectives even after they have proven unfeasible or irrelevant.

CAN NURSING SERVICE BE THE ONLY DEPARTMENT PRACTICING MANAGEMENT BY OBJECTIVES?

It is very likely that many hospital administrators do not practice management by objectives. It is also very likely that there are administrators who do not share their planning with other members of the management team. More seriously, there may be administrators who do not even plan five or even one year in advance. Does this mean that a director of nursing service cannot practice management by objectives? No, it does not. Ideally, so that all may function on a common base, there should be a written philosophy of nursing care and a written philosophy of nursing service which is understood by all members of the nursing service department.

If a director of nursing service wishes to incorporate management by objectives in her department, it is essential that those who will be practicing it likewise understand the principles involved. Perhaps she may wish to begin by involving only those personnel occupying the positions immediately beneath her in the department's organizational hierarchy and eventually strive to include head nurses.

Once the director has formulated her objectives for a given period of time, she is ready to brief her immediate subordinates and begin the cycle of management by objectives as discussed earlier. Because it is important that the director of nursing service keep the administrator up to date on the major operations of her department, she should review with him her objectives and keep him informed as milestones are reached. Following are examples of objectives which may be proposed by the director for her department for a one-year period: (1) Reduce medication errors by 50 percent during the next 12 months, (2) complete entire admission procedure on all patients within one hour after patient is admitted to the nursing unit, (3) reduce number of back injuries among nursing personnel by 80 percent, (4) do six-month pilot study of taping all change of shift reports on 1 North, 2 North, and 3 Middle, (5) convert to cyclical staffing on all nursing units. Following are examples of objectives for which the director may wish to set a three- or five-year target period (or whatever length of time best meets the needs of her department): (1) institute team nursing on all nursing units on all three shifts, (2) decentralize budget preparation so that each head nurse prepares her own annual budget.

Because objectives are statements of an expected outcome, note that none of the examples includes the "how to." Some of the example objectives, such as the ones regarding medication errors and back injuries, may be adopted as written even at the head nurse level, others, such as the example regarding team nursing, would be made more specific by, for example, the in-service personnel.

CREATIVITY

At first glance it may appear that management by objectives hampers one's creativity and ingenuity. It might appear that this style of management outlines one's responsibilities in detail then requires one to follow a step-by-step procedure to accomplish them. Perhaps the greatest advantage of management by objectives is that it allows one to control his own performance.

Even though higher management must reserve the power to approve or disapprove them, the subordinate is given a wide latitude to exercise his creativity and ingenuity in the formulation of his objectives. In addition, the superior has an ideal opportunity, while reviewing the subordinate's objectives and plans, to encourage creative ability. This creativity would not be encouraged, however, if the superior handed down objectives to the subordinate, the subordinate, thereby, becoming merely an instrument to achieve the objectives of his superior.

While the system of management by objectives establishes the accomplishments for which one is responsible, it does not spell out the methods to be used to achieve the objectives. One is accountable for results and is at liberty to choose the means which will best achieve that result.

Management by objectives does not infer an atmosphere in which "the boss is watching" to make certain that a job is being done and being done correctly. To the contrary, the objectives provide a vehicle whereby one is given certain duties and is held responsible for the ends and not the means. The system is not compatible with spoonfeeding those in a management position; rather, the creativity allows for introduction of new ideas from outside the organization and allows for discovery of new ways, combinations, or methods of doing a job.

Periodic Review of Objectives and Results
A Method of Evaluating Personnel Performance

As was mentioned earlier, a superior should review his subordinates' goals periodically throughout the year to make any necessary readjustments. However, at the end of the target period, which is usually at the end of the budget year, the superior and his subordinates measure the year's results against the goals. Odiorne suggests that these four steps be taken by the manager:

1) Each subordinate should be asked to prepare a written statement evaluating his performance—that is, a comparison of accomplishments to the objectives. The written statement should account for any deviation and list achievements which hadn't been planned.

2) A meeting should be set between the superior and the subordinate, at which time the two will go over the latter's statement in detail, looking for the reasons for deviations from the pre-set objectives. The superior should ask himself if the variance was his fault or the subordinate's, or if perhaps it was not in the power of either one to control. Then he and the subordinate should form an agreement on the quality of the latter's performance and note his areas of weakness.

3) At this meeting, the superior should give his employee time to explore such areas as relationships with others on the job, or opportunity for advancement, or whatever is important to him.

4) This is the time to set up the subordinate's performance budget for the ensuing year.[6]

The annual review of objectives and results provides a method of evaluating personnel performance. Appraisal should always be the direct responsibility of one's superior and should always focus on proven performance.

Although managerial appraisal should focus on proven performance, traditional measurement is largely based on personality or personal characteristics and traits such as initiative, health, grasp of function, ability to work with others, etc. These characteristics and traits are usually scored on a numerical rating scale or classified as "above average" or "average" or "below average", etc. It is virtually no more than a stab in the dark to evaluate performance in this manner.

Despite its advantages over other managerial appraisal methods, management by objectives also has its limitations in that it cannot appraise and completely identify potential. It is presumed that the superior and his subordinate will jointly formulate objectives that will best serve the organization. However, the system too often stresses results and does not outline methods for achieving those results. The aspect of creativity as discussed above should enter here.

Even with its limitations, management by objectives has the positive aspect of avoiding the potentially damaging effects and inadequacies of most annual performance evaluations particularly if this meeting is identified as one of objective setting rather than appraisal interview. Such an approach is positive and allows one to lay the groundwork for formulating future objectives. Such a review also allows one to review one's performance and determine what can be done, not done, or done differently to achieve better results in one's management job.

CONCLUSION

Management by objectives is a system whereby positive achievement can be planned, measured, and evaluated. Its multiple uses are proof that it is a total concept of management.

Can management by objectives be applied in a large or small department of nursing service regardless of whether the system is used hospital-wide? The answer is yes. Review of the literature reveals that many well known organizations successfully use this style of management. All enterprises are similar in that they require people, money, and a basic idea of what is trying to be accomplished. Because of these similarities, management by objectives may also be utilized in a department of nursing service.

NOTES

1. Odiorne, George S. *Management by Objectives.* New York, Pitman Publishing Corp., 1965, p. 54.
2. Odiorne, *Management*, p. 78.
3. *Ibid*, p. 71.
4. McConkey, Dale D. *How to Manage by Results.* New York, American Management Association, 1965, p. 42.
5. McConkey, *How to Manage*, p. 55.
6. Odiorne, *Management*, p. 113.

BIBLIOGRAPHY

Drucker, Peter F. *The Practice of Management.* New York, Harper and Row, Publishers, 1954.
Glasner, Daniel M. Patterns of Management by Results. *Business Horizons* 12:37–40, Feb. 1969.
Howell, Robert A. A Fresh Look at Management by Objectives. *Business Horizons* 10:51–58, Fall 1967.

Ivancevich, John M. The Theory and Practice of Management by Objectives. *Michigan Business Review* 21:13–16, March 1969.

Killian, Ray A. *Managing by Design—for Maximum Executive Effectiveness.* New York, American Management Association, 1968.

Killian, Ray A. Management by Objectives, First Visualized as a Rating Method, Proves Valuable as Approach to Management, NIBC Report Says. *Management Services* 6:11–12, March, April 1969.

McConkey, Dale D. *How to Manage by Results.* New York, American Management Association, 1965.

Odiorne, George S. *Management by Objectives.* New York, Pitman Publishing Corp., 1965.

Olsson, David E. *Management by Objectives,* Palo Alto, Pacific Books, Publishers, 1968.

Schlech, Edward C. Management by Objectives: Some Principles for Making it Work. *The Management Review* 48:26–33, Nov. 1959.

Stumph, Charles F. Administration by Objectives. *Hospital Administration* 6:43–50, Winter 1961.

Tingey, Sherman. Management Today. *Hospital Administration* 14:32–41, Spring 1969.

Wikstrom, Walter S. Management by Objectives or Appraisal by Results. *Modern Supervisory Techniques.* ed. by Jack F. Rhode. Minneapolis, Applied Management Science, Inc., 1967.

20 | # Hospital Organization Development: Changing the Focus from "Better Management" to "Better Patient Care"

Johannes U. Stoelwinder
Peter S. Clayton

Australian hospitals share many problems with their American counterparts. Their cost is increasing at an alarming rate. General hospitals account for 41% of the 7.1% of the Gross Domestic Product spent on all health services (1975–76 estimates). The proportion spent on these hospitals is growing faster than any other segment (an average of 16.5% annually compared to 14.3% of all other expenditures). After inflation this is mostly the result of an increase in unit cost (Scotton, 1977). In the absence of legitimate outcome measures, hospitals are not able to demonstrate in tangible terms the quality and appropriateness of the services they provide. They are also operating in an increasingly turbulent environment created by the rapid change in medical

The authors wish to thank the many people who participated, supported, and otherwise made this program possible.

Reproduced by special permission from *The Journal of Applied Behavioral Science*, "Hospital Organization Development: Changing the Focus from 'Better Management' to 'Better Patient Care'," by Johannes U. Stoelwinder and Peter S. Clayton, Volume 14, Number 3, 1978, pp. 400–414, NTL Institute.

care knowledge and technology, in demography, and in public expectations of health care services, and by the increasing interrelationships with other institutions including government, schools, regulative agencies, supply organizations and others. Workers in hospitals are also bringing with them increasing expectations about the quality of their working life. Their increasing drive for professionalism and the increase in unionism appear to be expressions of this.

As a result, much attention has recently focused on hospital management and on ways in which it can be developed to respond to today's problems. Such efforts have taken a variety of forms under the generic term of organization development (OD). Unfortunately OD efforts in health care institutions have not always enjoyed the success they have had in industrial institutions (Weisbord 1976). Is this because OD processes are inappropriate to health care settings, and/or, are there factors within the health care organization which inhibit them? This case study addresses these questions.

The subject is an OD intervention in an Australian teaching hospital. Despite initial success, the intervention floundered in not being able to penetrate effectively into the patient care areas. By altering the focus of the intervention from "better management" to "better patient care," and developing strategies congruent with the norms of physicians and other health professionals, the participation of these key organization members was enlisted. As a result, the intervention was successfully adopted by the hospital in patient care, support, and administrative departments.

THE SITE

The Sir Charles Gairdner Hospital was opened in 1958 as a 180-bed hospital for the treatment of tuberculosis. In 1962, with the declining incidence of this disease, it was decided to develop the hospital and its adjoining site as the major teaching hospital/medical school complex for the State of Western Australia. A major building program was instituted which has already increased the bed complement to 540 and has seen the Medical School move on site. The building program, scheduled for completion in 1981, will provide some 900 general beds and 120 geriatric service beds.

Apart from its general management problems, this hospital has had to deal with a major change in mission and very rapid institutional growth. The resultant organizational strain led the Board of Management to seek the assistance of management consultants, who contracted to review the structure and establish a management training and development program.

The Initial Intervention

The initial intervention, commenced in April 1973, was based on work previously developed in the Sydney Hospital (Crawford, Ritchie and Whyte 1971). A full-time resident consultant was provided to perform three basic tasks:

1. Conduct a management training program for all staff with managerial roles. The training program, based on Management-by-Objectives (MBO), consisted of 10 workshops.
2. Assist these managers in implementing the MBO principles they had learned.
3. Establish, within the hospital, an ongoing management training capability.

After an introduction to the hospital, the consultant commenced the training program with top managers as the first participants. This was not only to familiarize them with the training program but to invite them to utilize the MBO concept in their division. The exercise resulted in the establishment of a "Hospital Executive" consisting of Administrator, Matron, and Medical Superintendent—the heads of each of the distinct divisions that form the hospital's administrative structure (Figure 20-1). After defining their own role as one of coordination, policy formulation and forward planning, the group next reviewed their areas of responsibility. This resulted in the reshuffling of some departments within the division. The group also established a formal management information system which is now utilized in regular reports to the Board of Management. The "Hospital Executive" has not been institutionalized and continues to function as a tripartite of equals. But it has not been able to resolve the issue of leadership which remains a source of instability. The consultant's role with this group was to assist its members in the team-building phase and to provide technical assistance. His legitimacy as a peer was maintained by his ability to help the group achieve successful outcomes and also by his contractual relationship with the Board of Management. The success of this aspect of the program was crucial to the subsequent developments and its interdisciplinary nature helped set fertile ground for the subsequent innovations.

The next phase of the program consisted of two streams. First, department heads were invited to attend the training program on the nomination of the division head. A series of these programs were held. Most administrative department heads and heads of departments of therapy attended and were subsequently assisted in implementing the MBO format within their departments. The degree of implementation varied considerably between departments but most established some formal objectives and monitors of resource utilization, work performance, and, to a limited degree, outcome. Most also

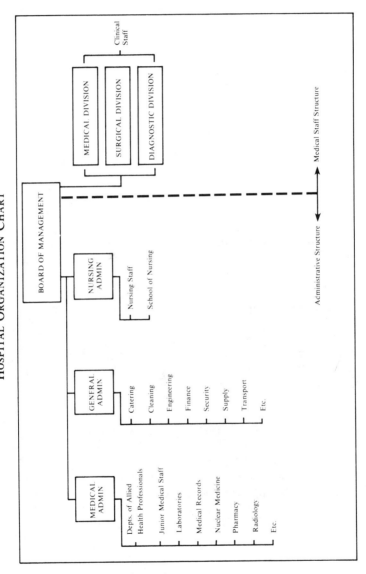

FIGURE 20-1

HOSPITAL ORGANIZATION CHART

BOARD OF MANAGEMENT

MEDICAL ADMIN
- Depts. of Allied Health Professionals
- Junior Medical Staff
- Laboratories
- Medical Records
- Nuclear Medicine
- Pharmacy
- Radiology
- Etc.

GENERAL ADMIN
- Catering
- Cleaning
- Engineering
- Finance
- Security
- Supply
- Transport
- Etc.

NURSING ADMIN
- Nursing Staff
- School of Nursing

MEDICAL DIVISION
SURGICAL DIVISION
DIAGNOSTIC DIVISION

Clinical Staff

Medical Staff Structure

Administrative Structure

established some formal mechanism of meeting with staff or supervisors to discuss problems and provide feedback. The second stream of activity was in the nursing division and included the management training program as well as a restructuring of nursing middle management. The MBO format was subsequently established within the nursing division with diffusion down to the ward charge level.

It was at this stage, 6 months after commencement, that some serious problems surfaced.

• The program was not reaching the medical staff and departments with medical staff heads such as radiology and laboratories.

• Implementation was reaching the wards only in the area of nursing staff. In this case, however, it was generating considerable conflict that was not being resolved. Utilizing the MBO format the nurses had set themselves objectives which naturally included good patient care. When they attempted to measure how well this objective was being achieved they aroused suspicion and even open hostility among other health care professionals in the ward who felt that the nurses were monitoring their performance. The nurses themselves soon became frustrated with the program. Although they were able to solve problems initially they soon found that they were left with the many difficult ones—most of them relating to their interdependence with doctors, other health care professions and other departments within the hospital. These problems could not be solved within the nursing division and there was no other hospital structure for their resolution. In this way, the program was creating more problems than the hospital had the capability to solve.

• The Board of Management was expecting this management training program to produce better management and, hence, cost containment. This was not being demonstrated.

PROGRAM REVIEW

At this stage the authors teamed up to review the program. The second author (PSC) was the resident consultant. The first author (JUS) had just joined the hospital's administrative staff after completing his specialty medical training there. It was felt that the two major problems with the implementation of the program were:

1. The organization structure of the hospital worked against effective management and, in the same way, against effective OD intervention.
2. The intervention had problems of entry into the professional structure, principally the medical staff, to whom it lacked credence and relevance.

The commitment to the overall strategy remained. A program of intervention was not prescriptive, but aimed at exposing and developing by participative and collaborative methods each individual's talent to identify and solve his own management problems.

THE ORGANIZATION STRUCTURE OF THE HOSPITAL

The organization structure of the hospital was typical (see Figure 20-1). In this model the administrative structure is organizationally separate from the medical structure. The administrative structure is a bureaucracy based on Weber's rational-legal model. It views the organization from the perspective of input and process. People are grouped in departments which either deal with input (e.g., Outpatient Department, Emergency Department) or, more usually, oriented to the division of labor associated with process (e.g., departments of nursing, physiotherapy, cleaning, catering, social work, etc.). Unlike in industry, the hospital's administrative structure cannot see input and process through to outcome because a major determinant of outcome, the medical staff, does not fall within its control. Furthermore, increasingly larger components within the structure are developing professional norms that cause individuals to feel accountable to their profession rather than to their administrative hierarchy for the work they do. This further reduces the authority of the administrative structure.

The medical staff structure is also a bureaucracy but varies in important ways from the rational-legal model. It is based on expert rather than hierarchical authority. It must also maintain the important characteristics of professionalism—particularly that of individual autonomy (Freidson 1970). Control is limited to giving advice, a characteristic that has led the structure to be termed an "advisory bureaucracy" (Goss 1961).

The primary task of a hospital is to achieve patient care outcomes. Applied to an individual patient this outcome is determined by three interrelated sets of factors.

1. Patient factors—including age, genetic make-up, attitude to disease and the investigative-therapeutic process, the presence of intercurrent disease, etc.

2. Environmental factors—including socioeconomic status, social support mechanisms, such as family, etc.

3. Organizational factors—This set is composed of (a) professional services, including the technical skills involved in doctoring, nursing, therapy and medication, as well as human skills, such as providing patients with information and psychosocial support; and (b) "physical services" patients require for the normal process of living, such as food, cleaning, linen service,

etc. These components form the organization's primary task. To achieve this primary task the hospital provides an array of supportive services such as laboratories, radiology, maintenance, supply and others. The final functional dimension is the staff, the coordinating and policy formulating mechanism.

The primary task is achieved mainly by a group consisting of doctors, nurses and various other health care professionals (including social workers, physiotherapists, occupational therapists, ward pharmacists and others) applying professional and human services. In doing so, the group members are utilizing the hospital's resources. They do this by determining the need for, and duration of, the patient's admission to the hospital and by the tests, medications and therapeutic and rehabilitative procedures they utilize.

How this group is structured is, therefore, of critical importance. The dual bureaucratic structure of the hospital can be represented by Figure 20–2. The ward structure is seen from the perspective of a patient receiving professional, human, and physical services. The characteristics of market division of labor and vertical integration are evident. There is no formal lateral integration at the work face. To be effective this structure should help the group deal with its organizational problems. At the technical level, there are problems of uncertainty—about cause and effect relationships in therapy, about patient arrival and departure from the ward, and about patient requirements of the care process (e.g., unknown diagnosis, latent disease, latent complications, etc.). In task performance there is a high degree of interdependence of a reciprocal nature among the group members. There are also problems within the social system. There is impact on the individual as a result of working with patients which expresses itself as high levels of stress and anxiety (Menzies 1960). Human interaction and exchange are limited because of the status differences among the individuals in the group and because, in the struggle for professionalism, the individual's desire for autonomy increases. This problem is enhanced in the socialization process during training which stresses the health professional's autonomy but fails to consider the interdependent nature of his future work experience.

It was the authors' belief that the organization structure of the hospital being studied was not effective and, therefore, inappropriate as it did not facilitate the resolution of technical and social system problems at the ward or work-face level. An alternative structure was developed (Figure 20–3) based on a sociotechnical systems approach (Emery and Trist 1960). It was determined by the need for coordination by mutual adjustment, for problem solving by active learning, for mutual support and respect among individuals, and for participative decision making in matters that affect the individual's work.

The patient care team, or "ward team," in each ward of 30 or so beds was

FIGURE 20–2

HOSPITAL ORGANIZATION STRUCTURE VIEWED FROM A PATIENT'S PERSPECTIVE

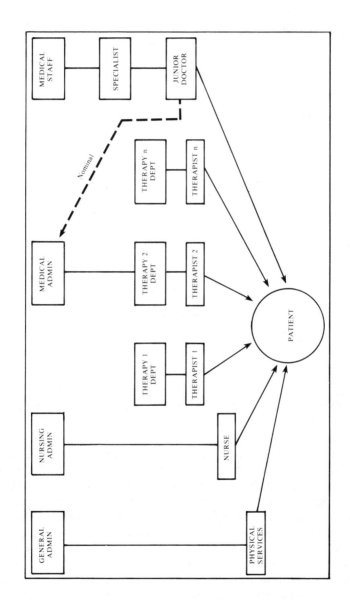

("Therapist" includes any health care professional.)

FIGURE 20–3

PROPOSED ORGANIZATION STRUCTURE OF A "WARD TEAM"

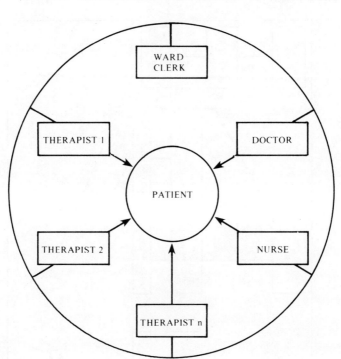

considered as a "corporate" identity forming the basic management unit. The method of bed allocation in this hospital allows each team to be readily identified. It was planned that each team would act as a self-regulating work group. Each would relate to the administrative structure of the hospital through a "Hospital Management Group" composed of the "second-in-charge" of each of the three administrative divisions. As such, this group has hierarchical control over all the departments within the administrative structure. The "ward teams" would relate to the medical staff structure via their specialist medical staff members. The professional departments within the administrative structure from which team members came would continue to exist (a) to perform tasks which were outside the "ward teams" activity, such as outpatient and specialty therapy, and (b) to maintain professional standards and ethics, education programs and career development for individuals. The "ward teams," medical staff structure and administrative structure would thus form a matrix organization.

Entry Into the Professional Structure

Implementation of this revised OD program required entry, not only into the formal medical structure, but into the overall professional structure of the health care professionals who would be involved. Having gained entry, it would require methodologies that would maintain its relevance and acceptance. The following strategies were developed:

• It was considered important that the change agents be perceived as having legitimacy to intervene in the patient care process and have acceptability among the health care professionals. It was, therefore, decided that the authors would act as an external-internal change agent team in the intervention. The external change agent would provide legitimacy in terms of having the skills, knowledge and experience to conduct such a program. It was hoped that the internal change agent, a physician who had recently undergone some of his training within the institution, would be perceived as sharing the values and norms of the health care professionals. He also represented a bridge between the disciplines of medicine and social science which formed the basis of the OD program. As a member of the hospital's administrative structure at the "second-in-charge" level and of the medical staff structure the internal change agent would add organizational legitimacy to the program. The teaming of external and internal change agents also would enable the protection of the program at all levels inside, and to some extent outside, the organization.

• To maintain acceptance, the OD program was developed to match the value system of the health care professionals involved. The emphasis of the program was on learning to use organizational skills to assist in achieving patient care goals rather than on better "management" of the hospital. The latter tends to "turn-off" health care professionals who see this as the administration's job—not theirs. The program was also redesigned so that it could be conducted within the ward environment eliminating the usual strategy of taking people away from their work setting in order to free them from workaday problems and interruptions. The strategy here was to fit the program to the professional's "home-base" and thereby gain greater acceptance.

• To aid its internalization the OD intervention was designed to be participative and based on mutual learning. The image of the "expert" model was to be avoided.

• It was recognized that this intervention would set off emergent processes in other areas of the hospital and, in particular, in the professional departments that would be most directly affected. The early involvement of these departments was incorporated within the program.

THE WARD TEAM MANAGEMENT PROJECT

The intervention in the wards was called the "Ward Team Management Project" (Clayton and Stoelwinder 1976). After gaining support from the "Hospital Executive" the project was explained to all managers in involved departments and their support sought.

A trial ward was selected on the assessed likelihood of success and relative status within the hospital. The critical factor determining the selection was the expected willingness of the ward's physicians to agree to, and actively participate in, the project. These physicians were also in influential positions within the medical staff structure. It was hoped that this influence would help in the subsequent diffusion stage.

The project commenced in January 1974 after gaining the commitment of the physicians to participate. The aim of the project was explained to the other team members (junior medical staff, senior nursing staff, physiotherapist, occupational therapist, social workers, ward pharmacist, and ward clerk) individually. They were invited to meet once a week to (a) discuss the care and progress of patients in the ward and (b) spend a further 15 to 20 minutes in an "Action Meeting" to take an overview of the ward's activities. The ward resident (called "registrar" in Australia) convened the meetings and nominally led the first section and subsequently the second section as well. During the first 10 weeks the latter section of the meeting was led by the change agents. This time was used to introduce the principles of MBO. The team during this period defined its objectives and developed performance measures. The change agents' prime orientation was not directed at these tasks per se but at using them for team building. The resident was also given special guidance in encouraging participative decision making and in containing the duration of the meeting. Unless action could be decided upon at the meeting (hence the name "Action Meeting") problems were referred to individuals or groups as appropriate to develop for future meetings. A simple form (Action Statement) was used to keep track of who in the team was doing what and by when in regard to decided action and unresolved problems.

After this initial phase, the "Action Meeting" was devoted to:

1. *Reviewing progress* (a) of the performance measures the team had developed—including average length of patient stay, avoidable patient days lost, the degree to which patients' medical problems were resolved on discharge (a self-audit using the problem-oriented medical record), nursing dependency, treatments given by the health care professionals on ward, etc., (b) of actions taken as a result of problems identification and solving.

2. *Problems identification and solving.* For example: Facilities and procedures were developed for outpatient endoscopies in the ward thus reducing the need for admission of these patients (the ward also contained the gastro-enterology unit); interteam-member consultation procedures were

reviewed and streamlined; the need for nonprofessional help for the occupational therapist on the ward was investigated (this revealed that such help would not be useful although it was initially considered desirable); major drug costs in the ward were identified and reviewed; inadequacies in the medical record and communication procedures with the patients' general practitioner were reviewed and improved; delays in patients' transfer to the geriatric service were highlighted and timesaving consultation procedures with that service were arranged; etc.

3. *Special projects which included further team-building exercises.* Examples included a special session to discuss the problem of the management of the dying patient, discussions of individual team members' roles, and a group review of the appropriateness of the project and its methods.

During this period at least one of the change agents attended the meetings in a supporting role. Support was also directed at facilitating successful outcomes of the groups' interaction with other areas in the hospital. Change agents also provided technical assistance in the mechanisms of collecting data about performance.

Over the initial 6-month period the trial ward team experienced a 9% reduction in length of patient's stay; a significantly improved patient undertanding of their medication regime 1 month after discharge (82% of patients from the trial ward were able to recount their medication regime correctly whereas only 66% of matched controls from other wards were able to do so. The observers were medical students who did not know which group the patients belonged to.). There was a 40% improvement, as measured by questionnaire responses, in team members' attitude to various aspects of their relationship with the team.

Three months into the trial it was decided to extend the project throughout the hospital wards. Similar interventions were also developed for the Outpatient Department, Emergency Department and Operating Theaters. Based on experience with the initial ward, the overall format and strategy remained unchanged. The initial phase was refined and shortened to 6 weeks on the average (depending on team progress). Each ward's final format varied in team membership, leadership, measures developed, and frequency and style of meeting. These factors were determined by the groups. The diffusion process took 18 months to complete. Sixteen of a potential 19 teams have been established and continue in operation.

RESULTS

The results lack specificity and changes should not be interpreted as directly caused by the OD program. They are subject to the effects of maturity as the program extended over a 2½-year time span. This introduces a number of variables, such as alteration of hospital financing mechanisms. The OD program intervened at all levels in the organization and in such a complex system it is rarely possible to pinpoint the locus of change responsible for the observed effect. Finally the data were collected primarily for the use of management decision rather than for rigorous scientific inquiry. The former allows for intuitive judgment, the latter attempts to avoid it.

In the authors' assessment, improvement in the hospital has been demonstrated in a number of areas.

OVERALL HOSPITAL PERFORMANCE

The financial performance of the hospital improved to the extent that it was able to reverse a trend and balance its budget in 1974–75 and 1975–76. The rate of increase in cost per admission had been increasing steadily in the 5 years preceding 1973–74. In that year it reached a high of 28.7% increase over the previous year. This was reduced to 15.4% in 1974–75.

Average length of patient stay was reduced by 10% in 1975 and this trend has continued. Although this does not deviate significantly from overall hospital trends, it has been achieved in the absence of a demand pressure which is the usual cause for a reduction in length of patient stay. In fact, occupancy was also increased slightly by the purposeful expansion of the hospital's emergency service.

PROBLEM-SOLVING ACTIVITY

It has not been possible to quantify the problem-solving activity generated by the program. Some examples will, however, show the significance of this activity to the hospital's performance.

• The ENT/Ophthalmology ward had had problems in scheduling admissions for elective surgery for many years. A sample measurement revealed an average four patients per month were sent home after being called for admission because beds were unavailable. Patients waited an average 3½ hours after arrival before reaching their beds in the ward. This frequently led to problems in preparing patients for surgery the next day. Morale was low, particularly among the nursing staff. Hospital administrators' attempts to solve the problem, including an elaborate information system, had all failed. This was the ward team's first problem after its introductory program. The team established a simple scheme which enabled the patient to arrive in the ward directly rather than to a central admissions area and reorganized the patient calling procedure. As a result, no patients were sent home in the first month trial period and patient waiting time from arrival to bed time was reduced to 10 minutes on average. The cost, apart from the time taken to evolve the solution, was $1,000 for equipment which is now shared with an adjacent ward. The scheme was so successful that it has been officially adopted and is being diffused throughout the hospital.

• Several surgical wards developed procedures for further streamlining admission for patients undergoing elective procedures. This included ambulant admission clinics and procedures for preoperative investigation. The result of these exercises was a smoother and less stressful patient admission, a reduction for laboratories in the out-of-hours work of routine preoperative tests and a reduction in stress on the admitting medical and nursing staff.

• The Emergency Department team was able to plan and commission extensive expansion of the department to cope with the development of this service. Within 3 years, the Department developed from a simple admissions receival area to a full emergency service for more than half of its designated region. This it was not scheduled to cover until the completion of the definitive department in the new ward building.

• The Outpatient Group was able to handle a 15% annual growth in attendances by redesigning procedures. Waiting times were also reduced. The group, with the assistance of the hospital's planning department, was able to commission its new definitive department. The building design required a complete restructuring of procedures. This, together with the physical move of the department, was achieved with the loss of only one clinic day.

STAFF ATTITUDE

The persistence of the change program is a reflection of its acceptance by the hospital in general. An example of the acceptance and enthusiasm of some of the health care professionals who were involved in the project was demonstrated in the ENT/Ophthalmology ward. They arranged for the commencement of the project in that ward without waiting for the change agents' intervention. These members overlapped with wards already involved in the project and saw it as a way to get the ward to deal with its chronic elective admission problem. They also felt it would help them deal with what they perceived as insufficient and inappropriate use of their skills by the medical staff on the ward.

Prior to commencing the project, team members answered a structured, anonymous questionnaire, which was again given 18 months later. The overall return rate was just under 80%. The results are shown in Table 20-1.

Senior medical staff involvement in the project has not been completely achieved. In about one third of the wards specialists directly participate. In another third they give support but do not actively participate. In the remaining wards tacit agreement only is given. Only one specialist has actively opposed the project. In view of the time constraints on these specialists (many of whom are part-time) this appears a reasonable acceptance of the project.

TABLE 20-1
WARD TEAM MEMBERS' ATTITUDE QUESTIONNAIRE

Question Groupings	1973-74 % Responding Satisfactory or Better	1975 Gain	% Gain 75 over 73-74
Attitude toward team membership	75	10	13
Clarity of role perception	86	4	5
Belief of other's under- standing of role	53	13	25
Understanding and influence on working environment	54	13	24
Communications	55	18	33
Relevance of job content	44	22	50

However, their more active participation remains a goal as teams with such involvement have, on the whole, performed more successfully.

HOSPITAL COORDINATION

The presence of multidisciplined "ward teams" has enabled the hospital to undertake its coordination task in a new and more effective manner. For example, a patient profile was established for planning purposes. On a single day teams gave information about the patients on their ward. Based on the acquired profile the need for alternative forms of patient accommodation was realistically assessed. Information was also derived in regard to nursing requirements and the dynamics of therapeutic process. Also established were studies on nursing dependency, hospital transportation system, food services, and others providing multifaceted information that cannot readily be collected without the team structure.

THE FUTURE

By the end of 1975, the internal change agent had moved to other duties within the hospital and the external change agent had withdrawn, thus concluding the intervention. Meanwhile, a department within the hospital had been established which was assigned the ongoing management training and development. This department has continued to provide support for the ward teams. One person has been responsible for facilitating team performance. For the first 2 years, this position was held successively by two physicians and now a pharmacist. Concepts and methodologies have continued to be reviewed on the basis of experience. It is hoped that this learning process will counteract some of the negative aspects of the program, particularly resistance to change associated with the program institutionalization that has occurred because of its success.

REFERENCES

Clayton, P. S., & Stoelwinder, J. U. Hospital management—the need for an alternative approach: Ward team management. *Australian Studies for Health Services Management.* 1976, 20 & 30, 43–56.

Crawford, L.E., Ritchie, F.L., & Whyte, H. M. Replanning Sydney Hospital: 3. An experiment in management. *Medical Journal of Australia.* 1971, 2, 1291.

Emery, F.E., & Trist, E. L. Socio-technical systems. In C. W. Churchman & M. Verhulst (Eds.), *Management science, models and techniques.* London: Pergamon Press, 1960, Pp. 83–97.

Freidson, E. *Professional dominance: The social structure of medical care.* Chicago, Ill.: Aldine Publishing Co., 1970.

Goss, M. E. W. Influence and authority among physicians in an out-patient clinic. *American Sociological Review.* 1961, 26, 39–50.

Menzies, I. E. P. A case study in the functioning of social systems as a defense against anxiety. *Human Relations.* 1960, 13, 95–121.

Scotton, R.B. Health costs and health policy. *The Australian Quarterly.* 1977, 49 (2), 5–16.

Wiesbord, M. R. Why organization development hasn't worked (so far) in medical centers. *Health Care Management Review.* Spring 1976, 17–38.

21 | Changing Perceptions of Organizational Communication: Can Short-Term Intervention Help?

Karlene H. Roberts
Nannette L. Cerruti
Charles A. O'Reilly III

Organizational change interventions have an effect on communication activities or at least on perceptions about them, job satisfaction, and opportunities to make job-related innovations for people subjected to the intervention (Blake et al. 1964; Campbell and Dunnette 1968; Morton and Bass 1964). Most opportunities for making interventions concerned with these factors are limited in the time they can take, particularly at nonsupervisory levels. Organizations do not usually permit their employees to be away from their jobs, and employees usually are unwilling or unable to attend training sessions in addition to their normal work. Therefore, knowledge of whether effectiveness of well-developed short programs warrants their cost is important. Careful evaluation of training programs is needed.

THEORETICAL FRAMEWORK

Most research concerned with such interventions presents obvious problems. First, communication, satisfaction, and other behavioral phenomena often are confused with one another, possibly because change agents are usually interested in altering simultaneously a whole zeitgeist of attitudes or behaviors. Second, the interrelationships among aspects of one phenomenon, such as facets of communication, are rarely considered. For example, it is often difficult to tell whether a discussion of gatekeeping in organizations is really an analysis of information change, or withholding of information, or summarization of information, or something else. Third, the distinction between organizational members' perceptions of their own and others' behaviors in their organizations and actual behaviors in those organizations is rarely made. Finally, most investigations of organizational change employ research designs from which it is impossible to infer whether results are caused by the intervention or by some other factor. Control groups are frequently missing. Situations in which change is the outcome of interest often fail to include preintervention measures or, if they do, there is frequently little attempt to account for measurement effects on posttests.

PURPOSE OF THE STUDY

The purpose of this study was to evaluate changes in perceptions about organizational communication, job satisfaction, and opportunities for innovative job behavior that result from a training program designed to improve the internal working situation in an emergency room of a large metropolitan hospital.

BACKGROUND OF THE STUDY

The need for training was brought to the attention of the hospital administration by a patient advisory board, which had been subjected to a series of ongoing diffuse complaints about problems and working conditions in the emergency room. Surveys, conducted on patients and emergency room personnel to determine the exact nature of these problems, indicated that patients were generally dissatisfied with the impersonal attitudes of the staff which often resulted in their being ignored or treated rudely. Emergency room staff often failed to understand what was expected of them, believed that changing the situation was impossible, and were dissatisfied with communication in general. Many staff members believed they had no influence on the organization, and most said their opinions were never solicited.

From this information and from numerous meetings with employees at all organizational levels, training goals were developed commensurate with the primary organizational goal of providing efficient medical care under what often were trying circumstances. These training goals included improvement in communication with particular emphasis on learning to listen, providing feedback and accurate information, building trust and teamwork among personnel by opening communication channels, and increasing self-esteem within the organization through encouraging feelings of independence, responsibility, and ability to take risks. The teamwork goal was particularly important because personnel in the emergency room represented a variety of disciplines and felt isolated from one another. There was little communication and interaction across functional groups. These goals were sanctioned by members at all levels in the hospital and were then translated into a training program.

Rather than assume that the training would "take," an evaluation was designed at the same time the program was being developed. Evaluation was considered in light of Campbell et al.'s (1970) designation of factors which should be included in any organizational training evaluation, i.e., evaluation should: 1) use multiple criteria, 2) be concerned both with interrelationships among criteria and with criteria to other relevant organizational variables. 3) include enough experimental control so that any change could be attributed to the training, 4) include provisions for making statements of practical and theoretical significance, 5) include a thorough analysis of the process and content of training, and 6) consider the systems aspect of training. (For example, how does some particular form of training fit with other components of the organization's activities?)

METHOD

RESEARCH DESIGN

The evaluation employed a modification of the Solomon four-group design (Campbell and Stanley 1963), which uses two experimental and two control groups.

It was not possible to assign employees at random to training (experimental) and nontraining (control) groups. Trained employees were all emergency room personnel. The control group consisted of outpatient department staff. These two units were similar in that personnel in both units see outpatients for short-duration visits (as opposed to the in-patient staff), and both are in the same organizational branch of the hospital. Both groups share the same staffing and space shortage problems, and patient complaints are similar in both areas. The critical difference in the two groups concerns the emergency aspects of the trained groups' work. Within the two training groups, people were randomly assigned to pre- and posttest only conditions. The same was true for the two control groups.

SUBJECTS

In both the training and the nontraining groups participants were registered nurses, licensed vocational nurses, nurses' aides, ward clerks, registration clerks, security officers, housekeepers, and social workers. No supervisors were included by vote of the training groups. Group 1 (emergency room training group with both pre- and posttests) included 16 persons; group 2 (emergency room training group, posttest) had 28 participants; group 3 (no training, pre- and posttest), 19 persons; and group 4 (no training, posttest only), 25 persons. To the extent possible the proportions of persons in each job function were the same across the four groups.

TRAINING CONTENT

Training content included discussions about related readings, and exercises concerned with one-to-one and group communication. Application of influence through communication and application of communication principles specifically to the work situations were discussed. Communications both within the staff and between staff and patients were discussed. The second content area emphasized group problem solving. Here proposals for action were considered, and the use of "task" and "maintenance" leaders discussed. Emphasis was based on the fact that changes in relationships with others in the organization are based on the willingness of individuals to explore new problem-solving alternatives. "New tools to solve old problems" was the underlying theme. All material presented was designed around the specific training program goals.

Two and one-half- to three-hour training sessions were held weekly for four consecutive weeks. Two sections were held to accommodate different work shifts, but the format for both sections was the same. Attendance was mandatory. Following each session, employees completed evaluation forms which were used as a basis on which to begin discussion at the next session. Trainers were from the Center for Interpersonal Development, a loosely knit organization of training facilitators.

MEASURES

A paper-and-pencil instrument that assesses three noncommunication and 11 communication variables was used to measure changes in perceptions of communication behavior in work teams after training concerned with these specific behaviors. The instrument assesses perceived trust in superior, the degree to which the respondent feels the superior has influence over him, and respondent's mobility aspirations. Noncommunication factors have been shown to impact organizational communications (Cohen 1958; Friedlander 1970; Mellinger 1956; O'Reilly and Roberts 1974; Read 1962).

Communication facets assessed were perceptions about desire for inter-action, directionality of information flow (upward, downward, lateral), accuracy of information flow, modality use (written, face-to-face, phone), summarization of information, perceptions about the amount of information passed, amount deliberately withheld, amount of information changed, overload, and general satisfaction with communication in the organization. These facets of perceived organizational communication have been shown to be relatively independent of one another (Roberts and O'Reilly 1974).

A variable closely associated with communication in previous studies and discussions (Lawler et al. 1968; Likert 1967) and one which should be influenced by organizational change efforts is job satisfaction. Consequently, job satisfaction was assessed on five dimensions: satisfaction with work, coworkers, pay, promotional opportunities, and supervision, using the Cornell Job Description Index (Smith et al. 1969). Overall satisfaction was measured, using the GM Faces Scale (Kunin 1955). Both measures show reasonable convergent and discriminant validity.

Finally, a number of questions were asked about employee's perceptions about their opportunities to try new things and generally to be more autonomous. These questions were drawn from the creativity and responsi-bility scales of the Minnesota Satisfaction Questionnaire (University of Minnesota 1966, 1967), another instrument which has undergone con-siderable development.

The pretest groups completed the instruments the day prior to the beginning of training. Posttest measures were taken four weeks after the training was completed.

RESULTS

A series of two-way analyses of variance showed that pretesting subjects did not substantially influence their posttest results. Results of t tests indicated that there were also no significant differences between experimental and control groups in such demographic characteristics as sex and age. (Job functions were approximately equally distributed across the four groups.) The group subjected to training was significantly lower in tenure than the control group.

Table 21-1 summarizes the significant results of the two-by-two analyses of variance (training and no training by pre- and posttest) for data concerned with communication, job satisfaction, and opportunities to be more innova-tive. Of the 3 noncommunication and 11 communication variables on the communication questionnaire, only 2 (desire for interaction and perceptions about information overload) were significantly altered by the training. Three

TABLE 21-1

SUMMARY OF SIGNIFICANT RESULTS OF TRAINING INFLUENCES
(N = 88) OF ANALYSIS OF VARIANCE FOR
DATA ON COMMUNICATION, JOB SATISFACTION, AND
OPPORTUNITY FOR INNOVATIVENESS FOR
TRAINED AND NONTRAINED GROUPS

	Groups			
Variables	Trained (TG)		Nontrained (NTG)	F-Ratio
Communication instrument				
Desire to interact with:				
All others (sum of three below)	TG	>	NTG	5.49**
Subordinates	TG	>	NTG	3.98**
Peers	TG	>	NTG	8.39*
Superiors		—		
Perceived information overload	TG	<	NTG	4.29**
Job satisfaction				
Satisfaction with work	TG	>	NTG	8.32*
Satisfaction with pay	TG	>	NTG	8.93*
Satisfaction with co-workers	TG	>	NTG	11.11*
Overall satisfaction	TG	>	NTG	7.71*
Opportunity for innovativeness				
To try new ideas	TG	>	NTG	4.21**
To try something different	TG	>	NTG	4.87**
To try own work methods	TG	>	NTG	4.63**
To be responsible for planning own work	TG	>	NTG	12.94**
To make own decisions	TG	>	NTG	10.57**
Freedom to use own judgment	TG	>	NTG	8.03**
More job responsibility	TG	>	NTG	4.83**

*$p < .05$
**$p < .01$

questions were concerned with desire for greater interaction (with superiors, subordinates, and peers). Desire for interaction with subordinates and peers appeared to contribute more to the significance level for the combined three than did the desire for interaction with superiors (which was not itself significant). After training, participants perceived that there was a general reduction of information overload.

Satisfaction with work, pay, coworkers, and overall job satisfaction improved significantly for employees who had been in the training program, but not for the control group. Finally, training improved emergency room personnel's perceptions about their opportunities to try new ideas, different things, and their own work methods. They also believed they were more responsible for planning and doing their own work and were allowed to make more of their own decisions.

DISCUSSION

It was somewhat surprising to find in this study so few changes in perceptions of organizational communication relative to changes in job satisfaction and perceived opportunities for innovativeness after a short intervention designed to bring about changes in all of these areas. Perhaps perceptions about communication are more firmly ingrained in employees and less changeable than their affective responses toward their jobs or their perceptions that they can broaden their own activities. Communication, even though measured perceptually, may be more a function of organizational structure than individual affect, that is, it may be more tied to the objective situation.

The training participants did not change on any variable relevant to their supervisors (trust, influence, desire for interaction with him or her, or upward directionality of information flow). This was probably because supervisors were not included in training and strongly argues for such inclusion, particularly in interventions designed to alter interactions with superiors. The posttraining experience is relevant here. Even though a separate meeting was held with all supervisors and trainers to explain the program, supervisors were generally not prepared to accept and promote the new attitudes and behaviors exhibited by the staff after training.

While some of the communication changes which occurred after training are encouraging (such as the perception that one is less overloaded with information), it is strange that these effects did not generalize to improved overall satisfaction with communication. The largest changes were in desire to interact with colleagues. This is understandable since one training goal focused on teamwork. However, if these desires for increased interaction are to persist, the organization must obviously make it possible for them to find expression. Follow-up measures, such as establishing employee action councils, might insure such implementation but did not occur in this organization. Too frequently organizational constraints prevent change in communication variables. An example concerned communication modality use. This may not have changed simply because it may not be possible to engage in more face-to-face or written information transmission after training in an organization in which standardized patient records are an important part of the intelligence system.

Job satisfaction changes after training may reflect the Hawthorne effect.

Increased satisfaction with coworkers and increased desire for interaction are understandable. Yet, members of the trained groups also reported higher satisfaction with pay. This leads to speculation that the changes in satisfaction could have resulted from the increased attention paid to the trained groups and their problems rather than to substantive alterations in their skills or work. A positive assessment of this possibility would require another measurement of job satisfaction several months after training.

Finally, the results suggest that the trained employees are significantly more optimistic about their opportunities to make a number of changes in their jobs. The training provided the catalyst for the affective change. This is clear. The lack of results for changes in communication, however, suggests that substantive changes which will permit innovations and teamwork to occur *must* be made by the organization.

IMPLICATIONS FOR NURSING

The evidence here indicates some success at changing attitudes through training but also suggests that respondents may not be able to change their behavior to reflect new attitudes. The persistence of changed attitudes may fade if substantive changes fail to support the affective ones.

REFERENCES

Blake, R. R., and Mouton, J. S. Breakthrough in organizational development: Part I. *Harvard Business Rev* 42:133–138. Nov. 1964.
Campbell, D. T., and Stanley, J. C. *Experimental and Quasi-Experimental Designs for Research,* Chicago, Rand, McNally and Co., 1963.
Campbell, J. P., and Dunnette, M. D. Effectiveness of T-group experiences in managerial training and development. *Psychol Bull* 70:73–104, Aug. 1968.
Campbell, J. P., and others. *Managerial Behavior, Performance, and Effectiveness,* New York, McGraw-Hill Book Co., 1970.
Cohen, A. R. Upward communication in experimentally created hierarchies. *Hum Relations* 11(1):41–53, 1958.
Cohen, A., and others. Experiments in organizational embeddedness. *Admin Sci Q* 14:208–221, 1969.
Friedlander, Frank. The primacy of trust as a facilitator of further group accomplishment. *J Appl Behav Sci* 6:387–400. Oct. 1970.
Kunin, T. The construction of a new type of attitude measure. *Personnel Psychol* 8:65–77, 1955.
Lawler, E. E. ed., and others. Managers' attitudes toward interaction episodes. *J Appl Psychol* 52:432–439, 1968.
Likert, Rensis. *The Human Organization.* New York, McGraw-Hill Book Co., 1967.
Mellinger, G. Interpersonal trust as a factor in communication, *J Abnorm Soc Psychol* 52:304–309, May, 1956.

Morton, R., and Bass, B. The organizational training laboratory, *J Am Soc Training Directors* 18:2–5, 1964.
O'Reilly, C. A., and Roberts, K. H. Information filtration in organizations: Three experiments. *Organizational Behav Hum Performance* 11:253–265. Apr. 1974.
Read, W. H. Upward communication in industrial hierarchies. *Hum Rel* 15:3–15, Feb. 1962.
Roberts, K. H., and O'Reilly, C. A. Measuring organizational communication. *J Applied Psychol* 59:321–326. June 1974.
Smith, P. C., and others. *The Measurement of Satisfaction in Work and Retirement.* Chicago, Rand-McNally and Co., 1969.
University of Minnesota, Industrial Relations Center. *Seven Years of Research on Work Adjustment,* by Ellen Betz and others. (Minnesota Studies in Vocational Rehabilitation: 20) Minneapolis, Univerity of Minnesota, 1966.
——— *Manual for the Minnesota Satisfaction Questionnaire,* by D. Weiss and others. (Minnesota Studies in Vocational Rehabilitation: 22) Minneapolis, University of Minnesota, 1967.

IV

A Contingency Approach
to Organizational
Change: Managerial
Actions and
Psychological Changes
Where Relevant

Introduction

This section describes the Hospital Internal Communications (HIC) Project, which encompassed nearly 40 different efforts at improving management in ten hospitals. In the course of the evaluation research on the project, data emerged on the two different and basic approaches to organizational improvement described in Parts II and III. One, "managerial action," emphasizes an authoritative approach to eliminating objective problems in the organization's structure and technology. The other emphasizes psychological change, learning in individuals, and improvement in interpersonal relations. As seen by the psychologist, these are "shallow" or "deep" change efforts, respectively. From the evaluation research, it became clear that the different shallow and deep interventions were being used in very different situations—in what came to be termed "action" and "understanding" systems.

ACTION AND UNDERSTANDING SYSTEMS

The psychologically shallow interventions were used to improve the procedures, structures, and technologies in action systems. These are characterized by a simple task, requiring relatively little information processing, and by an external management control system which emphasizes formal organizational structures and hierarchical controls. These are often managed by people who are somewhat authoritarian in outlook. In this kind of action system, the critical elements making the system work are procedures, structures, and technologies. Thus, it comes as no surprise that psychologically shallow interventions, i.e., managerial actions, such as the implementation of operations research or structural change, are often used and are often effective.

The psychologically deep interventions were used to change psychological characteristics in understanding systems. Such systems are characterized by complex tasks and by the internal controls possessed by professionals. Informal relations and other interpersonal psychological characteristics are the key organizational elements, not formal structures. Individuals are sensitive to these psychological elements and are open to new information.

Given the critical nature of these psychological characteristics in understanding systems, it is no wonder that OD and various psychological approaches are used and are relatively effective in creating change and improvement.

Those familiar with different medical specialities will recognize the close correspondence between what we call action and understanding systems and the practice of, respectively, surgery and internal medicine. As we shall see below (in Chapter 26), surgery provides an excellent example of an action system, and internal medicine, an understanding system. Surgery is relatively simple, and surgeons organize their wards in a hierarchical fashion, and they are often relatively authoritarian in attitude. Internists are faced with a more complex task requiring understanding, and, on the wards, they collaborate in a relatively egalitarian and informal fashion. They are also open to new information and sensitive about psychological matters.

Thus, it is no surprise that action-oriented interventions, managerial actions changing procedures and structures were found to improve surgical efficiency (surgical length of stay), while understanding-oriented interventions (i.e., discussion groups, sensitivity training, and survey feedback meetings) were found to improve efficiency in internal medicine. Here is evidence that different kinds of organizational settings require different approaches to change.

Hospitals in Charge of the Interventions

The account of the HIC Project also provides some suggestions for dealing with the issue of relative client power vis-à-vis an OD consultant. The HIC Project was successful, despite the physicians' high potential power in the hospital setting, because hospital staff were invited to take direct charge of the intervention. They did not merely participate; they themselves directed teams of college students who gathered a variety of data in the hospitals. Rather than attempting to overcome client resistance by using highly directive interventions in the small group setting as did the change agents at MLK (Chapter 16), the agency sponsoring the project invited the hospital staff members and ensured that they themselves were in charge of the interventions.

Because the intervention was truly nondirective, some of the hospital staff and teams of helpers undertook psychologically deep interventions (e.g., group meetings and discussions, sensitivity training, and interviews on patient anxieties about doctors' rounds). They took an understanding approach to change. Others commissioned psychologically shallow interventions (e.g., operations research studies of the scheduling in the surgical theaters or the flow of medical records). This was an action approach to change. The clients, in other words, selected the depth of intervention which they wished to experience.

A CONTINGENCY APPROACH TO CHANGE

Free client choice was clearly critical to the success of the HIC Project. The interventionist often uses one or the other of these two approaches in the belief that it is universally valid. The OD interventionist typically does a diagnosis and finds that the organization needs what he or she has to offer, and this is true also of the expert in one of the action approaches to change. In the HIC Project, both kinds of help were offered, and the clients could reject one to accept the other, or vice versa. Thus, the complete control of the client allowed a contingency approach to organizational change to develop. Clients saw that action and understanding approaches to change were not being pressed upon them by experts as universal panaceas. The hospital teams had a true choice, and they were able to select the approach that was congruent with their particular subsystem.

The HIC Project and the project successes and failures described in Part II together provide some evidence on the factors that seem to determine the success of OD efforts in health care organizations (see Table IV–1). OD or psychologically oriented (deep) change efforts seem to work if the target is a congruent—an understanding system—and the ratio of the change consultant power to physician power is high, as in the MLK study. Where these conditions do not obtain, alterations must be made in one or both factors. Margulies' intervention in a health maintenance organization (Chapter 18) used a more shallow OD intervention, survey feedback. This was more congruent with the relatively bureaucratic setting, and it was more acceptable to clients than a deep intervention. The HIC Project did not try to overcome physician resistance; it dispensed with outside expert consultants and harnessed the physicians' high power in the service of changing themselves.

READINGS ON THE HIC PROJECT

The first reading in this section (Chapter 22) provides a brief introductory overview of the HIC Project. The theoretical and research origins and the nature of the sponsorship all contributed to the basic thrust of the project— self-directed efforts by top hospital staff to improve communications. After brief training in data collection methods, these staff members proceeded to study and improve their hospitals.

Table IV-1
Factors Affecting the Success of OD: Intervention-Target Congruence and Consultant-Target Power

OD Study	OD Psychological Change Efforts Successful?	Depth of Intervention	Target an Understanding System?	Power of Physicians	Power of Consultant
Community Care Teams (MLK Study— Chapter 16)	Yes? (Perhaps only short term)	Deep	Yes, very high within teams	Low: Dependent on team; contract with organization	High: Small group (team) is target
Health Maintenance Organization (Margulies— Chapter 18)	Yes?	In between (surveys)	Yes? Comprehensive care (but community factors not important)	Medium: Dependent on contract with organization	Low? Organization or major, structured sub-systems as target
Hospital Internal Medicine Depts. (HIC— Chapters 22–24)	Yes	Deep	Yes—medical wards	High: Independently organized	Low: Organization or major, structured sub-systems as target
Medical Center (Weisbord study— Chapter 15)	No	Deep	Perhaps, but not between research teams	High: Organization dependent on research money acquired by researchers	Low: Organization or major, structured sub-systems as target

Chapter 23 provides some views of the HIC Project from within—from the administrators, nurses, and physicians who learned how to study and improve their organizations and then used either action or understanding approaches in those change efforts. The first part of the chapter describes the project activities at Lewisham Hospital, while the second and third parts describe some of the activities at Edgware and the London Hospitals. The excerpts were selected to illustrate some of the variety of techniques and approaches used. The first two hospitals were subsequently shown by evaluation research to have improved both medical and surgical lengths of stay, while the third improved surgical stays.

Chapter 24 reports a systematic evaluation of the effects of the project on the management of the participating hospitals, including length of stay. The evaluation uses a systematic, thirteen-year multiple time-series design. Change or improvement scores from the length-of-stay data are then used to show how managerial-action and psychological change occurred in the project hospitals.

The final reading (Chapter 25) shows how the concepts of action and understanding systems play a crucial role in organizational change. Most efforts at organizational improvement take either one or the other approach to change, not both. The HIC Project was an exception in that it provided both action and understanding orientations to change and allowed free client choice. This allowed congruent forms of help to be given. Since understanding and action approaches work in different situations, a contingency approach to organizational change seems required. There are no panaceas, but rather appropriate techniques for each case.

22 | The Hospital Internal Communications (HIC) Project

George F. Wieland

The Hospital Internal Communications (HIC) Project was initiated by Professor R. W. Revans to improve communication in ten London-area hospitals. The origins of the HIC Project lay in part in Revans' views of management and management education (Revans 1965, 1966). Management, as Revans sees it, is problem solving, and important to the process of problem solving is the acquisition of knowledge, in order to make decisions, and to evaluate the results of decisions. Management, furthermore, is best learned by doing, not by reading books or attending lectures, but by collecting information oneself, and by making decisions, acting on them, and evaluating the results.

LEARNING BY DOING OR SELF-HELP ORGANIZATIONAL CHANGE

Revans had earlier attempted to put his ideas into practice in a number of settings. When he was brought in to help the palm-oil industry in Nigeria, for example, he refused to give expert advice. Instead, he helped the local managers learn from one another by visiting one another's mills, discussing problems and solutions, and setting up practical trials and evaluations. Not only did the managers learn about their mills, they learned about their own personal methods and approaches to particular problems. Each helped the others learn about their respective shortcomings as well as how better to manage their little organizations. In this combination of the objective and subjective, and the structural and psychological, the Nigerian project foreshadowed the findings of the HIC evaluation study reported below.

After the Nigerian project, Revans also sparked off a similar effort at self-help organizational change in the U.S. Two communications professors at the University of Wisconsin helped top managers from six Milwaukee area firms to study and to solve problems in one another's firms (see Revans 1976, pp. 170–172). Finally, contemporaneously with the HIC Project, Revans was the catalyst for a self-help project in which senior managers from five very large Belgian firms used interviews and surveys to study and deal with problems in one another's firms (see Revans 1971, 1976, pp. 172–173).

RESEARCH ORIGINS OF THE PROJECT

The antecedents of the HIC Project are also to be found in Revans' research as well as in his views on management and organizations. Extensive research (Revans 1958) in the nationalized coal industry suggested that absenteeism, accident rates, and industrial disputes were related to quality of supervision and management. This work was extended into hospitals. Revans (1964) found that hospitals as a whole (i.e., across departments) tended to be relatively efficient or inefficient in terms of the average length of stay for the different kinds of patients. Using a sample of fifteen hospitals, he showed that the attitudes of supervisory nurses were significantly related to the average length of stay of medical patients. Specifically, he measured supervisors' attitudes on (1) whether there was time to instruct subordinates despite the pressures of ward duties, (2) whether conferences of the ward team were worthwhile, (3) whether it was necessary to explain instructions received from higher in the hierarchy, and (4) whether they felt high work standards could be set for subordinates without becoming disliked. If supervisory nurses felt these activities were feasible or worthwhile, then the hospital was more efficient in processing medical patients.

Further analysis by Revans seemed to implicate organizational functioning as a whole, from the top down. Poor interpersonal relations between supervisory nurses and the director of nursing, and also between supervisory nurses and physicians, seemed to be associated with impaired efficiency of hospitals. These findings led Revans to visualize the hospital as a learning system, with communications being vital for effective management.

In concluding his report of the hospital research, Revans suggested how hospitals could become "autotherapeutic organisms": "The hospitals themselves, personified by their administrators, their doctors and their nurses . . . must learn to conduct surveys, to interpret their findings, to seek the structure of the problems so revealed and to build the programs of participation by which these problems may be ameliorated" (Revans 1964, p. 98).

THE HIC PROJECT

This view led directly to the creation of the HIC Project. An official of The King's Fund Hospital Centre became interested in Revans' findings and organized a series of conferences between Revans and members of some of the hospitals in contact with the organization, with the hope that they might volunteer to participate in a project to make use of Revans' findings. The Department of Health and Social Security was also aware of Revans' research findings, and through participation at the conferences, also attempted to encourage volunteers to join a project. An important point agreed upon in these conferences was that the hospitals themselves would be in charge of the project and its direction, once they joined. Of some 30 hospitals expressing interest, 10 finally committed themselves to undertaking some experimental efforts along the lines worked out jointly in the meetings. The project was then funded by a research grant to Guy's Hospital Medical School.

THE HOSPITAL TEAMS

Probably the most important element in the HIC Project was the very active part played by hospital staff. Six of the most senior hospital staff (two each from administration, medicine, and nursing) made up the hospital team for each hospital. The three senior members of this team—usually a group secretary (administrator of a group of hospitals), a matron (director of nursing), and a consultant (senior hospital doctor)—attended a three-day residential course in which they were introduced to the project and presented with some important social science concepts and research findings. Their job was to support, as a "supporting team," the junior, operational members of the hospital team, usually a deputy group secretary or hospital secretary, a deputy matron or assistant matron, and another consultant or a registrar (junior doctor). This "operational team" attended a month-long residential course in which principles of group dynamics, organizational functioning, and interpersonal communications were covered.

A most important part of the month-long course included lectures and discussions on the construction and use of interviews and questionnaires and other methods of data collection, on data analysis, and on report writing. One whole week of the course was then spent entirely in "learning by doing," going into another team's hospital and doing a study.

After returning to their jobs, the teams started to plan a project in their own hospitals. Following Revans' approach to learning, the teams were encouraged to choose for themselves the topic to be studied and the methods to be used, and they tried to carry out as much of the work as they could themselves.

The Central Team

The work of assisting and facilitating project activity in the various hospitals, and the work of coordinating the overall HIC project, fell to a central team composed of two social science or management graduates, a nurse, and an expert in training. For the most part, these facilitators were hired after the basic orientation of the HIC project was set and even after some of the initial training had been carried out. In addition, about a dozen different students, taking university courses in the social sciences, were hired over the course of the last two years of the project. They spent up to six months attached to a hospital team, often residing in the hospital as they carried out project tasks for their respective teams.

The central team assisted the hospital teams upon request, but most of this assistance came at the middle stages of projects, in administering questionnaires and analyzing data. Much of the earlier planning stages, and the later stages of feeding back and discussing findings with those studied, fell to the hospital teams. Implementation of suggestions for action flowing out of the projects was usually done without any assistance from central team members. In all their work, the central team attempted to be nondirective and to avoid controlling the activities of hospital team members, as had been agreed upon in the planning conferences.

Hospital Projects

Nearly 40 different projects (employing surveys, observational studies, records analyses, etc.) were carried out in the ten hospitals (see Table 22-1). In

TABLE 22-1
Projects or Surveys in the HIC Project

Project Number	Nature of Project	Number of Staff Involved as Respondents or Objects of Observations
1	Survey of nurse attitudes	22
2	Study of the emergency department	43
3	Evaluation of internal management sources	53
4	Study of hospital corridor traffic	500
5	Conferences on moving to a new building	
6	Decentralization of nursing administration	
7	Study of coordination between supplies and engineering departments	18
8	Study of nurse preferences on duty schedules	432
9	Study of staffing, work loads, ward routines	60

TABLE 22–1, *continued*

10	Open-ended, "free" interview of hospital staff	141
11	Study of medical records department	
12	Study of journeys, admissions and discharges	
13	Emergency admissions project	139
14	Visiting hours project	141
15	Survey of ward sisters' (senior head nurses') attitudes	17
16	Survey of junior doctor attitudes	26
17	Survey of consultant attitudes	27
18	"Ease-of-contact" survey	400
19	Study of staff turnover in medical records department	43
20	Survey of staff attitudes on hospital amenities and welfare	14
21	Study of staff attitudes towards catering facilities	680
22	Study of contact between a pediatric ward and other departments	50
23	Study of contact between a "subnormal" ward and other departments	
24	Study of contacts between two wards and other departments (in a satellite hospital)	39
25	Evaluation of the emergency department	33
26	Follow-up study on x-ray, medical records and out-patient departments	
27	Survey of nurse attitudes	354
28	Survey of patient attitudes to drugs, etc.	96
29	Hospital management committees and senior hospital officer survey	11
30	Pilot survey of a pediatric and medical ward	64
31	Study of medical social work	
32	Project "paper chase"—examination of hospital forms and paperwork	114
33	Inquiry into the utilization of operating rooms	60
34	Student nurse counselling	50
35	Student nurse turnover survey	39
36	Medical ward observation study	
37	Study of patient anxieties on a medical ward	20
38	Attitude survey about housekeeping	135

a number of cases, several hundred staff members, covering every major group in the hospital, were surveyed, while in other cases, only a dozen or so key staff participated. The aims were sometimes quite broad, for example, to learn about the concerns of hospital staff, while sometimes the aims were as specific as learning how many nurses were in favor of straight or split shifts. Some collections of data led to a report but no further perceptible actions on the part of the hospital teams, while other projects resulted in administrative actions, or further discussions with respondents and even further related projects.

A final important element of the HIC project was a series of interteam meetings planned by the central team to help hospital team members to learn how to run and participate in discussion groups. In addition, hospital team members exchanged information on one another's projects and on general hospital activities.[1]

References

Conway, Mary E. Clinical research: instrument for change. *Journal of Nursing Administration*, 1978, *8*, 12 (December), 27–32.

Horsley, Jo Anne, Crane, Joyce, and Bingle, Janet D. Research utilization as an organizational process. *Journal of Nursing Administration*, 1978, *8*, 7 (July), 4–6.

Revans, Reginald W. *Standard for morale: cause and effect in hospitals.* London: Oxford University Press, 1964.

Revans, Reginald W. *Science and the manager.* London: Macdonald, 1965.

Revans, Reginald W. *The theory of practice in management.* London: Macdonald, 1966.

Revans, Reginald W. *Developing effective managers: a new approach to business education.* New York: Praeger, 1971.

Revans, Reginald W. (Ed.). *Hospitals: communication, choice, and change: The Hospital Internal Communications Project seen from within.* London: Tavistock, 1972.

Revans, Reginald W. *Action learning in hospitals: diagnosis and therapy.* London: McGraw-Hill, 1976.

St. Luke's Hospital Maternity Research Project Committee. Researchers? Of Course! *Journal of Nursing Administration*, 1975, *5*, 6 (November–December), 7–9.

Stevenson, Joanne S. Developing staff research potential, part 2: planning and implementation of studies. *Journal of Nursing Administration*, 1978, *8*, 6 (June), 8–12.

Wieland, George F., and Leigh, Hilary (Eds.). *Changing hospitals: A report on the Hospital Internal Communications Project.* London: Tavistock, 1971.

Note

1. For further details on the HIC Project, see Wieland and Leigh (1971) and Revans (1972). Revans' advocacy of learning by doing, or self-help improvement of management and organizations, was quite innovative for its time. However, especially among nurses, there has been a growing awareness of the efficacy of this approach in improving work behavior. See, for example, Conway (1978), Stevenson (1978), Horsley et al. (1978), and St. Luke's Hospital Maternity Research Project Committee (1975).

23 | Lewisham, Edgware, and The London Hospitals

I: LEWISHAM HOSPITAL
Marjorie Bell and Allan J. Brooking

The hospital is an acute hospital with 570 beds, an 87 per cent occupancy, and out-patient attendances numbering 129,000 each year.

The H.I.C. team concerned with the Project has remained the same except for two changes in the operational team. The original administrative member moved to a new post and was replaced in the team by his successor. Another administrative member joined when his department was being studied.

It would be fair to say that senior staff in the hospital were aware of the general problem of communication in management before the Project started. Although there have been no significant problems arising from the variety of nationalities of staff employed, the very presence of so many nurses from overseas has made the matron[1] very concerned that they should feel able to approach her about their problems. The hospital has also had occasional disputes, seemingly over catering arrangements but, in fact, partly over communication problems.

When the *Industrial Welfare Society* were seeking a hospital to carry out a short survey of communications in hospitals in the autumn of 1962, our hospital, therefore, volunteered. Their short report indicated that communications were not as good as they might have been, though probably no worse than in the majority of hospitals. The result of the survey was some discussion of the problem, but no concrete proposals as to how to improve the arrangements. Such a basically obvious factor as good communication required, it was felt, simply a greater determination by senior staff to spread adequate information downwards. The relationships at the top level were good, but it was decided that the only further formal effort needed to improve communication was a hospital magazine. This started in 1963 and, except for the

Reprinted by kind permission of King Edward's Hospital Fund for London.

matron's meeting with ward sisters, remained the chief means of communicating with staff generally, although it was not edited by the administrative staff, but by staff in the group laboratory. They produced a lively magazine, free from too much 'chief officer slant', but starting as a quarterly, it gradually became more intermittent.

JOINING THE PROJECT

The results of the IWS investigation, coupled with the general awareness of the need to improve the standard of hospital management, meant that the first letter about the H.I.C. Project aroused considerable interest. It offered not merely investigation of management problems in communication, but a 'do-it-yourself' exercise to put matters right.

At that time, as indeed throughout the Project to the present time, the problem had not been to recognize the need for good communication, but to judge whether the time and energy spent in 'improving' communication by means of more discussions, newsletters, conferences, and so on, is repaid by increased efficiency or, alternatively, to judge whether the same time and energy spent in another way would improve efficiency more. All the senior staff who attended the opening meetings in the autumn of 1964 were impressed by Professor Revans' exposition of the problem, but all felt the need for 'concrete' techniques for overcoming the difficulties outlined.

By spring 1965, having attended a series of meetings, we were sufficiently impressed with the statistical evidence and obvious belief in the Project to agree to send staff on an appreciation course, and on a month's course to learn techniques to deal with this problem of communication. A major difficulty, however, arose over the medical representation. We had foreseen this problem and, partly as a result of participating hospitals' comments on the position, the training course had been reduced from three months to one month. Nevertheless, the problem remained that no staff other than consultants were sufficiently permanent to give the necessary continuity to the project, and no consultants felt able to devote time to a month's course or to the investigations which were to follow, particularly as the latter had been estimated to take up to two days each week.

THE COURSES

The three-day appreciation course was a disappointment. It was attended by the supporting-team members. All went with the hope of gaining greater insight into the techniques likely to be used. Instead, they felt that they received simply further expositions of the problems without getting to grips with the possible means of their solution. It was now considered, even more strongly than before, that the key to success lay in the techniques to be taught in the month's course in September 1965.

The administrative and nursing members were chosen for the month's course and, although the nurse fell ill and her place was taken by another, this mattered less than the continuing failure to find a medical member. The chairman of the group medical advisory committee had agreed to attend for two days a week if none of his colleagues were willing to go, and indeed did so during the first week. Then, a senior surgeon, who hitherto had not been approached concerning the Project because of his known pressure of work, expressed an interest. After being given the background, he volunteered to attend as much as he could of the remaining two and a half weeks of the course. His subsequent attendance meant that a senior clinician was closely involved with the detail of the Project, although his very involvement in clinical work was to make it increasingly difficult for him to devote time to the Project in the following two years.

The techniques learnt were chiefly concerned with interviewing, conduct of discussion groups, the compilation of questionnaires and the evaluation both of the results of questionnaires and of statistics generally. There was considerable discussion of problems of human behaviour in the work situation and particularly of what constituted 'morale' in a hospital. Throughout ran the thread of the need for good communication up, down, and sideways, so that staff receive the information to enable them to do their jobs effectively and to feel secure in them. Those who attended returned feeling that they had some insight into the techniques of the social scientist, but not that they themselves were capable of doing more than conducting interviews and discussions.

THE ATTITUDE SURVEY

A week after the month's course finished, the three supporting members met the three operational members to decide on the future course of action.

The operational members felt strongly that any attempt to localize communication problems would mean that the senior staff would simply be acting from their own previous knowledge of the situation in the hospital, which might be completely wrong. It was suggested that a survey of the whole hospital by means of questionnaires to, and group discussions with, a representative sample of staff was necessary to identify the communication problems.

In discussion, this suggestion quickly evolved into interviews with staff to obtain their views, not merely on communication problems, but on general problems in the hospital, in order to make an assessment of morale which could then be compared with morale in three years' time by means of a similar survey. Such interviews would need to be carried out by outside interviewers, and the advice of the central team was sought.

Further discussion with the central team led us to decide that free individual interviews were needed so that staff could speak their mind without any guidance from the interviewer. This, in turn, meant not only outside help such as that which could be obtained from another hospital, but expert help from social science interviewers. This was quickly forthcoming, and, in December 1965, three interviewers spent three weeks conducting free interviews with nearly 150 staff of all grades.

Subsequent discussion of the methods used revealed three significant errors. First, the sample chosen, although for the most part at random, contained more senior staff than it should, as the lists were produced at a time when we were discussing the possibility of the interview work being cut down by having individual interviews only for heads of departments and above. In point of fact, the sample was large enough for the weighting of senior staff not to be particularly important. Secondly, the method of collecting the information in long-hand from free interviews meant that the chances of being able to carry out a repeat survey after three years were small.

The third problem also concerned the method of collecting data and was of much greater significance. In order to preserve anonymity, the longhand notes of the interviewers could only be placed in the categories agreed between central and local teams by the interviewers themselves. This, coupled with problems of reclassification and typing the vast volume of information, meant that the survey results were not available until mid-summer 1966.

This delay in obtaining results meant that the project went cold for nearly six months and the interest of the staff began to wane. Nor, when the team saw the results, were they particularly impressed. No dramatic new areas for investigation arose and the most significant points seemed to be that:

(i) human relationships and communication were the areas which gave most ground for criticism throughout the hospital;

(ii) most criticism about the service departments concerned the medical records, domestic, catering, and pathology departments. There was a considerable amount of comment about nursing staff problems because nurses formed a high proportion of those interereviewed, but the few junior medical staff interviewed produced an inordinate amount of comment;

(iii) The system for requisitioning for minor maintenance and supplies was criticized either directly or by implication.

As the summer holidays were just about to start, the team decided to feed back to each departmental head the comments concerning that department, together with the general section on human relationships and communication which affected everyone. This distribution was done, and meetings were held with all ward sisters and heads of departments at which the supporting-team members asked them to study the documents carefully, to discuss them with their staff in as objective a way as possible, and to take such action as they considered necessary to correct any faults implied by the criticisms. It was explained that after a few weeks, a project-team member would follow up to discuss matters with them but if, in the meantime, they required any further help, the project-team members would gladly give it.

NURSING STAFF

The supporting-nurse member of the team followed up the initial introduction of the document by meetings with sisters to discuss the comments, and then started a series of meetings with other nursing staff—something which had never been done before. Her comments give an indication of the way these meetings went.

'When I talked this over with the sisters, they were extremely good, they realized that some of the criticisms made were justified and were due to perhaps their being very busy or not spending that little time with the student nurses that they might have done. They felt that there were a number of ways in which they could help to make the staff feel happier about these things. But they also felt that some of the things the student nurses and the staff nurses had said were not justified, and perhaps they did not quite understand. But one of the chief things that was brought up by the nursing staff was that the matron had meetings with the sisters every month, but had no meetings with the rest of the nursing staff; and I must confess that this was perfectly true. It was something that I had decided many, many times I ought to, but I hadn't done, and I felt very guilty indeed when I read that the nurses realized as well as I did that this was something that should take place.

'Now, I discussed this with the sisters and said, "You know, it is very difficult getting all the nursing staff together to talk to me and discuss things *en masse*. So if I can arrange to have two meetings on two days running, will you release half your staff one day and half the next day, so that everybody gets an opportunity of coming?" We decided that this could be done, and, about a fortnight after my meeting with the sisters, I asked all the nursing staff to attend these meetings.

'I was amazed at the number, even the night nurses (I had it at 9 o'clock in the morning so that the night nurses could come), a very large attendance. I talked to them of the attitude survey, and I went through it with them. I tried, as best I could, to explain the reasons for these criticisms. I agreed that sometimes I was a little impatient with the sick staff, but I explained why. I said, "Very often, you know, there are a number of nurses who have a day off sick every week, and perhaps they are out on Wednesday, they come in on Thursday, and say, 'Sorry I was out yesterday, but I was ill all day', when somebody else has seen them shopping in the supermarket."

'Everyone agreed that I had never been impatient with someone who was ill in the nurses' sick bay. They have also said they didn't like being moved from one ward to another, and I pointed out again the reason why they were moved: if two nurses went sick in one ward, there is still the same number of patients to be looked after, and somebody has to look after them. I felt at the end of that meeting that, perhaps, I got a little way with them.

'Another thing they brought up was social life. "Why can't we have more social life?" I said, "You can have more social life, you can have just as much social life as you like, but you must do something about it." I explained, "Not very long ago, only a year or two, I arranged for a dramatic society to give plays in the hospital and on the day the party arrived to give their play, there were about three people in the recreation room, and I and my staff were running round the nurses' home begging people to come, so it was decided that it wasn't wanted, but if you want it, you can have it. I will help you in any way I can, but you must do something about it yourselves." And I have found since then that they have done more about it. I have had more nurses coming to say, "I have a 21st birthday next week, may I have a party?" And we have supplied refreshments, or they have come and asked for equipment. They put on a play at Christmas time which they haven't done for a number of years, and I do feel that, in a sense, it is doing quite a lot of good to do things for themselves.

'Then, I have tried to keep up the meetings with the nursing staff. I think this is very important indeed. I have met them every other month since the survey. About a year afterwards, I talked at both meetings, for quite a long time and then asked, "Do you really think that these meetings that you asked for are worth while?" And there was silence just for a second or two and I felt very despondent and thought "No", and then one nurse said, "Well, I think they're very worth while." Then there was a murmur of assent among the rest of them, and I said, "I don't want these meetings to be a lecture and I don't want to come here and just talk to you while you sit here and listen. This meeting has got to be a two-way traffic. When I come I want to discuss things with you, to criticize, but to suggest as well. It is not going to help any of you at all for me to just come and talk to you. I can come along to the classroom and do that, but I want us all to discuss things and to hear your suggestions." And immediately there were quite a number, some of them minor and some very worthwhile points. We have opened a new operating theatre and one of the nurses said to me, "Do you know there is no bell in the recovery room to summon the anaesthetist?" I didn't know, and I was very pleased to know and to be able to do something about it, and said so. Later, I made a point of telling the nurse who put the suggestion forward that it was now done.'

Medical Records

One department which came in for much criticism from the nurses was the medical records department, a very busy and devoted group of staff who suffered from overwork and sickness, and who were characterized by high turnover.

They had their criticisms too; they mentioned the problems created by medical staff who cancelled clinics at short notice or altered timing of appointments, thereby causing 600 letters to be sent out altering appointments, or those consultants who took case notes away—and then complained bitterly because the 'records staff has lost them'. These points were made in a discussion with the supporting-medical member of the H.I.C. team, who took them to a full meeting of the medical staff committee.

Feedback from the records department in autumn 1967 indicated that matters were much improved. Nevertheless, since the meetings with the records staff a year before, the team mounted, with the help of the central team, studies into admission and discharge procedures, messenger services, and the problems of missing case notes. These statistical assessments of the current situation produced a number of surprises, not least the fact that admission procedures were generally satisfactory, whereas the timing of discharges and the delays in sending out notes to the patients' general practitioners were often unsatisfactory. These matters were followed up with the staff concerned, to produce a system which, it is hoped, will be generally more satisfactory.

It also became clear that the money spent on agency staff, to relieve staff shortage in the department, would be better spent on employing junior clerical trainees who could be trained in all aspects of the department's work. This was done.

Requisitioning Procedures

During 1967, requisitioning both for supplies and maintenance was completely reorganized. Centralization of stores has taken place, with a determined effort to give all users a complete catalogue of what is available. The old maintenance requisitions have also been redesigned to give a better follow-up of uncompleted jobs. By the time of the ward sisters' and heads of departments' meeting in September 1967, there were 'no complaints'.

General Communications

Four developments, besides matron's meetings with her nursing staff, are:
1. bi-monthly meetings of heads of departments and ward sisters' representatives;

2. the intermittent magazine, *Pulse*, has been replaced by a regular monthly *Bulletin of Internal News* under the same editors;
3. a staff suggestions scheme;
4. a thriving staff club, perhaps the most significant innovation of all.

The developments certainly seem to add up to much greater flow of information through the organization and a friendlier atmosphere which, unfortunately, is impossible to evaluate. We are currently trying to further this by improving the staff's first introduction to the hospital by means of conducted tours, and a handbook, while making it clear that the most effective introduction which the newcomer gets is from his head of department.

EVALUATION

For those of us closely concerned with the project, evaluation is impossible. A trained social scientist may be able to provide objective means of assessment; the team members can only reckon the time and energy it has cost against what appears to be a 'better atmosphere' in the hospital. Even this may be self-delusion.

In our own personal assessment of our experience of the H.I.C. Project, we make the following comments:
1. The initial decision to conduct the attitude survey was the right one, because it has formed the mainspring for further action.
2. Delay in obtaining the results, though almost unavoidable to preserve anonymity, was nearly disastrous.
3. The original multidisciplinary team has become largely administrative and nursing, with the occasional willing co-operation of the medical members. The working pressures on consultant clinicians seem to make this inevitable.
4. It is impossible to treat the Project as a special study apart from the day-to-day running of the hospital. Therefore those concerned must be chief members of the three staff groups, the matron, secretary, and chairman of the medical staff committee or his equivalent. Even so, it is extremely difficult to maintain momentum.
6. The essential centrality of the subject in general administration has meant that involvement of other staff has been intermittent. The educational value of the Project has, therefore, largely been absorbed by the comparatively few H.I.C. team members.

Initially, the hope that the heads of departments' meetings might be vehicles for the full discussion of management problems was not realized, in that although the heads of departments claimed that they found the meetings 'interesting' the team were disappointed at the lack of contribution from the heads of departments themselves. As an experiment some changes were made:

(a) a rotating chairman was appointed from the departmental heads;

(b) the seating arrangements were made more informal, and

(c) syndicate discussion groups were occasionally used.

It is pleasing to report that following these changes there has been a marked improvement in the usefulness of the meetings and in the content of problems discussed.

II. EDGWARE HOSPITAL. 'TRAFFIC SURVEY'—
A STUDY OF CONGESTION IN THE CORRIDORS
H. S. C. Marsh

The supporting-administrative member initiated this project, because he was disturbed by the amount of traffic in the main hospital corridor, situated in the surgical block. It was often extremely congested, and although the supporting-administrative member felt that some of the crush was due to the layout of the surgical block, he was eager to discover the extent of, and reasons for, the traffic, and also some means of reducing it.

A previous work study report had shown that domestic staff were used to run messages. Perhaps some of the traffic was due to this. The formal network of communication was evidently not working well, and people would go and see the relevant person in order to get things done more quickly. At this stage, the possibility of introducing an efficient messenger service to cope with difficulties in communication was suggested.

The supporting-administrative member called in the central team to help in defining the problem, and to discover the nature and extent of all hospital staff journeys. A central-team student came to work in the hospital, and she was later joined by another student.

The central team and the hospital team decided to run a pilot survey in order to find out what problems would occur when undertaking a survey of traffic throughout the hospital, getting the staff to collect their own data, so that right at the beginning they would be involved. Students and central-team members went to departmental meetings and talked to ward sisters about the objectives of the study. These were: to discover the extent and nature of the traffic; whether this was related to a breakdown in the formal messengering network; if so, to attempt to provide solutions.

THE PILOT SURVEY

While publicity and preparation for the main study were going on, using both formal and informal methods of communication (personal contact and

Reprinted by kind permission of King Edward's Hospital Fund for London.

departmental meetings), a pilot survey was carried out in two wards and three departments. An attempt was made to record on data sheets all journeys made to and from these wards and departments, the reasons for them, and the time spent on them. The data seemed to bear out of the original view that journeys by staff were mainly connected with departments providing clinical services, i.e. pharmacy, X-ray, and the pathological laboratory.

The pilot survey showed also that attempts to get the study publicized were not very successful. Very few doctors knew about the proposed survey and the porters were also unaware of the purpose of the study. The data sheet was tidied up and made more intelligible. It was intended that the staff should record every journey they made and all the callers who arrived at their ward or department.

THE MAIN SURVEY—DATA COLLECTION

More attempts to publicize the study were made. The medical member of the team saw the mess president, the nurse members contacted assistant matrons and ward sisters; the students visited the porters individually to explain the purpose of the study, and central-team members and students spoke at the departmental heads' meeting.

The pilot survey seemed to suggest that benefit might be obtained by concentrating on those areas which involved the largest number of journeys and staff time. The focus of the study was to be on those journeys related to clinical services to patients, thus confining the sample to all wards, and the following departments: pharmacy, X-ray, pathological laboratory, medical records, hospital secretary, and theatre.

The study also included the collection of data, by the central-team students, on existing official messenger systems (e.g., pathological laboratory, porters, postmen) and by the hospital team on the type and size of wards and the staffing of departments. It was hoped that the caller-return sheets would show how much time was spent by ward and departmental staff on either replacing or supporting official messenger systems, by giving figures on the number, nature, and frequency of journeys, the time spent on them, and the type of staff undertaking them, together with some idea of peak journey times in order to help plan a more efficient messenger service.

The data collection was carried out over two weeks, and attended by as much publicity as possible. The response to the survey was almost a hundred per cent in the first week, but, predictably, there was a falling-off in the second week.

DATA ANALYSIS AND INTERPRETATION

A preliminary analysis of data was carried out by the central team, to discover the peak times for all journeys and callers to wards and departments.

The data were also analysed to show the time spent on journeys for each ward and department by each grade of staff. The information was presented in the form of simple histograms or graphs.

Eventually, it was decided that the data collected about ward staff journeys should be discussed by the hospital team with ward sisters, and that relating to departmental journeys with departmental heads. This was done, and the chief pharmacist suggested that the journeys should be represented in the form of density graphs. A density graph constructed later by the chief pharmacist and the operational-administrative member showed an excessive number of journeys to pharmacy. The students, operational-administrative member, and the chief pharmacist continued to analyse the data and present it more comprehensibly using density graphs with frequency of journeys and callers marked, to show up peak periods.

During the next fortnight, the operational-nurse member discussed the data with ward sisters at the sisters' meeting. A team meeting was held, consisting of the departmental heads involved in the survey, sisters' representatives, the central team, and the hospital team. All these groups had considered the data, and all had comments to make upon them. The sisters, noting that the greatest number of callers came between 8.0 a.m. and 9.0 a.m., suggested that one person collecting everything from the wards would be much easier to cope with and that journeys could be saved from the wards to pharmacy if the wards could have a twenty-four hour antibiotic stock. It would be a good idea, they felt, to put a printed slip in patients' medical records to say whether or not they had been X-rayed before. Would it not save time if porters collected X-rays when they collected patients? These and many similar points were discussed and the hospital team decided that they would spend several weeks trying to estimate the need of wards and departments for a 'central porter' for collection and delivery — an idea which had caught everyone's imagination.

At a meeting a few days later, the hospital team drew up an information sheet which was designed to discover more about the type of service required by ward and departmental staff. Membership of this team, now called a 'working party', included the hospital secretary, two ward sisters, and all heads of departments involved in the survey. Each member of the working party made it his responsibility to gather information about collection and delivery times from the staff with whom he was most closely concerned. Within a two-week period, most of these data were collected and analysed.

TENTATIVE IMPROVEMENTS

At this stage, the hospital team decided that it might prove useful to do a dummy run of a messenger service to see what problems came up. The run would involve all areas in the hospital, and would include collecting and delivering specimens, all paperwork, and postal services. The trial run was a great success. The hospital team acted as messengers noting times of collection and delivery as they went along.

Two messengers would be needed to cover the entire hospital, one operating in the surgical block and departments immediately adjacent to it, and the other in the medical block and the remainder of the hospital. The team did two rounds during the day collecting all the messages. Sisters had been asked not to send anyone out on messages on that day, but to leave the collection to team members, and this was done.

The introduction of a messenger service would in some ways affect the present portering system in the hospital and the team felt this should also be considered in relation to a messenger service. The student went back to the original data that had been collected on the portering services, to see those areas which a messenger service could effectively take over. There was a proposal that the two present post porters should be used as messengers, but it was felt that they were too old for such a strenuous job. However, by some reorganization of the gate portering staff (two had retired) certain duties could be transferred from the post porters to the gate porters, thus allowing the required number of hours to be available for the messenger service. The dummy run had demonstrated the need for some form of trolley to carry post, requisitions, and specimens. The student designed a trolley to cope with all such requirements. (This was a modified form of a trolley designed by members of the hospital staff taking part in one of the internal management courses.)

A female messenger has now been appointed for the medical block complex, and it is intended that the existing post porter will cope with the surgical block. The response to the trial run was extremely favourable but much remains to be completed before a comprehensive messenger service, as envisaged by the study, can be introduced.

III: The London Hospital
Michael J. Fairey

The London Hospital is a teaching hospital which also has a district responsibility. It has the largest out-patient department in the country (430,000 clinical attendances annually) and its out-patient load is a little under two per cent of the total out-patient load of England and Wales. The hospital has 717 beds and discharges between 16,500 and 17,500 patients per annum. The bed occupancy overall averages between 91 and 93 per cent on

Reprinted by kind permission of King Edward's Hospital Fund for London.

four days out of every seven in every week of the year. The bed occupancy of the main hospital exceeds 94 per cent.

In addition to the medical school (approximately 470 students) and the dental school (approximately 220 students), the hospital has training schools not only for nurses and physiotherapists, but also for radiographers (both therapeutic and diagnostic), domestic science students, dieticians, and dental surgery assistants, and it participates in training schemes for laboratory technicians, social workers, EEG recordists, and cardiac technicians.

Seven members of the hospital staff participated in the H.I.C. Project. The house governor, the deputy matron, and a consultant psychiatrist took part in the three-day appreciation course; and an assistant matron, a consultant psychiatrist, the lecturer in social medicine, and the deputy house governor took part in the month's training course.

The hospital first became aware of the H.I.C. Project through the King Edward's Hospital Fund for London. It is difficult to say what members of the team expected of the Project, since its purpose was not entirely clear. It might well be, however, that this was because they were not able to attend the two briefing sessions held at the beginning of the Project. The mystery was not noticeably dispelled during the progress of the month's course at Hastings, where a similar confusion was apparent. Members of the team formulated a working hypothesis that the aim of the Project was to instil methods by which to perceive and study problems within a large organization; and that the success of this attempt would be evaluated. In the event, this hypothesis proved to be not too far from the truth.

CHOICE OF A PROJECT

On the team's return from Hastings, one of the medical members was absent from the hospital for a further three months. The remaining three members of the operational team discussed a number of projects and the following were those most seriously considered:

1. *Attitude Survey of a Complete Cross-Section of the Hospital*
   This project was considered to be impracticable because of the size and diversity of the hospital; and the *immediate* practical value to be derived from such a survey did not seem to be commensurate with the work involved.

2. *The Role of One of the Major Service Departments of the Hospital*
   One of the major service departments of the hospital appeared to be suffering, both geographically and socially, some degree of isolation from the hospital. It was considered that a survey of the staff's perception of the department might demonstrate how closer integration might be effected.

3. *Survey of Senior Medical Students' and Junior Medical Staff's Attitudes*

   Though this problem has been extensively studied elsewhere, the team considered that it might be fruitful to study in their own hospital the difference in attitudes towards authority between senior medical students and junior medical staff a year or two years after qualifying. It was considered that the survey of overall attitudes of those within this spectrum might point up factors significant in the change. If this were the case, it might well be that some of these factors could be ameliorated by administrative measures.

4. *Medical Records Department*

   At the time, morale within this department was causing some concern and a survey of the staff might, it was thought, suggest methods by which morale could be improved.

5. *Attitudes of Those Involved with the Emergency Admission of Patients*

   The emergency admission of patients had posed a severe problem for some years and the nursing staff in particular found the continual strain trying and not in the best interests of nurse training. An operational research survey was already in progress and an attitude survey would complement its findings.

These projects were discussed by all the members of the team and with the matron. It was considered that the hospital had sufficient overt problems to make it unnecessary at this stage to look for hidden problems that might emerge in a general attitude survey.

The survey of attitudes of senior medical students and junior medical staff, while perhaps interesting sociologically and capable of suggesting meaningful improvements, was not immediately applicable to any urgent problem facing the hospital at the time.

The major service department had been a source of some apprehension for a number of years. The reduction of its isolation would, undoubtedly, have been of benefit to the organization of the hospital. A number of problems, to some degree based on personal relationships, existed, however, and it was felt that the time was not appropriate to bring these relationships to a crisis.

Morale in the medical records department was a source of much concern and in other circumstances this would have been the survey of choice. The department had, however, been surveyed by a team from another hospital as part of the Hastings course. It was considered inexpedient to repeat a survey within the same department so shortly after the training survey.

On the other hand, a survey covering the whole field of emergency admissions would touch on one of the major problems facing both the medical and the nursing staff. For this reason it was felt that it was this survey which should be pursued, since it would be dealing with a problem of immediate concern to a large section of the hospital. It would be complementary to an existing survey; and the problem surveyed was of considerable importance.

ORGANIZATION OF THE EMERGENCY ADMISSION PROJECT[2]

The final choice of a project was made known in the first instance through the team's approach to those members of the staff included in the full survey. At the same time announcements were made to the consultants, and to other members of the medical staff, telling them of this new approach to a longstanding problem. No initial efforts were needed to attract the interest of those whose work was affected by the project. Interest in the problem was already widespread and, indeed, members of the team were struck throughout by the willingness of all those approached both to discuss the problem and to pose solutions, usually of a most practical nature.

The organization of the project devolved upon the four members of the team who had attended the month's course on social research techniques. Following the choice of project, the team met to discuss the form the inquiry should take. It was decided to undertake a pilot survey, which would be organized by the nursing and administrative members of the operational team. When they, with one of the medical members, had completed the interviews for the pilot survey (early April 1966), the team met to consider the results. From these results one of the medical members devised a questionnaire to be used in the major part of the survey. After discussion among the team, this was amended slightly and the questionnaire printed. Advice on the study design was then sought from the members of the Medical Research Council's Social Medicine Research Unit, and at this point our other medical member rejoined the team.

The nursing and administrative members determined the population to be surveyed by reference to the records, drew the appropriate sample in the one instance where this was necessary, and organized the dispatch of a preliminary letter to those chosen as respondents. In the period late April to mid June 1966, 116 interviews were carried out by the four members of the team. During the latter half of this period, the administrative member discussed with the operational research department the processing of the data collected. The computer program for analysing it was devised and the program tested. The information contained in the completed questionnaire was coded for the computer and the result subsequently analysed by the administrative member. The results were then discussed with the members of the team, who unanimously nominated him to write the report. The draft report, complete save for the concluding section, was completed with assistance from a medical member by mid July.

Both the house governor and matron were kept in touch with the progress of the inquiry by the members of their staff on the operational team. An interim report, setting out the ground covered by the pilot survey, was submitted to the house governor in mid April.

One object of the survey was to seek, from those who experienced the problems associated with the emergency admission of patients, their own solutions to the problems posed. To this extent, the survey mirrored the ideas of those involved. It should, however, be remembered that the object of the study was the description in depth of a problem, partly to solicit suggestions and partly to inform those who had the responsibility for finding a solution.

At no stage during the survey did any member of the team experience any reaction from those interviewed which could be remotely described as unco-operative. Indeed, many of those interviewed welcomed the interviewers, and expressed hopes that their efforts might result in some radical solutions to the problems described.

ACTION TAKEN IN THE EMERGENCY ADMISSION PROJECT

In describing the action taken upon the report, it is first necessary to consider the part played by the attitude survey, the details of which have just been described. The problem to which the talents of the team were applied was one that had troubled the hospital for a number of years. The survey was complementary to a study, by the operational research unit, of bed usage and of the various phenomena associated with the pressure of emergency admissions. The role of the attitude survey, therefore, was to provide further information on a problem, the existence of which was known, and of which some aspects had already been investigated.

The findings of the attitude survey were fed back to most of those who had taken part. They were presented at two study days for staff nurses (thus covering all the staff nurses) and two study days for sisters (thus covering all the ward sisters involved). A copy of the survey was given to all the senior registrars undertaking full duty and most of the junior registrars; and a summary of the report went to every member of the consultant medical staff and the board of governors. On subsequent reflection, there was a rather startling omission in this feedback process, in that house officers as a body were not offered access to the results. A number of copies were circulated, however, to individuals known privately to members of the team.

In the discussions with the nursing staff about the results of the survey, the major points of interest lay in the social and ethical problems involved in refusing patients when the hospital was full, or alternatively, of not refusing them and the subsequent necessity of putting up extra beds in the wards. Many of the sisters, in particular, appeared to be impressed by medical staff arguments for extra beds; and there was a noticeable absence of inter-disciplinary recrimination. In discussing the results of the survey with medical staff, there was a similar absence of this reaction.

Overall, both in the results of the survey and in the feedback discussions, it was encouraging to observe that both medical and nursing staff were profoundly concerned with the same problem and attempted, in general, to meet the same aims—although their respective professional spheres gave them different perspectives on essentially the same process.

During the period of the feedback meetings (September to December 1966), a multidisciplinary working party convened by the house governor, with the approval of the medical staff, had been considering what remedial measures could be taken. The members of the working party had the findings not only of the attitude survey but also of the statistical study carried out by the operational research team. A number of measures were considered and suggestions were formulated for discussion by the standing committee of the medical staff. At this point, however, events overtook this ordered process of consideration.

In the latter half of December 1966 and more particularly in the early part of January 1967, the pressures had been extremely high (on 11 January the occupancy in the hospital was 99.04 per cent). The combination of this continuing pressure and shortage of nursing staff was such that it was considered that the problem should be discussed with the chairman of the hospital. At a series of discussions between the chairman, the matron, and the house governor, it became apparent that if some control could be exercised on admissions from the waiting-list, it might be possible to alleviate the pressures arising from the high but unpredictable level of emergency admissions. The nursing and administrative members of the team were instructed to devise a system using the simple principle that the number of patients to be called for admission should not exceed the number of patients who would be discharged on any given day. This principle could be further refined in that an allowance could be made representing the average number of patients who might be admitted as emergencies on a given day.

They devised a system in which the ward sisters, in consultation with the registrars of the firms concerned, would predict the number of patients to be discharged for each one of the seven days in advance of the day on which the prediction was made. No firm could send for more patients than the number predicted as due for discharge three days ahead. On the basis of the predicted discharges three days ahead, patients on the waiting-list were warned that they were coming near the time of their possible admission into hospital. As a further safeguard, patients were asked to telephone the hospital, at first on the day of their admission, but latterly on the afternoon preceding the admission, to check whether their bed was still available.

This system was introduced gradually throughout the hospital from mid February to mid July 1967. It was introduced in this piecemeal fashion to enable the two operational members to discuss the scheme and its implications individually with every member of the medical and nursing staff directly involved (a total of approximately ninety-five medical staff and twenty-six nursing staff).

NOTES

1. English terminology for hospital positions differs somewhat from American terminology. The reader should keep the following points in mind:
      The supporting hospital team consisted of three very senior members of the hospital, one each from administration, nursing, and medicine. On the administrative side, the supporting team member was usually a group or hospital "secretary" (administrator), on the nursing side, a "matron" (director of nursing), and on the medical side, a "consultant" (most senior level of hospital doctor). The operational hospital team often consisted of the deputies or assistants of members of the supporting team. On the administrative side, the operational team member was often a hospital or deputy hospital secretary (administrator), on the nursing side a deputy or assistant matron (director of nursing), and on the medical side, a junior-level hospital doctor.
      Two other points on terminology should be noted: A ward "sister" is the nurse in charge of a ward—comparable to a senior head nurse in the U.S. In the teaching hospital, the most senior administrator is termed the "house governor." ———Ed.
2. For a short account of this project see Webster, B., 1967, Problems of the Admission of Patients. *Nursing Times* 63, 885–886. A detailed report of this project is given in Fairey, M., Barber, B., and Webster, B., 1970, Admission Procedures in a London Teaching Hospital. *British Journal of Hospital Medicine*, 4, 800–820.

24 | An Evaluation of the Hospital Internal Communications (HIC) Project

George F. Wieland
Amos Bradford

A number of research studies suggest that length of stay can be reduced by more efficient and effective care in the hospital. One surgeon (Lahti 1970) found that he could send home three-quarters of a group of 1000 consecutive patients by the second postoperative day. He did this by communicating reassurance and expectations that it was normal to go home quickly. A nursing experiment (Skipper and Leonard 1968) to mitigate anxieties in mother and child resulted in reduced physical and psychological problems and shortened pediatric length of stay. Another controlled experiment (Lindeman and Van Aernam 1971) showed how nurses communicating the "stir-up routine" to patients reduced surgical length of stay (see also Janis and Leventhal 1965).

Internal medicine length-of-stay has also been reduced. Grant and Cohen (1973) used patient education and physical therapy to reduce the length of stay for acute myocardial infarction from an average of 26 to 23 days. Similarly, Hutter and associates (1973) describe an accelerated program for recovery from acute myocardial infarction with patients walking by the twelfth or thirteenth day and having only about a two-week hospital stay.

The research reported here was supported by grant #3–ROI–HS–01739 from the U.S. Department of Health, Education and Welfare. Earlier phases of the evaluation research were funded by a USPHS Post-doctoral Fellowship, a grant from the Department of Health and Social Security (Great Britain) to Guy's Hospital Medical School, and the Faculty Research Fund at Vanderbilt University. Statistical advice for the analyses was provided by Professor William A. Ericson. An earlier version of this paper was presented at the Academy of Management national meetings, Atlanta, 1979.

Another hospital (Royston 1972) emphasizes the communication of reassurance and reports sending 62 percent of the acute myocardial infarction patients home at the tenth day. Finally, a study of acute medical wards shows that long stay was attributable to the failure on certain wards to provide physiotherapy early enough (Sutherland 1972).

Given these suggestive findings that better communication could shorten length of stay, we expected that the two largest categories of patients in these project hospitals, general medicine (19,000 patients per year) and general surgery (21,000), would experience improved efficiency as a result of the communications and efficiencies instituted by the Hospital Internal Communications (HIC) Project. These "directly targeted" patient categories should have had shorter lengths of stay because internists and surgeons participated on the hospital teams and because these kinds of wards were the focus of study by hospital projects. Three smaller categories of patients, pediatrics (4,000), traumatic and orthopedic surgery (5,000), and urology (2,000), could also show some indirect, diffused project effects. Two large nontargeted patient categories, gynecology (13,000) and obstetrics (18,000), were expected to show no project effects because of lack of participation by gynecologists and obstetricians and because studies were not targeted on these wards.

METHODS AND FINDINGS ON PROJECT SUCCESSFULNESS

A quasi-experimental research design was used, measuring average length of stay for five years before (1961–65), three years during (1966–68), and five years after (1969–73) the project, and comparing project hospitals with a comparison group of all other hospitals in the same administrative region. That is, the basic data consist of a thirteen-year time series for each patient category in each of the ten project hospitals. Each time series shows relative standing year by year compared to the average length of stay in the comparison group of hospitals. A summary of these data (for all ten project hospitals) is provided in Figures 24–1, 24–2, and 24–3.

Two kinds of statistical tests were made on these data. The first, Clayton's test[1] (Campbell 1963) was used to discern if the project intervention served to break, and subsequently to improve, the length-of-stay trends observed over the thirteen years. An overall best-fit regression line for the entire thirteen years was compared with two partial best-fit regression lines. The time period 1961–65 was selected to display the trend before the project, and a second period, beginning two years after the project began (1968–71) was selected to display the contrasting trend resulting from the impact of the project efforts. If the partial lines are significantly different from the overall lines, and if the

FIGURE 24-1

EFFICIENCY OF HIC HOSPITALS:
GENERAL MEDICINE, GENERAL SURGERY

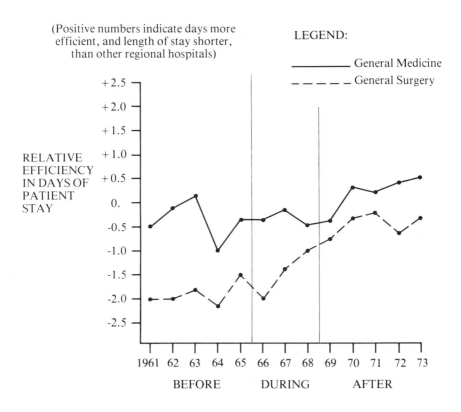

(Positive numbers indicate days more
efficient, and length of stay shorter,
than other regional hospitals)

LEGEND:

——————— General Medicine

— — — — — General Surgery

RELATIVE
EFFICIENCY
IN DAYS OF
PATIENT
STAY

+ 2.5
+ 2.0
+ 1.5
+ 1.0
+ 0.5
0.
-0.5
-1.0
-1.5
-2.0
-2.5

1961 62 63 64 65 66 67 68 69 70 71 72 73

BEFORE   DURING   AFTER

"after" trend is better (in terms of level and slope) than the "before" trend,
then there is evidence of positive project effects.

A total of 52 analyses was conducted, one for each category of patient in
each of the hospitals. The remaining 18 time series contained some missing
data or were totally absent because the particular hospital did not treat
certain categories of patient.

The overall results for the 52 comparisons of trends before and after the
project provide support for the conclusion that the project did have a positive
impact on patient care efficiency. Both of the large categories of patients
which were expected to show positive effects, general medicine and general
surgery, show more positive than negative changes in trend (4 versus 3 for
general medicine, with 1 nonsignificant; 5 versus 2 for general surgery, with 2

FIGURE 24–2

EFFICIENCY OF HIC HOSPITALS:
PEDIATRICS, TRAUMATIC AND ORTHOPEDIC SURGERY, UROLOGY

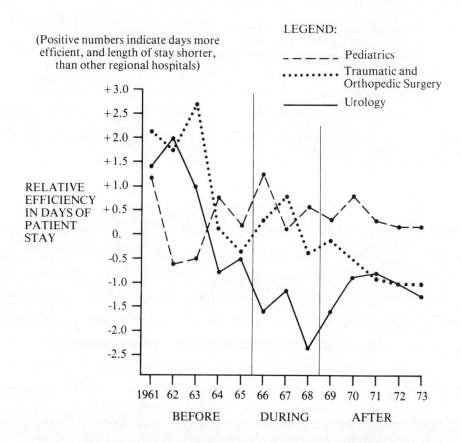

nonsignificant). The indirectly targeted categories also show generally positive effects (3 versus 2 and 2 for pediatrics, 4 versus 1 and 2 for traumatic and orthopedic surgery, 4 versus 1 and 1 for urology). Finally, the two nontargeted categories show either no project effect (gynecology: 3 versus 3 and 2 nonsignificant) or an apparent negative project effect (obstetrics: 1 versus 6).[2]

A second statistical test used analysis of variance contrasts (pooling all five years of "before" data and contrasting them with the similarly pooled "after" years). This test was feasible for several of the patient categories, those which had no rising or falling trends in the before period. Using the basic data from a

FIGURE 24-3

EFFICIENCY OF HIC HOSPITALS:
GYNECOLOGY, OBSTETRICS

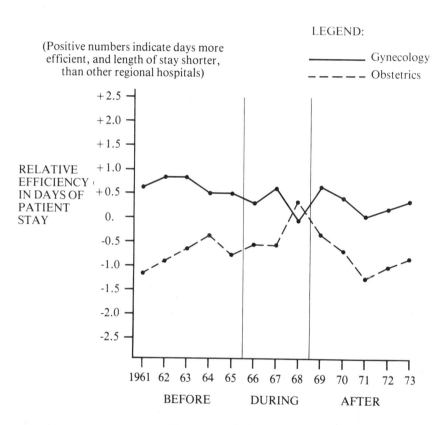

LEGEND:

(Positive numbers indicate days more
efficient, and length of stay shorter,
than other regional hospitals)

————— Gynecology
— — — — — Obstetrics

RELATIVE
EFFICIENCY
IN DAYS OF
PATIENT
STAY

1961 62 63 64 65 66 67 68 69 70 71 72 73

BEFORE   DURING   AFTER

two-way analysis of variance (hospitals by years) and following Winer (1971), 1961–65 (before) was contrasted with several combinations of after years (1969–71, 1969–72, 1970–73).

The results for 1970–73 as after years (the other combinations being quite similar in results) are highly significant and positive for general medicine and general surgery, but not significant for pediatrics (see Table 24–1 for details). Thus the analysis of variance-procedures testing for contrasts in the pooled before and pooled after years seems to support the analysis using Clayton's test. The HIC Project was successful in improving the performance of project hospitals in their processing of medical and surgical patients.

The other categories of patient could not be tested by contrasting pooled

TABLE 24-1
CONTRAST EFFECTS BETWEEN 1961-65 AND 1970-73

Patient Category	Contrast observed	SS contrast	df	MS error	F
General Medicine	146.15	948.48	1,84	198.6	4.78*
Pediatrics	32.161	40.23	1,72	470.63	.09
General Surgery	287.97	4472.85	1,105	207.01	21.61**

Mean 70-73 minus mean 61-65
*$p < .05$
**$p < .01$

before and after levels of efficiency because of the existence of changing trends in the before data. However, in the case of obstetrics and gynecology these trends were not major. Further contrast analyses disregarding these trends yielded evidence of a positive project effect for obstetrics, but only initially and temporarily, with a quick return to levels of efficiency expected from the extrapolation of earlier trends. (This temporary improvement accounts for the apparent subsequent negative effect found using Clayton's test.) Gynecology, however, shows apparently no project effects whatsoever.

In summary, taking into account both the tests for changes in efficiency trends and the tests contrasting levels of efficiency before and after the project, there seems to be good evidence of improvement in both of the large, directly targeted categories of patients, general medicine and general surgery. There is mixed evidence for the smaller and indirectly targeted categories of patient, traumatic and orthopedic surgery and urology show improvement but pediatrics apparently does not. Finally, the evidence seems to indicate no major effects on the large, nontargeted categories of patients, obstetrics and gynecology.

It should be emphasized that these demonstrated improvements are over and above the improvements "naturally" occurring in all hospitals as part of their efforts toward shortened length of stay. The improvements in all other hospitals in the same administrative regions had been subtracted out of the project hospitals' scores before statistical tests were made. The multiple time series design used here is quite powerful, allowing one to eliminate most alternative explanations for the improvements achieved (see Appendix 24-A for further details). Furthermore, in the few cases in which project hospitals showed significant negative project effects, there seem to be plausible reasons. These were hospitals which "rejected" the project early on and decided not to participate further (see Appendix 24B).

Under conservative assumptions, shortened length of stay reduces hotel and capital costs, but not treatment costs. Hotel and capital costs at the time totalled $25 per day for these English hospitals. Thus, during the five years after the project (1969–73), the observed 0.6 day and 1.4 day saved for medical and surgical patients, respectively, yield a total savings of $5 million. This amount of savings is impressive, since reducing length of stay was not a major thrust of the project. There were no project activities specially aimed at this criterion. Instead, hospital teams focused on specific management problems as well as on interpersonal problems. Because the project was self-directed, the focus of efforts in each hospital, and in each specific project, was very idiosyncratic, dealing with the immediate concerns of the hospital team. In short, the demonstrated effects on efficiency of patient care are probably only the tip of the iceberg as far as the achievements of the HIC Project are concerned.

THEORETICAL RATIONALE FOR THE IMPROVEMENT PROCESS

Two theoretical models, "action" and "understanding" systems, help explain how the project came to have these demonstrated effects. The action system is characterized by simple tasks, requiring relatively little information processing, by external management controls (formal organizational structures and hierarchical controls), and by people with relatively authoritarian orientations. The understanding system is characterized by complex tasks, by internal (professional) controls, and by people who are relatively sensitive to psychological variables and open to new information.

There seems to be a rather direct correspondence between surgery and action, and between internal medicine and understanding. We found that surgery and internal medicine are relatively simple or complex tasks, respectively, in terms of the new information needed to perform the task of medical care.

Surgery generally consists of simple cases which are similar from patient to patient. The cases are "cold" (nonemergency), and the patients generally are healthy and recuperate on schedule. Surgeons can specialize and perfect certain techniques. Finally, surgeons often are able to use external control systems. They have decision trees for procedures, and they can use planned admissions and discharges.

The practice of internal medicine, in contrast, often entails more difficult cases with multiple complaints, acute conditions, patients in general ill health (often because they are elderly), and physical conditions which often involve interactions with complex psychological factors. Internists may specialize, but a breadth of knowledge is required to take into account all the possible interacting factors. Finally, in internal medicine, decisions are made on the basis of interaction with the task (feedback from tests and results of therapies) and on the basis of discussions among all those in contact with the patients. Internists and internal medicine departments make use of an internal control system.

The social structures on surgical and medical wards also reflect the difference in task complexity (Coser 1958, 1962; Hawkins and Selmanoff, n.d.). The surgeons organize their department in a pyramidal, hierarchical fashion, with work controlled by orders and directives. They centralize authority and limit participation in decision making at lower levels. The internists organize in a more decentralized fashion. They delegate authority and exchange information with colleagues so as to reach more consensual decisions. The organization of nurses on the surgical ward also reflects relatively simple and routine work requirements, while nurses in internal medicine participate more with the doctors in coping with the complexities of patient care (Davies and Francis 1974). Surgical nurses perform routine procedures, the events on the ward are predictable, and problems have defined procedures. Surgical nurses have greater definition of duties and definition of authority than do nurses on internal medicine wards. These latter are, in contrast to surgical nurses, more able to influence diagnoses and therapy, and to consult with junior doctors.

Finally, surgeons and internists differ in psychological makeup in ways which are congruent with the different task requirements. A review of fifteen studies of medical students and practicing physicans shows that internists are intellectuals and prefer to develop rapport with people, while surgeons are doers, best described as authoritarian (Wieland 1979; see also Wechsler 1976). Specifically, a surgeon's self-image derives from working with the hands and being decisive and the specialty is relatively narrow and technical. Surgeons have a low tolerance for ambiguity, they place a low value on patient rapport, they are politically conservative, and they have a need to dominate, persuade, and influence others.[6] In contrast, internists see themselves facing intellectual challenges and emphasizing mental operations. They face the broadest of all medical specialties and prefer this ambiguity, they have a high concern for people, and they are politically liberal.

Given these differences between surgery and medicine, we expected that action-system effects, i.e., improved surgical performance, might be determined by one set of improvement procedures, and understanding-system effects, i.e., improved internal medicine performance, by another set of procedures. Specifically, we wondered whether surgery might be improved by an approach to change akin to traditional management consultancy. The managers (administrators, nurses, and physicians) in the project would use surveys to gather data, which would lead to recommendations for action—for managerial actions, modifying policies, procedures, techniques, etc. These would ultimately impinge on surgical ward performance.

Internal medicine might benefit from an organization development (OD) approach. That is, the managers could use the survey projects to gain a better understanding of the psychological dynamics of their organizations. They would change in attitude and in their work behavior with others, helping to create a better interpersonal system which would ultimately impinge on the performance of the medical wards.

METHODS FOR FINDING OUT WHY THE PROJECT WORKED

Criterion scores for each hospital were constructed, showing the relative amount of project-created improvement in general medicine or surgery. The relative standing of a hospital before the project was eliminated by using residualized scores. In other words, the criterion scores reflect how a hospital's relative efficiency standing is different from what it might have been if there had been no HIC Project and the hospital had continued as before.[7]

Correlational analyses were then conducted to ascertain the prior determinants of improvement in action-system functioning (as measured by surgery) and in understanding-system functioning (as measured by internal medicine). Hospital scores for these prior determinants were obtained by averaging the observations, ratings, attitudes, etc., of hospital team members on two sets of interviews and survey questionnaires, administered during the active period of the HIC Project (in mid–1967) and at its end (January 1969). The correlations were based on $n=10$ hospitals.

Suchman's (1967) process evaluation was used to order the possible factors leading to project success. Ultimate project success in terms of improved length of stay was seen as due to penultimate success, or certain immediate project outcomes in the hospital. These immediate project outcomes were viewed as the possible result of project inputs, which, in turn, might vary according to differences in the preexisting nature of the hospital organizations participating in the project. All of these different aspects of the improvement process were directly correlated with the "hard" criterion data for improvement in average length of stay.

DETERMINANTS OF ACTION- AND UNDERSTANDING-SYSTEM IMPROVEMENT

Correlating these survey data with the amount of improvement in surgery and medicine, we found that certain project outcomes were related to action-system improvement, and certain others, to understanding-system improvement. For example, what we term "managerial actions"—the solving of managerial problems and the taking of administrative action (to institute new procedures, routines, or structures, or to alter technological arrangements)—are associated with improved action-system functioning (but not with understanding-system improvement). Thus, the correlations on the right half of Table 24–2 are mostly positive and large enough to be statistically significant, but those in the left hand are not significant. Other correlational evidence using the change in level of efficiency is found in Wieland (1979) and yields the same pattern of results.

On the other hand, improved understanding-system functioning is associated with "psychological changes," by which we mean (1) the reported acquisition of significant new information, (2) reported change in the patterning of team member (and close associate) work behavior, and (3) psychological change in hospital team members, as perceived by the central team (see Table 24–3 for some examples of the correlations found).

Further correlational analyses were conducted in order to learn why some hospital teams emphasized managerial actions and subsequently improved

TABLE 24–2

RELATIONSHIPS BETWEEN MANAGERIAL ACTION OUTCOMES AND
IMPROVEMENTS IN UNDERSTANDING AND ACTION SYSTEMS

Managerial Action Outcomes	Improvements in Understanding and Action Systems	
	General Medicine	General Surgery
1. Hospital problems solved or reduced	–.22	.51
2. Team members helped to correct a number of problems	–.26	.65*
3. The people studied were gotten to work on their problems	.03	–.03
4. Worthwhile actions taken in hospital	–.32	.71*
5. "Right" changes made in the *hospital*	.26	.84*
6. Enduring effects of the project	.02	.61*

*Significant at $p < .05$

TABLE 24–3
RELATIONSHIP BETWEEN PSYCHOLOGICAL CHANGE AND
IMPROVEMENTS IN UNDERSTANDING AND ACTION SYSTEMS

Psychological Change	Improvements in Understanding and Action Systems	
	General Medicine	General Surgery
1. Team given more knowledge about problems existing in the hospital	−.07	.31
2. Team given information about functioning of hospital	.50	−.31
3. Team given information about functioning of work associates	.30	.24
4. Team members improved their work	.46	.43
5. Team members improved quality of work	.05	.39
6. "Right" changes made in team members' work	.78*	.20
7. Important accomplishments in the hospital, including psychological changes	.35	.59*
8. Team members jobs changed— made harder by extra project work	.83*	−.35
9. Jobs of others around the team made harder	−.15	−.06
10. Team members' jobs made harder or easier	.82*	−.14
11. Central team rating of psychological changes in hospital team members	.66*	.22

*Significant at $p < .05$

general surgery, while more or less independently, some teams emphasized psychological changes and improved general medicine in their hospitals. We found that variation in the amount of effort (time) spent by the hospital teams or by the central team at various project activities (e.g., administering surveys, analyzing data) had little or no effect on subsequent improvements in general medicine or general surgery. There was only one area of exception to these negative findings. Hospital team participation in meetings led to subsequent improved understanding-system functioning. The more the hospital team members discussed project data among themselves and with others in the hospital, and the more they attended the special interteam discussion meetings, the more medicine efficiency improved in the hospital.

Next we tried to look at the style with which hospital teams carried out project activities, to pinpoint a distinction between an action or under-standing orientation. Those taking an understanding orientation were generally critical and saw psychological and interpersonal difficulties in their organizations. They also had a critical concern about the data collected in hospital projects, and they critically examined HIC Project goals, too. They had relatively clear perception of the goals of the early, course portion of HIC when psychological concepts were presented and a cohesive team was created. Finally, they said that their jobs were concerned with many different interests. In short, these teams had an intellectually critical and psychological approach to the project.

In contrast, teams with an action orientation emphasized identifying important problems or topics for study and getting clear data on underlying causes. They wanted data with action implications, and they used it to take administrative action. They thought that post-course project aims (i.e., acting to improve their hospitals) were clear, and they tended to strike out con-sciously and explicitly at a series of specific hospital problems. In the same vein, they reported that their jobs consisted primarily of problems which others brought to them. In short, action-oriented teams were concerned with the gathering of clear, problem-oriented relevant data which would enable them to act on, and rectify, the problems "out there."

We found that teams taking on action or an understanding orientation tended to improve action-system functioning (i.e., surgery) or understanding-system functioning (i.e., internal medicine), respectively. Table 24-4 provides some illustrative findings. The effects of these orientations were mediated by managerial actions and psychological changes, respectively. (We also found that teams with an understanding orientation tended to get considerable central-team help, and to participate a lot in meetings, while those with an action orientation did not; instead they expended a lot of time in planning and launching their hospital projects.) It seems, then, that the orientation that one takes to organizational change is a very important determinant of what very different kinds of organizational changes can result.[8]

TABLE 24-4
RELATIONSHIPS BETWEEN HOSPITAL TEAM ACTION AND
UNDERSTANDING ORIENTATIONS AND IMPROVEMENTS IN
UNDERSTANDING AND ACTION SYSTEMS

Hospital Team Action Orientation:	Improvement in Understanding and Action Systems:	
	General Medicine	General Surgery
1. Importance of topic studied	−.07	.57*
2. Clarity of data obtained	−.40	.38
3. Causal data obtained	−.28	.45
4. Data with action implications	−.57	.71*
5. Took action	.20	.50
6. Clear about later HIC	.55	.55*
7. Struck out in new directions	−.34	.66*
8. Considered other projects	.28	.69*
9. Work consists of problems	−.32	.90*
Understanding Orientation:		
10. Desired change in hospital	.22	.15
11. Felt needed HIC	−.09	.17
12. Felt others needed HIC	−.13	.03
13. Had concern beforehand	.23	−.38
14. Obtained already known data	.65*	−.16
15. Obtained invalid data	.74*	.37
16. Compared data to other units	.45	.14
17. Clear about early HIC	.27	.46
18. Compared HIC/hospital goals	.82*	.03
19. Breadth of work interests	.35	−.15

*Significant at $p < .05$

WHICH ORGANIZATIONS CHOSE ACTION AND WHICH CHOSE UNDERSTANDING APPROACHES TO CHANGE?

Next, going one step further back, we tried to find out if certain kinds of hospitals and hospital teams seemed to be predisposed toward taking either an action or an understanding approach to change (and were predisposed toward actually improving these respective systems when a chance appeared).

We found that action-systems tended to improve in organizations that were

TABLE 24–5

RELATIONSHIPS BETWEEN ORGANIZATIONAL RESPONSIVENESS,
INFLUENCE, AND INTEGRATION AND IMPROVEMENT IN
UNDERSTANDING AND ACTION SYSTEMS

Organizational Responsiveness	Improvement in Understanding and Action Systems	
	General Medicine	General Surgery
1. Success	−.49	.62*
Influence in the Hospital		
2. Nurses	.05	.50
3. Administrators	−.36	.64*
Organizational Integration		
4. Mutual knowledge, or awareness of the problems of each other, between administrators and others in the hospital	.15	.66*
5. Awareness, physicians—others	−.26	.31
6. Awareness, nurses—others	−.70*	.67*
7. Awareness, within top echelons of each profession	−.56	.55*
8. Awareness, between top and middle echelons	−.05	.71*
9. Awareness, between top and lowest echelons	.54	.38

*Significant at $< .05$

already well organized or well structured. These organizations were already responsive to internally instituted changes and had influential hierarchical structures. They also were well integrated; different groups and different levels in the organization agreed about priorities and were mutually aware of each other's problems. (For examples, see Table 24–5.) We found that these successful organizations tended to take a no-nonsense approach to change.

Their teams were relatively authoritarian in attitude—valuing authority and being closed minded, not interested in discussing matters or learning about the views of others. These hospitals achieved managerial action outcomes and improved action-system functioning.

In contrast, an understanding orientation and subsequent psychological change and improvement in understanding systems seemed to be related to preexisting distress at the highest level in the hospital team (the supporting team), and to its taking an active part in the project. For example, the negative correlations in Table 24-4 show that poor existing hospital integration is associated with subsequent improvement in the efficiency of internal medicine functioning. We also found that the extent to which hospital team members rated the supporting team members as poor communicators was associated with the hospital subsequently improving internal medicine efficiency. These distress factors seemed to predispose the hospital teams to an understanding orientation and to participation at meetings for psychologically deep intervention (sensitivity training).[9]

Those at the very top of the hospital structure, the supporting team members, were very important in this process of improving internal medicine. The supporting team facilitated an understanding orientation and high participation in meetings by being emotionally committed, active, and influential in the project and by providing psychological support for the project work of their subordinates.[10]

Table 24-6 provides a summary of the correlational findings described here. Each of the factors in columns 1, 2, and 3 is significantly associated with the improvement listed in column 4 of each row—improvement in action-system functioning or improvement in understanding-system functioning, as the case may be. In addition, almost all of the relationships between factors in columns 1 and 2 and between columns 2 and 3 are significant, suggesting the process by which improvement occurred. That is, certain kinds of hospitals (column 1) selected certain kinds of help (column 2). Those receiving these certain kinds of help reported different kinds of outcomes (column 3). Finally, these self-reports of different kinds of outcomes were associated with different kinds of improvement, according to our analysis of length-of-stay data (column 4).

DISCUSSION AND CONCLUSIONS

Perhaps the most important outcome of this evaluation study is the demonstration that Revans' self-help approach to management improvement is indeed effective. In more specific terms, this evaluation study shows that hospital management efficiency can be systematically improved in hospitals, no small matter in these times of spiraling health care costs.

A key to improvement in efficiency was the participation of physicians in

TABLE 24-6
SUMMARY OF THE IMPORTANT FACTORS FOR IMPROVING ACTION AND UNDERSTANDING SYSTEMS

(Factors in columns 1, 2, and 3 are significantly correlated with a project effect in column 4.)

1 Pre-existing Organizational Conditions	2 HIC Project Activities and Processes	3 Outcomes during the Project	4 Subsequent Project Effects
Well-Structured Organizations Responsive to internal change, influential hierarchies, well integrated (agreeing and aware of problems), authoritarian culture (24-5)*	*Action Orientation to the Project* Important topics, clear data on causes and for action, taking action, striking out on a number of different problems, being problem-oriented in their work (24-4)	*Managerial Actions* Solving problems, instituting new procedures or techniques (24-2)	*Improved Action System Functioning* Improved efficiency in treating surgical patients
Distressed Organizations Poor organizational integration, poor communication at very top (24-5)	*Understanding Orientation to the Project* Generally critical, seeing psychological and interpersonal problems in their organizations, critical about data & goals of HIC, having a breadth of interests in their work (24-4) Going to meetings, getting central team help Very top is emotionally committed, active, and influential toward HIC; provides psychological support to juniors doing project work	*Psychological Changes* Acquiring new information, changing behavior in the team or with others, individual psychological change (24-3)	*Improved Understanding System Functioning* Improved efficiency in treating internal medicine patients

*Figures in parentheses indicate the number of the table providing correlational data for the relationship between the particular factor and improved action or understanding system functioning.

the project hospitals. Many of the physicians in the HIC Project did not feel that they had enough time to participate or were not so inclined. But those who did participate supplied sufficient medical expertise and medical legitimacy to make the project a success. Comparing this effort at improving the efficiency of hospitals with similar efforts indicates that self-direction was essential to the success of the HIC Project. Physicians not only were able to say "yes" or "no" when asked to participate, they were able to decide on the nature of the change effort. The central team of the HIC Project then provided the different kinds of help physicians and others on the hospital teams requested, or, in some cases, they put the hospital teams in contact with outside experts (from colleges or universities), who possessed capabilities that they did not themselves have.

More specifically, physicians could decide whether they wanted assistance with an action orientation or with an understanding orientation, depending on their own personal perspectives and the requirements of their own jobs, roles, etc. For example, an internist could get help interviewing his patients regarding their anxieties on the wards and help in surveying the sources of interpersonal conflict between housekeeping and nursing staffs. A surgeon might not be interested in such kinds of psychological or understanding approaches to improvement. But in a change project run by psychologists, those might be the only kinds of help available. The surgeons in the HIC Project, however, were provided help in studying the causes of missing lab and x-ray reports, help in designing new work schedules for operating rooms, and the like. They were helped to do the action-oriented kinds of projects which most surgeons seem to prefer.

The general point is that physicians vary considerably in the kinds of work that they do as well as in their personal predilections toward their work, and an improvement project that is to be truly comprehensive must address these different requirements. A narrow or one-sided effort at change and improvement is doomed to failure.[11]

In conclusion, evaluation research on the ten hospitals of the HIC Project shows that major improvements in hospital efficiency are feasible. Furthermore, comparisons of hospitals within the project as well as with other projects seem to show that a successful effort at improving management efficiency must include a variety of forms of help, including help which facilitates psychological change and better understanding, as well as help which facilitates managerial action. Provision of different kinds of help and the opportunity to control and direct the providers of help would seem to be essential in encouraging physician participation, without which relatively little can be done to improve hospital management. Being able to choose and control the methods of help will allow physicians—and nurses and administrators—to select those forms of help which they need and which they feel are congruent with their own styles of organization and management.

Appendix 24-A

Attempts at Explaining the Positive Findings Away—Threats to Validity

The multiple time-series design used here is one of the strongest designs for eliminating alternative possible explanations for the observed relationship between the change project and the improved efficiency noted in the study (Campbell and Stanley 1963; Campbell 1963; Cook and Campbell 1976). The use of the multiple time-series design allows one to eliminate all of the eight frequently encountered plausible alternatives to the desired experimental effect sought.

(1) "History," or another contemporary causal factor (e.g., new National Health Service policies), is here eliminated by the use of the controls, the other hospitals in the same administration regions as the experimental hospitals. In addition, special analyses showed that the demand for beds (i.e., high waiting lists and high occupancy levels) or increased expenditures for medical staffing were not correlated with subsequent improvement in length of stay (for details, see Wieland 1979). (2) "Maturation," or the improvement (e.g., learning) of an organization over time, was eliminated by use of control hospitals. (3) "Testing," or change in measures due to repeated measurement, was similarly eliminated by use of control hospitals. (4) "Instrumentation," or change in the nature of the measuring instrument, was eliminated by use of the same instrument (Form SH3) for both experimental and control groups. (5) "Statistical regression," or the natural movement of unreliably measured extreme scores toward the mean, was eliminated by the use of time-series data. Examination of length-of-stay data for the project hospitals shows that they were for the most part near (within one day of) the regional averages during the baseline period before the project. In cases such as surgery, for which hospitals were not within one day of regional averages, there is no movement toward the mean over the five-year base period. In the cases of urology and traumatic and orthopedic surgery, at the time the hospitals were selecting themselves into the project the scores drifted from relatively more efficient downward to reach the mean clearly precluding regression toward the mean as an explanation for subsequent improvement during and after the project. (6) "Experimental mortality," or the differential loss of participants from experimental or control groups, is eliminated by using all hospitals in the regions for the control group and by using all ten project hospitals. Even though two of the ten project hospitals discontinued active participation (the "rejecters"), they are treated as project participants so as to provide a conservative estimate of project effects.

(7) "Selection," or the differential recruitment of project or control group hospitals, is assessed by examination of the project hospitals' standing before the project. As indicated above, the project hospitals were, at the time of

selection into the project, close to average in patient length of stay, except for general surgery stays, which were longer. However, Clayton's test data (see Wieland 1979) show that two of the three hospitals which were *above* average in efficiency subsequently showed improvement as a result of the project. Thus the hospitals seemed to be average in length of stay to start with, while in the case of surgery, for which they were sub-par, "good" as well as "poor" hospitals improved as a result of the project.

In a further test for spurious selection effects, correlations were run between a variety of project variables and relative hospital efficiency (for both general medicine and general surgery) before and during the project. Project variables included the amount of time put in by hospital staff, amount of help received from the central team, and so on. These project variables were not significantly correlated with relative efficiency before or during the time of the project (see Wieland 1979). In other words, relatively "good" (or "bad") hospitals did not receive more (or less) project help because they were relatively "good" (or "bad"). If this had been true, the improvement in length of stay could have been a simple spurious effect of "good" hospitals' getting more project help and at the same time improving length of stay (with a resulting spurious correlation between project help and improvement in length of stay). Such is not the case. However, the project variables did show significant correlations with improvement in length of stay after the project.

In another sense, there is a selection bias, but not in a way that obviates the conclusions regarding the efficacy of this bootstrap approach to change. The hospitals are a biased group in that they volunteered for the HIC Project. This would seem to be essential in any project based on the tenets of self-help. If the volunteering of hospitals is to be cited as an explanation of improved efficiency, so much the better. Subsequent projects will ensure success by taking only volunteers and not coercing participation.

(8) Finally, there is the possibility of certain interactions between any of the above threats to validity. This would most likely take the form of selection combining with another threat to validity. This threat to validity implies that the hospitals may have been initially no different from others in their regions, but that they selected themselves into the project because of some prospective differential factor which was to occur during the period of the project. That is, a hospital could have been selected into the project because of some prospective change which was to occur in its history, maturation, and so on. The hospital officials' awareness that an occurrence beneficial to the hospital was going to coincide with the project (the history case), or that the hospital was going to start learning more rapidly over the next few years during the project, but for some reasons unrelated to the project (the maturation case), might have led to their volunteering the hospital for the project.

The defenses against this threat to validity are two: (1) Any subsequent project would want to use the same process of volunteering so as to maximize the demonstrated length-of-stay effects, whether or not the threat to validity existed. (2) Any argument about selection-interaction effects must be extremely convoluted and specially tailored for each hospital, leaving one with the more parsimonious explanation of a "project effect" which operated systematically across the entire group of project hospitals, but not in the comparison group.

In summary, there would seem to be no plausible alternative explanation for the observed relative improvement in length of stay in the ten project hospitals. Taking a systematic "worst case" approach to the experimental findings yields only the project effect as a parsimonious account of the findings.

APPENDIX 24–B

Explanation of Negative Project Effects

While expectations of general project success in improving medical and surgical efficiency are confirmed, there are still some doubts regarding specific areas of improvement. Clayton's tests show, for example, that several of the hospitals had negative changes in efficiency trends for general medicine or general surgery. Did the project cause this apparent deterioration in efficiency?

One explanation seems to rest in the nature of the project participation by three of the ten hospitals. First of all, Revans has argued that two of the general hospitals did reject the basic assumptions and requirements of the project, and that their negative attitude toward the project is quite clear when one examines the ten reports written by the hospitals (Revans 1971).[12]

The official report on HIC Project participation by one of these two rejecting hospitals concludes as follows:

> So although our use of HIC methods has not been very extensive, we are not entirely disenchanted, but would prefer not to undertake more than we can cope with, even though the help of experts is at our disposal. As to the future, we have hopes of being able to continue to do something to meet staff wishes in the catering field, and there are plans for a small departmental project upon which our thoughts have not yet fully crystallized.
>
> Beyond this, we shall continue along the path already mapped out, but perhaps with diminished enthusiasm and no longer any great belief in the theory that a problem has only to be evaluated to be solved. (Alderson 1971, pp. 51–52)

In an addendum to the report by the hospital team, the senior doctor on the team expresses similar negative attitudes:

> To sum up: As far as I am concerned, there have been few positive results to get excited about so far. Staff of all grades tend to be uninterested or suspicious. Unless there is some money available to make the necessary changes that are suggested by an investigation, further effort is a waste of time. (Knowles 1971, p. 53)

It is not clear how these negative attitudes arose, although there is some evidence that early help by an understanding-oriented central team member was incompatible with the basic action orientation in this hospital (for some details, see Wieland 1979). In any event, the key hospital team members were not very enthusiastic about the project.

Similar negative attitudes toward the project were found in the other hospital. The team provided a very brief, three-page report stating:

> My own view, for what it is worth, is that the HIC Project suffered from too much pressure to produce results by its techniques, when in the hospitals there may have been more pressing problems which had to be solved by other methods. This, I believe, was the case at our hospital where, during most of the Project period, we were concerned with the overriding task of completing, equipping, moving into, and commissioning the new hospital building. It is only since the move has been completed that we have begun to use HIC techniques to solve a real problem, the one concerning nursing staff described by my colleague.
> . . . One further criticism I have to make, with the benefit of hindsight, is that there was a lack of definition of the purpose at the Hastings course. (Bardgett 1971, pp. 20–21)

Perhaps even more important was the fact that this second hospital, during its supposed participation in a program of self-directed learning, engaged an outside group of consultants for an extensive change project based on a highly structured program for improvement. One must question the desirability of two diametrically opposed change programs being undertaken simultaneously by the same organization.[13]

In addition to taking on this structured program for change, the hospital was also building a major new physical facility. It has been argued (Sarason 1971) that a major cause of failed attempts at social innovation is the involvement of the chief administrator in the multitude of activities that arise when one attempts to house the innovative activities in a new facility. The planning and controlling activities for the facility invariably come to dominate the time and energy of the administrator, to the detriment of the different and sensitive issues of building a new social organization.

If these two rejecting hospitals are eliminated from the analyses for general medicine and general surgery, the results are highly positive: for Clayton's test, 1961–65 versus 1968–71, general medicine shows four positive hospitals and one negative, general surgery has five positive and zero negative. For

Clayton's test, 1961–65 versus 1966–73, general medicine shows four positive, zero negative, and general surgery shows six positive, zero negative hospitals.

The single remaining negative finding for general medicine is found in the teaching hospital. In this hospital, efficiency and short lengths of stay, while important, had to share the limelight with student teaching as determinants of how patients were handled.

There is another possible reason why this hospital did not show a positive improvement in general medicine stay and in fact showed a significant decrement: the project was viewed by the hospital staff as being primarily an extension of operations research and other similar activities already existing in the hospital. Furthermore, while the hospital team members were not rejecting, they held themselves aloof from Revans and the central team. They felt that their own facilities, such as the operations research department and computer, would enable them to proceed quite on their own.

The fact that in this hospital pediatrics and obstetrics also seem to have been negatively affected by the project (according to Clayton's test, 1961–65 versus 1968–71) as well as general medicine, is suggestive. These are all departments for whose patients the social and psychological components of the process of care are important. One may speculate that an overemphasis on operations research studies for management action, together with the hospital's absence from the project meetings organized by the central team, may have slighted the social changes needed for improvement in general medicine and the related patient categories.

The three rejecting or aloof hospitals account for all of the apparent project-caused decrements in the directly targeted patient categories. One might eliminate these hospitals from the evaluation of project efficacy, as Revans (1976) has done, arguing that including rejecters of the project is not a fair test. Be that as it may, the significant positive findings of the contrast tests employing all of the hospitals, even rejecters, clearly and in a very conservative and cautious fashion demonstrate the efficacy of the bootstrap approach to organizational change and improvement.

REFERENCES

Alderson, W. North Middlesex Hospital. In Reginald W. Revans (Ed.) *Hospitals, communication, choice, and change: The Hospital Internal Communications Project seen from within.* London: Tavistock, 1972. Pp. 46–52.

Armenakis, Achilles, and Field, Hubert S. Evaluation of organizational change using non-independent criterion measures. *Personnel Psychology*, 1975, *28*, 39–44.

Bardgett, W. E. Hillingdon Hospital, Additional Comments. In Revans (Ed.) *Hospitals, communication, choice, and change.* Pp. 20–21.

Campbell, Donald T. From description to experimentations: interpreting trends as quasi-experiments. In Chester W. Harris (Ed.) *Problems in measuring change.* Madison, Wisc.: University of Wisconsin Press, 1963. Pp. 212–242.

Campbell, Donald T., and Stanley, J. C. Experimental and quasi-experimental designs for research on teaching. In N. L. Gage (Ed.) *Handbook of research on teaching.* Chicago: Rand McNally, 1963.

Cook, Thomas D. and Campbell, Donald T. The design and conduct of quasi-experiments and true experiments in field settings. In Marvin D. Dunnette (Ed.) *Handbook of industrial and organizational psychology.* Chicago: Rand McNally, 1976. Pp. 223-326.

Coser, Rose L., Authority and decision making in a hospital: a comparative analysis. *American Sociological Review,* 1958, *23*, 56-63.

Coser, Rose L., *Life in the ward.* East Lansing, Michigan: Michigan State University Press, 1962.

Davies, Celia, and Francis, Arthur. *Hospital organization research project final report.* London: Imperial College of Science and Technology, 1974.

Franklin, Jerome L. Characteristics of successful and unsuccessful organization development. *Journal of Applied Behavioral Science,* 1976, *12*, 471-492.

Grant, A., and Cohen, B. S., Acute myocardial infarction: effect of a rehabilitation program on length of hospitalization and functional status at discharge. *Archives of Physical Medicine and Rehabilitation,* 1973 *54*, 201-206.

Hage, Jerald. *Communication and organizational control: cybernetics in health and welfare settings.* New York: John Wiley, 1974.

Hawkins, James L., and Selmanoff, Eugene D. Authority structure, ambiguity of the medical task, absence of the doctor from the ward, and the behavior of nurses. Indiana University Medical Center (mimeo, undated).

Hutter, A. M., Jr., Sidel, V. W., Shine, K. I., et al. Early hospital discharge after myocardial infarction. *New England Journal of Medicine,* 1973, *288*, 1141-1144.

Janis, Irving L., and Levanthal, Howard. Psychological aspects of physical illness and hospital care. In Benjamin B. Wolman (Ed.) *Handbook of clinical psychology.* New York: McGraw-Hill, 1965. Pp. 1360-1977.

Knowles, G. S. A. North Middlesex Hospital, Additional comments. In Revans (Ed.) *Hospitals, communication, choice and change.* Pp. 52-53.

Lahti, P. T. Early postoperative discharge of patients. *Michigan Medic,* 1970, *69*, 755-760.

Leigh, Hilary, Wieland, George F., and Anderson, John A. D. The Hospital Internal Communications Project. *Lancet,* 1971, 1005-1009.

Lindeman, C. A., and Van Aernam, B. Nursing intervention with the presurgical patient—the effects of structured and unstructured preoperative teaching. *Nursing Research,* 1971, *20*, 319-332.

Nadler, David, Mirvis, Philip, and Cammann, Cortlandt. The ongoing feedback system: experimenting with a new management tool. *Organizational Dynamics,* 1976, *4*, 4(Spring), 63-80.

Revans, Reginald W. *Action learning in hospitals: diagnosis and therapy.* London: McGraw-Hill, 1976.

Roberts, Karlene R., Cerruti, Nannette L., and O'Reilly, Charles A. III. Changing perceptions of organizational communication: Can short-term intervention help? *Nursing Research,* 1976, *25*, 197-200.

Royston, G. R. Short stay hospital treatment and rapid rehabilitation of cases of myocardial infarction in a district hospital. *British Heart Journal,* 1972, *34*, 526-532.

Sarason, Seymour B. *The creation of settings and the future societies.* San Francisco: Jossey-Bass, 1972.

Skipper, James K. Jr., and Leonard, Robert C. Children, stress, and hospitalization. *Journal of Health and Social Behavior,* 1968, *9*, 275-287.

Suchman, Edward A. *Evaluative research: principles and practice in public service and social action programs.* New York: Russell Sage Foundation, 1967.

Sutherland, A. *A study of long-stay admissions to the acute medical wards of the Aberdeen hospitals.* Edinburgh: Scottish Home and Health Department, 1972.

Ullrich, Robert A., and Wieland, George F. *Organization theory and design,* rev. ed. Homewood, Ill.: Richard D. Irwin, 1980.

Wechsler, Henry. *Handbook of medical specialties.* New York: Human Sciences Press, 1976.

Weisbord, Marvin R. Why organization development hasn't worked (so far) in medical centers. *Health Care Management Review,* 1976, *1,* 17–28.

Wieland, George F. Action research and change in ten hospitals. Manuscript, Ann Arbor, Mich., 1979 (Washington: National Technical Information Service, 1981).

Winer, B. J. *Statistical principles in experimental design,* 2nd ed. New York: McGraw-Hill, 1971.

Wise, Harold, Beckhard, Richard, Rubin, Irwin, and Kyte, Aileen. *Making health teams work.* Cambridge, Mass.: Ballinger, 1974.

NOTES

1. The following F ratio is computed: In the numerator is the variance of the points predicted by the two partial trends from the points predicted by the single overall trend; in the denominator is found the variance of the observed values from the two partial trends. The degrees of freedom are (a) one, and (b) the number of the time-series points minus one. For examples of the use of this test, see Campbell (1963) and Armenakis and Feild (1975).

2. Using a longer span of years for the second partial trend (1966 to 1973) yields the same pattern of results over all seven categories of patient.

3. A component of a sum of squares was calculated, based on a squared comparison (which is the difference between the means, or two sets of means, in the present case), divided by N times the sum of the squares of the coefficients used in the comparison. This component of the sum of squares then serves as the numerator (with 1 degree of freedom) of an F-test and is divided by the residual variance from the basic analysis of variance.

4. Because efficiency is correlated year to year, the required assumption of homogeneity or symmetry of covariance matrices is violated. However, the conservatively biased Greenhouse and Geisser test (Winer 1971, p. 523), which involves treating the observed F as having fewer degrees of freedom (1 and N–1), still shows general surgery to be significant, and general medicine is nearly significant at this level. If one removes the teaching hospital from this analysis (because its goal of improving efficiency may not have been as strong as in the other hospitals), the contrast for general medicine is highly significant (F=10.8), even after the quite conservative Greenhouse-Geisser procedure is used.

5. For the details on the differences between internal and external controls, see Ullrich and Wieland (1980).

6. In fact, Wechsler (1976) reviews a number of studies of surgeons, and terms them "authoritarian and stubborn, believing strongly in physician authority in patient care as well as emphasizing the physicians's need to control patient behavior" (p. 109). Also see Wechsler for summaries of most of the fifteen studies cited here.

7. The hospital's standing (either level or slope) "before" (i.e., 1961 to 1965) was used

to predict subsequent hospital standing "after." Then, this predicted score was subtracted out of the actual subsequent score (level or slope), leaving a residualized score. Without this correction, those hospitals which were, in 1961 to 1965, relatively more efficient than their regions, or trending toward better efficiency than their regions, would be likely to "look good" after the project. That is, the correction is needed because there are high correlations from year to year in the relative performance of hospitals.

8. For additional evidence that an understanding orientation leads to psychological change, see Franklin (1976). He found that fourteen successful OD projects, but not eleven unsuccessful projects, had organizational members who wanted to experiment with new ideas.

9. For additional evidence on "distress" leading organizational members to choose a psychological approach to change, see Nadler et al. (1976). In a most unusual OD intervention, organizational members were allowed to use survey feedback or not, as they wished. High use was made by those departments showing distress. Departments that were well functioning did not.

10. Franklin (1976) also found top management "support" was present in successful OD projects, but not in unsuccessful ones.

11. For a project which attempted to use an understanding approach to improve the functioning of internists and surgeons, but was successful only with the former, see Hage (1974), a summary of which will be found in Chapter 25.

12. A graduate student, knowing nothing of the project beyond the article by Leigh and colleagues (1971), easily selected the two hospital reports which display a rejecting attitude.

13. An examination of the performance of this hospital over all of its patient categories shows a profoundly negative record (e.g., for Clayton's test 1961–65 versus 1966–73, there are only two positive categories and four negative ones).

The Significance of Action and Understanding Systems

George F. Wieland

The most significant implication of the study of action and understanding systems is that these orientations affect the way individuals should view one another and their organizations. Each person must begin by studying his or her own goals and determining whether they are action- or understanding-oriented. Depending on which approach is preeminent, individuals and organizations behave very differently. In this chapter we shall attempt to show some of the implications that flow from distinguishing between action and understanding systems.

ACTION AND UNDERSTANDING AS GOALS

When we speak of action and understanding goals we mean that the ultimate intentions of the individual or the ultimate aims of the organization are primarily action or understanding.[1] If one or the other of these goals is preeminent, then it would seem that the particular organization is best organized in one way or the other. Action systems seem to take on simple, readily understood tasks that require little information processing. They use routines and a hierarchical structure, with an external control system, and they tend to employ individuals comfortable with the use of, or compliance to, authority. Such organizations are well suited to achieving action, or as Hage and Aiken (1970) put it, they are geared for production, turning out larger quantities of some product or service.

An understanding goal leads to complex tasks which are not readily understood, to an informal structure emphasizing exchange of information with an internal (professional) control system, and to the employment of individuals who have broad interests and who are open to new information. Such organizations are more concerned with the quality of a product or service, and with achieving a new and unique answer to a problem or need.

In the parlance of organizational study, we propose a "contingency" approach to management and organizations, weighing whether the primary goals center around action or understanding. It is for this reason that one may speak of action and understanding "systems." They are systems in that the kinds of goals, technologies, structures, and personalities tend to covary, providing a relatively good fit which is conducive to the ultimately effective functioning of the organization.[2]

TWO KINDS OF PEOPLE

A contingency approach for organizational change should be as commonplace as is the contingency approach for organization design. But it isn't. It may well be that the change agents, who are people, have problems in going beyond their own personal predilections toward action or understanding. There is, in fact, psychological research showing a clustering of personal predispositions which are conducive to action and a clustering of those conducive to understanding.

Caine and colleagues (1973), for example, asked people admitted to a psychotherapy clinic about their preferences for type of treatment, group psychoanalytic therapy or behavior therapy (behavior modification). The former, analytic approach, we would categorize as an understanding approach to change, while behavior modification, with its emphasis on quick results without understanding, we would categorize as an action approach to change.

The study of a sample of 130 consecutive admissions to the clinic shows that the preference for one or the other approach is predictable in several ways. It is no surprise, for example, that the conservatism of the patient predicted a preference for the action over the understanding approach. As the researchers point out, group therapy is more "democratic," the patients are encouraged to challenge the therapist and they are expected to take an active role in helping other patients. This is in contrast to the authoritarian relationship between therapist and patient in behavior modification. The findings in this study are congruent with the Hospital Internal Communications (HIC) evaluation data showing that authoritarians tend to view change in terms of an action approach.[3]

Another dimension differentiating preferences for these two therapies is the inward/outward direction of interest of the patient. Just as we found in the

HIC evaluation that managers taking an interest in psychological matters would tend to pursue an understanding approach to change, Caine found that inwardly directed persons tend to focus on their own feelings and attitudes as objects of change. They also tend to involve other people (in addition to the therapist) in the therapy, just as we found in the HIC evaluation that managers with an understanding orientation would engage in meetings and discussions with others. In addition, the researchers found that inwardly directed patients tended to question attitudes and assumptions in the group, just as one component of the understanding orientation in the HIC Project was the comparison and questioning of the goals of the project.

The third dimension concerns divergence/convergence in style of thinking. Caine and colleagues found that divergent thinkers, like managers who have a wide breadth of interests, preferred the understanding approach to change. The divergent thinkers were open to explore a range of possibilities in therapy; they were open to group therapy and to the plenitude of material likely to be dredged up in analytic therapy. In contrast, the convergent thinkers, like relatively closed minded, "no-nonsense" managers, were more interested in an action approach to change, in this case, the direct modification of behavior without examining basic causes.[4]

Different Goals Coordinate with Different World Views

MacGregor's (1960) contrast between Theory X and Theory Y is most suggestive in this regard. A key element in these two basic world views is how one perceives human nature. Theory X is predicated on a conservative view, a negative view of human nature. Because humans are perverse—they are lazy and acquisitive—a Hobbesian approach to management follows. Individuals are controlled by using external controls, by external structures and rewards and punishments.

In contrast, the Theory Y of humanistic psychology, and, generally of organization development (OD), too, takes a positive and optimistic view of human nature. Individuals are basically good, and organizational structures of various kinds only hinder this goodness from emerging. A Rousseauian approach is used to organize individuals: good human emotions and spontaneity are encouraged. Organizing individuals consists of helping them get in touch with themselves (their positive human natures), and helping them to get in touch with the goodness in one another, too.

Action and understanding systems make considerable sense when they are viewed as based on Theory X or Theory Y, respectively. Thus, Argyris (1976), for example, has argued for the greater use of understanding systems. He advocates deutero-learning or double-loop learning. One learns not merely how better to reach a given goal (single-loop learning) but also questions the very goal itself (double-loop learning). (This kind of questioning in the HIC Project was part of an understanding orientation to organizational change.)

It is no surprise, then, to find Argyris' work rejected out of hand by more conservative researchers, who, we would speculate, have a world view based on rather different assumptions from Argyris. For example, a sociologist from a conservative college (which refuses on ideological grounds to take HEW grant money) says in a review of Argyris' *Increasing Leadership Effectiveness*, "Emperor Chris, if not unclothed, has his scholarly pants down. To paraphrase H. L. Mencken, no leadership theorist has gone broke by underestimating the gullibility of readers of books about leadership" (Haga 1978, p. 187).

Another sociologist (Gross et al. 1971) displays the essence of the action approach to change, in his criticism of psychologists and in his contention that a change program in a school is not really contingent on the teachers' degree of willingness to change or similar psychological characteristics. Instead, he sees managerial action as the key, in this case, support by the principal and other administrators in the form of physical resources and structures to free time and eliminate conflicting demands.

DIFFERENT VALUES

Proponents of understanding or action systems often take a strong moralistic stance, that one is "right" and the other is "wrong." This is only natural given the close grounding of these systems in one's view of ultimate reality, a grounding in values and in what Kant termed the "categorical imperative."

Some implore managers to switch to Theory Y because it is more "effective," and organization development is advocated as a means of improving the "effectiveness" of organizations, while, in fact, the evidence is not yet in. There are even cases of apparently decreased organizational effectiveness as a result of organization development. Managers at TRW Systems, for example, devoted considerable effort to improving relations with one another, while changes in the economy went unperceived and led ultimately to major layoffs and organizational retrenchment (*Business Week* 1973).

All this is not to say that organization development as an end is "bad" or that it is "good." It can be either, depending on one's basic assumptions and values. The point is that justifications of OD as a means to certain ends, such as effectiveness,[5] must be made under the canons of scientific evidence. If such evidence is not available, then a reasoned advocacy should be made on value grounds alone.

The HIC evaluation has shown for understanding systems, OD is a means to better organizational performance. However, for action systems, OD may not be effective. When given a choice, persons in action systems do not make use of OD, probably because of the deep value incongruities, as well as incompatibilities with the technology and structure of the system. In such a system, managerial action would be more effective.

There is evidence that an analogous situation holds for humanistic psychology, for its advocacy of certain behaviors as being more desirable and effective. When judged against criteria of individual effectiveness (personality integration and mental health), behaviors such as openness and spontaneity are sometimes effective, but sometimes just the opposite kinds of behavior, more ordered and controlled orientations, are more appropriate. This was what Coan (1974) found when he took an inductive approach to studying personality and applied multivariate analysis to see how a very large number of personality variables covaried in a large number of subjects. He obtained "no evidence . . . of a unitary dimension that might be properly viewed as a general factor of personality integration, self-actualization, or positive mental health" (p. 197).

Coan criticizes the circularity of Maslow's concept of self-actualization. Maslow apparently valued creativity and admired creative people. Thus in selecting the optimal personalities for study, he tended to select creative individuals and he proceeded to find creativity, spontaneity, openness, and other similar factors to be characteristic of very effective persons. But it has yet to be proved that more open, spontaneous people are more effective people.

In summary, then, we have argued that much of what passes for rigorous scientific research is barely concealed advocacy on value grounds. Certainly, we allow that research efforts may be directed by values, and as such they may even be more effective in grappling with important (i.e., value-relevant) problems. But the values of the researcher and the values of the subjects of the research (including organizational values) should be clarified, and their role in basic research and its application should be more clearly specified. The concealment of values is liable to give practitioners some nasty surprises when they go to apply the research findings in their own organizations.

CHANGE EFFORTS CONGRUENT WITH
ORGANIZATIONAL CHARACTERISTICS

A contingency approach to organization design is now commonplace. Starting with the seminal work of Burns and Stalker (1961) and Lawrence and

Lorsch (1967), managers are advised to structure their organizations in one way or another depending on the basic characteristics of the relevant organizational subsystems, usually on the basis of the technology or (closely related) environmental uncertainty. Analogously, the present research, we have suggested, seems to support a contingency approach to change and improvement efforts. Change efforts should be congruent with the type of organization being changed.

However, the present study differs from the work of the above contingency theorists in one important respect: no primacy is given to any single determining or differentiating factor on which change efforts are to be contingent. We assume that action and understanding systems comprise interdependent goals, technologies, structures, and people. As far as we know, none by nature takes priority. The goal of an action system is to act and such a goal is compatible with a simple task, a high reliance on formal structure, and a preponderance of authoritarian human characteristics. But any one of these elements may lead to a shift toward more congruence in the other, contingent elements. Authoritarian individuals may be selected into (or self-select into) an organizational system with predominantly action goals, but the converse is possible, too. Individuals in the organization may select goals (or structure, technology) according to their authoritarian preferences or basic views of the world. As Child (1972) so aptly puts it, there is "organizational choice." That is, organizational members can modify structure, technology, and goals according to their selective perceptions of what is needed.

The implications, then, are that managers, and those helping managers improve their organizations, need to diagnose not only the technological (or environmental) constraints on organizational systems and subsystems, but also the goals, structure, and, especially, the human element, to see if an action or understanding approach to change is more appropriate to the system in question.

A number of recent developments support the view that managers must also take into account people and structure, as well as technology, in efforts at contingency management. With regard to the human element, psychologists have learned that not all people are Theory Y types. They have begun to differentiate people with Theory X views of work from those with Theory Y views (see, for example, Hulin and Blood 1968). Furthermore, there is increasing advocacy of the idea that work and organizational environments should be more individualized (Kahn 1973) and that some workers may not prefer enlarged or enriched jobs, even if many do.[6] In the same vein, managers are advised to fit their control system (internalized or externalized) to their own management styles (Camman and Nadler 1976).

The structural component of the organizational system is highlighted in a recent paper (Schein and Greiner 1977) in which researchers on organizational change recommend that OD be modified when it is used in the highly structured bureaucracies which we have termed action systems. These researchers discuss how OD can be modified to fit the requirements of such action systems. However, we would suggest that OD needs more than the "fine tuning" that Schein and Greiner advocate, if bureaucracies are to benefit. More than "a more positive attitude" and "more thorough knowledge" will be needed, because there is a basic value incongruity between OD and action systems.

The third organizational component, goals, has received little explicit recognition by researchers and practitioners of organizational change. One exception is the Blake and Mouton grid approach to change. However, while their phase 4 requires organizational members to discuss the substantive nature of organizational goals, there is no recognition that the type of goal, whether action or understanding, makes OD or some other approach to change more or less appropriate.

Organizations probably come to emphasize action or understanding goals by the operation of what Thompson (1967) has termed the "inner circle," a coalition of powerful individuals who wittingly or unwittingly make decisions and take actions out of which organizational directions evolve. Guth and Tagiuri (1965) provide an illuminating example in which the vice-presidents of a research and development firm argued over organizational strategy in terms of 1) rapid growth by researching new products, 2) rapid growth by increasing readily marketable products, and 3) slower growth with continued emphasis on quality. After a number of fruitless meetings over the "objective" merits of each strategy, it emerged that different strategies were being advocated because of the differing personal values of the top executives involved. The first strategy was advocated by a vice-president who seemed to be a "businessman-scientist," valuing profits and growth but also valuing the intellectual stimulation of a research environment. The second and third strategies were defended by vice-presidents who valued business achievement or research creativity, respectively. When all these values were clarified, a strategy integrating the values of all three executives became feasible.[7]

Probably most organizational members, including top executives, are less than fully conscious of the organization's goals and strategies. Over time, a certain way of looking at important issues, as well as at everyday matters, evolves. Basic premises are not questioned (Perrow 1972), but nevertheless they exist. They are hard to change; they are part of the basic "culture" of the organization (see Chapter 14 of Jay 1971, for insightful clinical descriptions of organizational cultures). Harrison (1972) is perhaps the only practitioner of planned organizational change who has given explicit recognition to different basic types of organizational culture, his distinctions being the power-oriented, role-oriented, task-oriented, and person-oriented organizations.[8] More important than the typology is Harrison's emphasis that the change agent or management consultant should diagnose the organizational or subsystem cultures and decide whether his or her recommendations are congruent or in conflict with the culture.

It would seem, then, that those wishing to facilitate organization improvement should learn to discern the varied emphases in the goals, strategies, and even cultures, of organizations. As in Guth and Tagiuri's illustration, most organizations are likely to combine an emphasis on action and understanding, but one is likely to predominate to a greater or lesser degree. Congruent help depends on the change agent's discerning the basic nature of the client system.

CHANGE-AGENT BIASES IN PERCEPTIONS

Research evidence seems to suggest that change agents tend to see organizations in terms of either action systems or understanding systems, not both, and they try to change organizations in ways compatible with their own particular perceptual bias (Tichy 1974, 1975; Tichy and Hornstein 1976). In this research, the change agents using an action approach (a structural approach, external to the social system of the organization) are described in terms of "analysis for the top" (AFT). Tichy found these change agents to be very different from OD consultants (who took an "internal" or understanding orientation) in background, goals, diagnostic procedures, and techniques used for change.[9]

In terms of the characteristics they brought to the consulting situation, the AFT change agents were quite conservative while the OD consultants "labeled themselves as liberals." The latter saw much more change needed in society, and they saw society so structured that "alienation is inevitable." They saw more need for relatively radical change ("strike at the roots") and disagreed more that compromise was desirable, compared to the AFT consultants. The OD consultants' main goal in consulting was to improve the problem solving of the client system, while for the AFT consultants it was improved system efficiency and increased output. The OD consultants emphasized the organizational culture in their diagnosis, while the AFT consultants emphasized work processes, resources, and performance.

In both cases, the change strategies tended to correspond to their respective diagnostic approaches. There seemed to be a "self-fulfilling cycle," as Tichy put it. The OD consultants introduced confrontation meetings, sensitivity training, team development, and individual counseling in an effort to change the culture. The AFT consultants concentrated on job training and technological innovations much more, and they generally worked on formal structure and work process more (they had a "systems analysis and operations research bias"). In general, OD consultants looked at the culture of the individuals and their organization and that is what they tried to change,[10] while the AFT consultants looked at the work process and that is what they tried to change. Tichy advises managers looking for consultants: "consumers beware!"

CLIENT CHOICE FACILITATES CONGRUENT HELP

We suggested above that much research and much practice of organization change seems to be based on one or another system of values and assumptions about the world. If this is true, it may often be difficult for an organization to get help that is congruent and compatible with its basic character in terms of action or understanding. Better diagnostic skills on the part of practitioners may be one answer, but until these are common, a greater emphasis on informed choice by the client may be of great help in avoiding incompatible forms of help.

Specifically, organizational clients should be given free choice of both action and understanding forms of interventions—free choice of OD and also of the more traditional forms of help facilitative of managerial action. While traditional OD practitioners report use of free choice, there is less than complete freedom, since to decline OD help usually means declining all help by the consultant. Most OD consultants are not prepared to offer the help predicated on the conservative values with which an action system is comfortable. Free choice means offering both action and understanding kinds of intervention and allowing the client, or client subsystems, to choose either.

The HIC Project was most unusual in its provision of free choice in this form. Revans emphasized that only hospital staff knew their own problems and could solve them, and having said this he withdrew from active management of the project. Although he continued to play an inspirational and motivational role, he refrained from pushing his theories, models, or ideas onto the hospital staff. Thus it was up to the hospitals and to individual hospital team members to decide what their problems were (psychological difficulties or structural ones requiring managerial action), and it was up to them to invite central team help. Some hospital teams waited months before inviting central team help (to the great dismay and intense frustration of the central team members). One team proceeded to work without any direct central team help at all.

The freedom of the hospitals to choose help or not was enforced by the strong norm established at the beginning of the project. The sponsoring Department of Health and Society Security asked the hospitals to "get on board" but promised that they would be able to "steer," too. This was supported by the other sponsor, The King's Fund Hospital Centre, a voluntary organization with the main purpose of supporting hospital innovations and improvements that seemed to be outside the scope of the nationalized health service. The officials from both these organizations held the bulk of the power on the advisory committee which steered the project. Their members chaired the committee and they numbered a majority on the advisory committee as well. This power was used throughout the project period to enforce a strict norm of hospital control.[11]

In addition to deciding when to invite the central team, if ever, to their hospital, the hospital teams also exerted control over the nature of the central team help provided. This was shown by a study of the central team's change-agent role (Wieland 1979). While central team members desired to make psychologically deep interventions, their actual behavior was in general quite discrepant: it was usually shallow. To learn the cause of the discrepancy, we compared the profile (i.e., differential emphasis) for these behaviors with the desires of the central team members themselves, the desires of the two sponsoring agencies, and the desires of the hospital teams. The resulting correlations demonstrated that the hospital team desires were most likely the cause of the actual configuration of central team behaviors. This was possible because central team work in the hospitals was very dependent on continual legitimation by the hospital team. The compartmentalized nature of hospitals made continual legitimating introductions necessary as the central team members moved to new departments or levels in the organization. Thus the hospital teams were almost always in a position to halt or redirect projects in their hospitals.

The real proof of the hospitals' power in choosing central team help is given by the refusals of further help. As part of the evaluation interviews, we asked central team members to recount their "worst mistakes" while working in the hospitals. In answering this question, one of the central team members reported introducing an understanding orientation to change at a hospital rating very high in authoritarianism, an approach which was incongruent with the character of the hospital and which led to her not being invited back again.

> V: . . . I think I antagonized the X hospital team quite early on when we had a small (hospital project) group. . . . (The hospital team members) gave a very good presentation of what they were doing. . . . Then they said "we don't know what to do now," and they were expecting some kind of direction about how to handle the feedback (of project results) and what to do about it. We didn't give them this (i.e., any answers or directive forms of help).

This central team member was never invited back to the hospital.

In What Sense Was the HIC Project an OD Effort?

One might well ask if the HIC was organization development. As mentioned above (see also Wieland 1979), the HIC Project was, in general and on the average, more shallow than the usual OD effort. Many of the hospital team members did not want a deep intervention, and the physicians in particular were in a position of sufficient power to prevent such interventions whenever they were undesired.

But there is a more positive reason for choosing such a relatively shallow approach to OD: there is likely to be more "carry over" as Strauss (1976) terms it. More individual change is carried over into organizational change. To understand this, one may array OD efforts along a continuum of individual to organizational focus, with T-groups (especially "stranger" labs or ones with collections of individuals who are organizationally unrelated) at the individual end of the continuum. Process facilitation and team building, i.e., work on the interpersonal problems of organizationally related individuals, are in the middle of the continuum. HIC is further toward the organizational end of the continuum, since it deals with relations among the top staff members of the organization as well as with their more distant organizational responsibilities (interpersonal relations of near and distant subordinates, as well as structural and technological problems in distant corners of the organization).[12]

By directly involving organizational concerns (following Revans' prescriptions for learning by doing or action learning) the HIC Project would seem to have dealt with the problems of carry over. Critics of OD and especially the individually oriented T-groups have pointed out that individuals may change, but that this is no assurance that they will change the organization when they return to their everyday work efforts (Strauss 1976). As one book asked, "After the turn on, what?" (Houts and Serber 1972). Other, unchanged persons and the general inertia of norms and other structures may be difficult to change and may cause the changed person to regress and revert to former behavior.

As we see it, there may be a trade-off between the depth of an OD effort and the pervasiveness of organizational change. Deep efforts can be very successful by removing an individual from his organizational context (that is, the individual is "unfrozen" by the absence of usual organizational support). But by failing to devote attention to the organizational context, such efforts leave organization norms and structural-technological arrangements untouched. On the other hand, a more shallow OD effort, such as HIC, can cover more organizational matters, but individuals are often basically unchanged. In the short run, anyway, the choice of deep or shallow change efforts may depend primarily on whether one values individual or organizational change more (as well as depending on whether the client will permit a deep intervention or not).

But we have been speaking of the HIC Project *in general* as being relatively shallow. As we have seen, some interventions were quite deep. Team members were confronted with survey data, or with perceptions of training group members, that questioned their attitudes, styles of management and the like. With support from superiors, as well as peers and central team members, they made efforts to assimilate these data, and psychological change apparently ensued.

Other hospital teams did not make heavy use of central team help. They had managerial action in mind, and as (limited) help from the central team they received data which aided in designing problem-solving actions.

The former process, in which central team members facilitated psychological changes and these in turn affected the functioning of others in the organization, is very similar to traditional OD focused on individual change. The latter process, in which very shallow, cognitive forms of help are devoted to facilitating managerial action, is not OD, it is the antithesis. Rather than being "concerned with understanding, appreciation, and the exploration of possibilities" as is OD, it is "concerned with the world as it is now and how it can be managed" (Blackler and Brown 1978). In encompassing both the main schools of practice in changing organizations, OD and managerial action, the HIC Project is best viewed as a project in "organizational change."

HIC Evidence for a Contingency Approach to Organizational Change

The HIC Project was in part an effort in organization development, but because it made provision for client choice (by avoiding high consultant power and also by providing a variety of change program alternatives), it was also an effort in traditional management consultancy aimed at managerial action. Normally the OD consultant is highly committed to his or her humanistic values and world view (an understanding view in which psychological and interpersonal problems are important) and is quite antipathetic toward an action-oriented approach to ameliorating "external" structural or technological problems. Because the HIC Project allowed both approaches to organizational improvement (and thereby caused some conflict and confusion), it provided the potential for learning about the situations in which one or the other approach was more appropriate.

The analysis here is not, by any means, definitive. The evaluation study was not designed to test a contingency model. It was, in fact, focused on the psychological and OD-like processes of organizational change (see Wieland and Leigh 1971, Chapter 3). But in an attempt to evaluate what was really going on—from a nonideological curiosity about what Revans and the hospitals had really set in motion—we have acquired some data that is at least very suggestive about the differential appropriateness of OD and traditional management consultancy.

These two approaches to change, understanding and action, seem to be differentially appropriate in two senses. First of all, understanding and action were chosen by two different kinds of individuals and organizations. The understanding approach was selected by distressed organizations and by top staff who not only had psychological problems but also seemed committed to a psychological approach to change. The action approach to change was chosen by highly integrated organizations that were well structured for action and by individuals who were authoritarian (hierarchical and closed-minded in outlook).

Secondly, and most important, the two approaches to change were differentially appropriate in terms of their effects. Use of the understanding (OD or psychological) approach to change resulted in improved functioning of an understanding subsystem in the organization (improvement in a system with a complex task, with a high degree of informal structure and interpersonal collaboration, and with individuals valuing knowledge and intellectual stimulation).

But an understanding approach to change did not improve functioning of the action subsystem, it was the action approach to change that did. Managerial action on technical and structural matters improved the action subsystems comprising relatively simple tasks, a strong and hierarchical formal structure, and individuals valuing authority and action rather than knowledge. Furthermore, the action approach to change not only did not improve understanding system functioning, the data give some indications that it even had a deleterious effect.

THE CRITICAL NATURE OF CONTROL SYSTEMS

The existence of two approaches to organizational change and their differential effectiveness in different organizational settings may be linked to the existence of two fundamentally different approaches to organization itself. Organizations are different from other social collectivities such as families, informal groups, and communities in that there is a very large element of conscious, purposive design involved in the organization. Organizations may be viewed as the conscious coordination of various elements, including most importantly, people, toward some purpose or goal.

People are organized ("coordinated" or "controlled" depending on various writers' terminologies) in two different ways: from "outside" or from "inside."

Internal control systems consist of procedures which individuals have internalized, the attitudes, norms, roles, etc., which individuals have been socialized to feel are obligatory. External control systems consist of arrangements external to individuals, such as formal rules and regulations and authority structures which provide "orders."

In organizations with internal control systems, the critical elements are "inside" of people, and a psychological or understanding approach to change is required. In fact, external, action-oriented approaches to change tend to be resisted because organizational members have been socialized to "make up their own minds," to "do what is right" according to their internalized (often professional) standards. Internal controls are used when each organization member has many different response capabilities (described as "redundancy" within each individual by Emery [1974]), and each is expected to select the appropriate response according to his or her perception of the (usually very complex) task requirements.

Psychological forms of help, such as the "talking cure" will allow individuals to reorder their thinking and develop new ways of looking at things. In addition, groups of collaborating individuals can exchange views and share information, and they can build up commitments to new ways of working that enhance the informal collaboration which is often so critical in understanding systems. For successful change, the organizational members need to change themselves, rather than rely on an external change agent (see, for example, Franklin 1976).

In contrast, in organizations with external control systems, the critical elements are "outside" of people, and an action approach to change, modifying "external" structure, is more efficient. In this approach, change is "engineered" in a mechanical fashion. The external control system is, of course, characteristic of bureaucracies or organizations designed according to the traditional classical management designs, with formal authority and formal roles predominant. Individuals are treated as objects and assigned to relatively specialized roles. (According to Emery [1974] "redundancy" is not found within an individual but between them. Individuals are treated as easily replaceable parts.) Such structures are often found where the technology is relatively simple, as in the production department of many manufacturing firms. The different elements of the task are known and can be split into specialized jobs and then combined in a rational, preordained process.

Other organizations have external control systems because a potentially complex task has been defined as simple. Many governmental bureaucracies are faced with multiple, conflicting values, and even ends and means are often inextricably interwoven (Braybrooke and Lindblom 1963). But the task has been defined as simple: deliver certain services, to certain categories of client, using a limited number of standardized procedures. Various formal structures (rules, formal procedures, standards) determine, in the main, how individuals and the organization as a whole function. The critical element, it seems, is not whether the task is simple or complex, but how the organization goes about defining the task and organizing its staff.

The most direct way of dealing with problems in an organization with an external control system is thus to change some of those external factors. The factory worker, for example, is subjected to Taylor's time-and-motion study, and work procedures are modified. Jobs may be redesigned and assigned differently, and entire production systems may be changed on the basis of management science studies using work methods or operations research techniques. The same techniques are applied to bureaucratic paper shuffling and even to client processing in governmental service agencies.

OTHER RESEARCH SUPPORT FOR A CONTINGENCY APPROACH TO CHANGE

The available research evidence from health care organizations seems to support the contingency approach to change advocated here. Consider, first of all, the hospital emergency department, which uses a relatively simple technology to process patients with great dispatch. It is an action system par excellence. Psychological subtleties are relatively unimportant, quick decision making and even authoritarian brusqueness are the rule. The use of an understanding approach to change in such a setting can be expected to yield relatively little improvement in performance. This is, in fact, what Roberts and colleagues (1976) found when they examined the effects of OD training, using an excellent control-group and before-and-after experimental design.

An understanding approach to change did apparently work in a hospital project described by Hage (1974). However, this effort at improving the quality of patient care, a program among physicians, was only acceptable to a portion of the physicians—those in understanding systems. According to Hage, the hospital in question suffered from a "loose medical organization," i.e., there was little organizational coordination or professional control. The specific changes in the hospital were to add several new medical subspecialists to the staff (in hematology, endocrinology, infectious diseases, and neurology), and to add a number of socialization mechanisms (teaching rounds, grand rounds, and subspecialty rounds). There were also new assistant directors of medical education in medicine, surgery, obstetrics/gynecology, and pediatrics.

The aim of these changes was to create a better quality control system for patient care. There would be better supervision and education of the house staff and through them, the practicing physicians. In other words, a "high feedback system" would be created. This then would be an understanding approach to change. The information and behavioral skills of some new specialities would be added to the hospital in the hopes that psychological changes would transpire in various kinds of meetings and discussions.

It comes as no surprise that the educational intervention that Hage describes—one more suited to an understanding system than an action system—was more or less accepted by the internists and, almost as much, by the pediatricians (who essentially practice internal medicine on children), but rejected almost totally by the surgeons.

In addition, it is interesting to find that internists took an understanding orientation to change while others, including especially the surgeons, took an action orientation. The senior internists, for example, used conferences to introduce the new program and they talked to everyone about it, including the nurses. Others, especially in obstetrics and gynecology, used a more formal approach—the chain of command. A significant response among the surgeons was that they would suffer a loss of authority if the new educational program were implemented.

In short, Hage describes an intervention which could improve the functioning of understanding systems, an intervention which would facilitate the exchange of information and would enhance learning and psychological change. For these reasons it was accepted by the internists, and for the same reasons it was rejected by the surgeons. The former, we have come to see, are organized to work on complex tasks requiring understanding. The structure is informal, relying on discussions with exchange of information, and controls are based on this internalized information. In contrast, the surgeons are organized in an action system, to work on a relatively simple task. They are relatively closed to new information and they rely on authoritative action—a formal chain of command and external controls.

Unfortunately, there is apparently no other rigorous research evidence on the efficacy of OD in health care settings. The anecdotal evidence by Beckhard and others (Wise et al. 1974) on the success of sensitivity training, process facilitation, and team building in the community health care teams at the Dr. Martin Luther King, Jr. (MLK) Health Center and the apparent failure of similar techniques among the central management staff at MLK support a contingency view. The community health teams belong to understanding systems, while central management is organized entirely differently, in a formal hierarchy, with a concern for formal procedures and other appurtenances of a bureaucracy.

Margulies' (1977) study of OD at Kaiser Permanente similarly fails to provide rigorous evaluation data, but the anecdotal evidence also supports the contingency perspective. Psychologically deep interventions, or understanding approaches to change, were not used in this bureaucratically structured setting. Relatively impersonal questionnaires and feedback were used to focus on action system characteristics, on structural matters such as staff assignments and on procedural changes in the kinds of formal reports submitted. In short, this OD effect used a relatively action-oriented intervention, and because the setting was an action system, the change effort was apparently successful.

In a similar vein, Weisbord (1976), in reporting why his OD efforts had not (so far) been successful in a medical center, advocates more shallow, action-oriented intervention, such as work on budgeting procedures, clarifying goals, and resource planning. Weisbord's characterization of the medical center as being composed of independent subunits ("feudal fiefdoms," some administrators have called them) indicates that the organization as a whole could not be characterized as an understanding system and thereby is not an appropriate setting for OD.

Stoelwinder and Clayton's (1978) account of OD in an Australian teaching hospital supports these views on the differential appropriateness of understanding and action-oriented interventions. A management-by-objectives (MBO) program was useful for top management but not effective in reaching down into the wards. When entry was obtained at the ward level, the approaches to change apparently varied according to a contingency model for change. Stoelwinder and Clayton describe successful team building (including "participative decision making") in a ward which was apparently for medical patients. More action-oriented approaches to change predominated in the surgical wards (procedures for "streamlining admission" and a "reorganized patient calling procedure"), in the emergency department (planning and commissioning an extensive expansion of the department), and in the outpatient group (redesigned procedures).

Finally, evidence in favor of the contingency approach to change is found in the carefully documented success of action-oriented change by means of industrial engineering (Ludwig 1971) and operations research (Griffith et al. 1976). These approaches can be used in nonmedical, routinized areas of the hospital (e.g., laundry, housekeeping) or in the action system components of medicine (e.g., admissions scheduling and preadmission testing procedures).

THE EVIDENCE FROM NON-HEALTH SETTINGS

Research in non-health settings is also supportive of a contingency approach to change. The classic Morse and Reimer (1956) study concerned the clerical staff in a large insurance company. Controls were removed from members of an experimental group, their supervisors were eliminated, and their jobs were enriched. They were given autonomy in deciding about many matters including work methods and processes.

Given a bureaucratic organization with relatively simple tasks (including a steady, dependable flow of work), these changes seem inappropriate for enhanced organizational effectiveness. The hope was that improved morale would increase productivity, and such was the case, but the productivity increase was less than that in another group of staff members subjected to a greater amount of centralized control. The results seem to be congruent with our assertion that in certain kinds of organizations (action systems, with external controls), external changes are more likely to be effective in improving productivity than internal, psychological changes. The improved morale created in the Morse and Reimer experimental group did improve productivity, but less so than did the direct approach of structural change.

Passmore and King (1978) studied the hourly work force in a food processing plant and found that a combined program of survey feedback and also structural and technological changes in one unit improved that unit's productivity while survey feedback (as well as minor job redesign to improve motivation) in the other unit yielded little improvement in productivity. The evaluation design used by Passmore and King is limited in that probable interaction effects are unknown, but the results of the study seem to support the view that technical and structural interventions (i.e., managerial action) are more effective than psychological changes in improving the productivity of an action system such as a manufacturing plant.

A number of studies done by the Tavistock Institute have modified "socio-technical systems." These changes are primarily in the form of reassignment of job duties and altered work flows, although some consideration is also given to psychological matters such as the compatibility of work group members. The studies do not include experimental controls, but time-series data do provide some evidence of success in the form of improved productivity. It is no accident that most of these projects have been conducted in organizational units which seem to be action subsystems: groups of coal miners (Trist et al. 1963); cotton mill workers (Rice 1958); and airplanes and terminal staff, dry cleaning shops and plants, and automated steel mills (Miller and Rice 1967). These are primarily action subsystems, and individuals are generally coordinated by external, structural controls.

In some contrast, most of the interventions using a primarily psychological approach are successfully conducted in systems which emphasize understanding. To take one widely used approach, we find that Likert's interventions to create a participative organizational system have been conducted primarily with managers, those who must deal with considerably more uncertainty than the workers on the shop floor or than those in situations where technological constraints are considerable (Parsons 1960). Indeed, many of the managers in these studies have been employed in marketing departments, where the work entails considerably more uncertainty (in dealing with a complex environment) than in production departments (Lawrence and Lorsch 1967).

Some comparative evidence supportive of a contingency approach to organizational change may be inferred from an extensive evaluation (Marrow, Bowers, and Seashore 1967) of the change program at Harwood, a pajama factory. Harwood used a team of behavioral scientists to improve interpersonal relations from managers down to supervisors and machine operators and to encourage participative management. This program included extensive sensitivity training. In addition, two teams of engineering consultants worked on technological and structural changes. The work flow throughout the plant was reorganized and supervisory and management controls were altered accordingly. Job specifications, methods, standards, and incentive plans were altered, and an induction program was begun for new machine operators, helping them acquire the techniques needed to operate the equipment.

In an independent evaluation study, an effort was made to assess the apparent resulting improvements in a very defined area, the level of machine operator performance, and to indicate the relative contribution of different change program elements by looking at the correlations in timing. By an admittedly crude but insightful procedure, the evaluators attributed some of the improvement to managerial action or structural changes and some to psychological changes, but most to the former.[13] In an action system such as a manufacturing plant, it is no surprise that productivity can be greatly affected by structural and technological interventions.

The implication of all this for the psychologist who would be an "organizational" consultant is that many jobs (even jobs done by some professionals, such as surgeons or surgical nurses) can be improved by management consultancy on "external" structure and technology, as well as, or perhaps even more than, by OD. Of course, one can argue on humanistic value grounds that OD should be used, but on grounds of improving the effectiveness of the organizational system management consultancy may be preferable to OD. It must be noted that efficacy is contingent to some degree on the kind of organizational system involved.

Finally, we should point out that a self-help approach to change (with the client in control of the help) does avoid treating the contingency model for change as completely deterministic. The self-help aspect allows the client to choose on a variety of grounds—not necessarily based on a good "fit" with existing organizational structure or technology, but perhaps on the basis of other values (Millar 1978).

Some Conclusions

Three major conclusions may be drawn from this research:

1. *Organization development, or an understanding approach to organization change, works. That is, OD can achieve improved organizational functioning.* There is continuing controversy about the efficacy of OD, perhaps in part, we have suggested, because the basic value differences between proponents and opponents make an objective, data-based evaluation seem unnecessary to them. In addition, incongruent use of OD on action systems, rather than on a congruent subsystem as in the HIC Project, may account for failures in affecting organizational outputs. Whatever the dynamics, to date there is little evidence on the effectiveness of OD in organizational change (Strauss 1976). Using a tight experimental design, we have demonstrated major subsequent organizational improvement in the processing of internal medicine patients, and we have linked the degree of such improvement to the extent of prior psychological changes in key organizational staff during the project. These changes in turn are linked by correlations to (1) the hospital team's taking an understanding approach to change and (2) to the extent of help from the central team, including psychological forms of help.

2. *An action approach to organizational change works, too. That is, the traditional management consultancy approaches focused on organizational technology or structure are also effective.* We have demonstrated a considerable amount of improvement in organizational functioning with regard to surgical patients, and this improvement was found to be correlated with earlier managerial action: the solving of managerial problems and the taking of administrative action (to institute new procedures, routines or structures or to alter technological arrangements).[14]

3. *A contingency approach to organizational change seems appropriate. OD (a psychological approach to change) and managerial action (to change structure or technology) are chosen, and are effective, in different organizational settings.* We found that effective OD, which is to say the above demonstrated psychological changes and improved functioning of understanding organizational subsystems, tended to occur where there was poor organizational integration and poorly functioning senior staff and where the senior staff were emotionally committed and influential in the change work. In contrast, managerial action and subsequent improved action-system functioning occurred in organizations already well organized or well structured for actions. In addition, the focus of efforts was different for the psychological and the action or structural approaches to change. The former was focused on understanding subsystems and the latter on action subsystems in the organization. In short, both approaches to change are effective, but each must be used in the appropriate setting.

REFERENCES

Ackoff, Russell L., and Emery, Fred E. *On purposeful systems.* Chicago: Aldine-Atherton, 1972.

Argyris, Chris. *Increasing leadership effectiveness.* New York: John Wiley & Sons, 1976.

Blacker, Frank, and Brown, Colin A. Organizational psychology: good intentions and false promises. *Human Relations,* 1978, *31,* 333-351.

Blake, Robert R., and Mouton, Jane S. *The managerial grid.* Houston: Gulf Publishing, 1970.

Braybrooke, David, and Lindblom, Charles E., *A strategy of decision.* New York: Free Press, 1963.

Burns, Tom, and Stalker, G.M. *The management of innovation.* London: Tavistock, 1961.

Business Week. Where being nice to workers didn't work. *Business Week,* 1973, no. 2263 (January 20), 98-100.

Caine, Thomas M., and Leigh, Rosaline. Conservatism in relation to psychiatric treatment. *British Journal of Social and Clinical Psychology,* 1972, *11,* 52-56.

Caine, T.M., Wijesinghe, B., and Wood, R.R. Personality and psychiatric treatment expectancies. *British Journal of Psychiatry,* 1973, 122, 87-88.

Cammann, Cortlandt, and Nadler, David A. Fit your control systems to your managerial style. *Harvard Business Review,* 1976, *54,* 1 (January-February), 65-72.

Casey, David, and Pearce, David (Eds.) *More than management development: action learning at GEC.* New York: American Management Association, 1977.

Child, John. Organizational structure, environment and performance: The role of strategic choice. *Sociology,* 1972, 6, 2-22.

Coan, Richard W. *The optimal personality: an empirical and theoretical analysis.* London: Routledge & Kegan Paul, 1974.

Emery, Fred E. Bureaucracy and beyond. *Organizational Dynamics,* 1974, *2,* 3 (Winter), 3-13.

Franklin, Jerome L. Down the organization: Influence processes across levels of hierarchy. *Administrative Science Quarterly,* 1975, *20,* 153-164.

Getzels, Jacob W., and Jackson, Philip W. *Creativity and intelligence.* New York: John Wiley & Sons, 1962.

Golembiewski, Robert, Billingsley, Keith, and Yeager, Samuel. Measuring change and persistence in human affairs: Types of change generated by OD designs. *Journal of Applied Behavioral Science,* 1976, *12,* 133-157.

Griffith, John R., Hancock, Walton M., and Munson, Fred C. *Cost Control in Hospitals.* Ann Arbor, Mich.: Health Administration Press, 1976.

Gross, Neal, Giacquinta, Joseph B., and Bernstein, Marilyn. *Implementing organizational innovations: a sociological analysis of planned educational change.* New York: Basic Books, 1971.

Guth, William D., and Tagiuri, Renato. Personal values and corporate strategy, *Harvard Business Review,* 1965, *43,* 5(October-November), 123-32.

Haga, William James. Review of *Increasing leadership effectiveness* by Chris Argyris. *Contemporary Sociology,* 1978, *7,* 186-187.

Hage, Jerald. *Communication and organizational control: Cybernetics in health and welfare settings.* New York: John Wiley & Sons, 1974.

Hage, Jerald, and Aiken, Michael. *Social change in complex organizations.* New York: Random House, 1970.

Hage, Jerald, and Dewar, Robert. Elite values versus organizational structure in predicting innovation. *Administrative Science Quarterly,* 1973, *18,* 279–90.

Harrison, Roger. Understanding your organization's character. *Harvard Business Review,* 1972, *50,* 3 (May–June), 119–28.

Houts, Peter S., and Server, Michael (Eds.). *After the turn on, what? Learning perspectives on humanistic groups.* Champaign, Ill.: Research Press Company, 1972.

Hudson, Liam. *Contrary imaginations: A psychological study of the young student.* New York: Schocken, 1966.

Hudson, Liam, *Frames of mind.* London: Methuen, 1968.

Hulin, Charles L., and Blood, Milton R. Job enlargement, individual differences, and worker responses. *Psychological Bulletin,* 1968, *69,* 41–55.

Inkeles, Alex, and Smith, David H. *Becoming modern: individual change in six developing countries.* Cambridge, Mass.: Harvard University Press, 1974.

Kahn, Robert L. The work module—a tonic for lunch and lassitude. *Psychology Today,* 1973, *6,* 9(February), 35–39.

Kolb, David A. Individual learning styles and the learning process. M.I.T. School of Management, Working Paper # 535-71, Spring 1971.

Lawrence, Paul R., and Lorsch, Jay W. *Organization and environment: managing differentiation and integration.* Boston: Division of Research, Harvard University Graduate School of Business Administration, 1967.

Likert, Rensis. *New patterns of management.* New York: McGraw-Hill, 1961.

Likert, Rensis. *The human organization: its management and value.* New York: McGraw-Hill, 1967.

Ludwig, Patric E. *Dollars and sense: an approach toward hospital cost containment and quality improvement through management engineering programs.* Battle Creek, Mich.: W.K. Kellogg Foundation, 1971.

MacGregor, Douglas. *The human side of enterprise.* New York: McGraw-Hill, 1960.

Margulies, Newton, Managing change in health care organizations. *Medical Care,* 1977, *15,* 693–704.

Marrow, Alfred J., Bowers, David G., and Seashore, Stanley E. *Management by participation: creating a climate for personal and organizational development.* New York: Harper & Row, 1967.

Millar, Jean A. Contingency theory, values, and change, *Human Relations* 1978, *31,* 885–904.

Miller, Eric J., and Rice, Albert K. *Systems of organization: the control of task and sentient boundaries.* London: Tavistock, 1967.

Morse, Nancy C., and Reimer, Everett. The experimental change of a major organizational variable. *Journal of Abnormal and Social Psychology,* 1956, *52,* 120–129.

Parsons, Talcott. *Structure and process in modern societies,* New York: Free Press, 1960.

Parsons, Talcott, and Bales, Robert F. *Family, socialization, and interaction process.* Glencoe, Ill.: Free Press, 955.

Parsons, Talcott, Bales, Robert F., and Shils, Edward A. *Working papers in the theory of action.* Glencoe, Ill.: Free Press, 1953.

Passmore, William A., and King, Donald C. Understanding organizational change: a comparative study of multifaceted interventions, *Journal of Applied Behavioral Science,* 1978, *14,* 455–468.

Perrow, Charles. *Complex organizations: a critical essay,* 2nd ed. Glenview, Ill.: Scott Foresman, 1979.

Rice, Albert K. *Productivity and social organization: the Ahmedabad experiment.* London: Tavistock, 1958.

Roberts, Karlene H., Cerruti, Nannette L., and O'Reilly, Charles A., III. Changing perceptions of organizational communications: Can short-term intervention help? *Nursing Research,* 1976, *25,* 3 (May–June) 197–200.

Schein, Virginia E., and Greiner, Larry E. Can organization development be fine tuned to bureaucracies? *Organizational Dynamics,* 1977, *5,* 3(Winter) 48–61.

Stinchcomb, Arthur L. *Creating efficient industrial administration.* New York: Academic Press, 1974.

Stoelwinder, Johannes U., and Clayton, Peter S. Hospital organization development: changing the focus from "better management" to "better patient care." *Journal of Applied Behavioral Science,* 1978, *14,* 400–414.

Strauss, George. Organization development. In Robert Dubin (Ed.) *Handbook of work, organization, and society.* Chicago: Rand McNally, 1976. Pp. 617–685.

Tichy, Noel M. Agents of planned social change: Congruence of values, cognitions and actions. *Administrative Science Quarterly.* 1974, *19,* 164–182.

Tichy, Noel M. How different types of change agents diagnose organizations. *Human Relations,* 1975, *28,* 771–799.

Tichy, Noel M., and Hornstein, Harvey A. Stand when your number is called: An empirical attempt to classify types of social change agents. *Human Relations,* 1976, *29,* 945–967.

Thompson, James D. *Organizations in action.* New York: McGraw-Hill, 1967.

Trist, E.L., Higgin, G.W., Murray, H., and Pollock, A.B. *Organizational choice.* London: Tavistock, 1963.

Ullrich, Robert A. *A theoretical model of human behavior in organizations: an eclectic approach.* Morristown, N.J.: General Learning Corporation, 1972.

Ullrich, Robert A., and Wieland, George F. *Organization theory and design,* rev.ed. Homewood, Ill.: Richard D. Irwin, 1980.

Weisbord, Marvin R. Why organization development hasn't worked (so far) in medical centers. *Health Care Management Review,* 1976, *1,* 2(Spring), 17–28.

Wieland, George F. *Action research and change in ten hospitals.* Manuscript, Ann Arbor, Mich., 1979 (Washington: National Technical Information Service, 1981).

Wieland, George F., and Leigh, Hilary (Eds.) *Changing hospitals,* London: Tavistock, 1971.

Wise, Harold, Beckhard, Richard, Rubin, Irwin, and Kyte, Aileen L. *Making health teams work.* Cambridge, Mass.: Ballinger, 1974.

NOTES

1. Goals are not always easy to ascertain—there are problems of conceptualization as well as measurement (see, for example, Ullrich and Wieland 1980, Chapter 6).
2. An objective for further research is to ascertain the causal dominance of the various elements in the system. Hage and Aiken, for example, see the technology as the critical determinant in what we term understanding systems, and structure in action systems.
3. See also Wieland (1979) for full details on this and other evaluation findings.
4. Caine's research provides succinct, empirical evidence regarding these dimensions which have, in fact, received major theoretical attention elsewhere. Ackoff and Emery (1972), for example, have highlighted the internal-external dimen-

sion, and they have characterized individuals, and cultures, according to whether they tend to perceive and react more to external or internal phenomena. Parsons (Parsons et al. 1953; Parsons and Bales 1955) has categorized change processes according to whether the external or internal receive initial, and thereby primary, attention (for application of Parsons' model to the HIC Project, see Wieland and Leigh [1971] Chapter 19).

A divergence-convergence dimension has been viewed as basic to understanding creativity (Getzels and Jackson 1962), and is more recently seen as a significant factor in experiential learning and the differential skills needed for various occupations including management (Kolb 1972). Hudson (1966, 1968), starting with convergence-divergence and using it as a central element, has conducted numerous empirical studies of school children and their choice of scientific or liberal arts majors and future professions. He feels there is a single very general system of values related to convergence-divergence:

Convergent thinking:	Divergent thinking:
Respect for authority and self-control	Freedom of expression and behavior
Masculine virtues	Feminine sensitivity
Choice of scientific vocations	Choice of arts, humanities

Conservatism-liberalism has, of course, been much studied. Recent investigation and theorizing suggests that modernity and the ability to work in large, formal organizations may be intimately related to liberal rather than conservative values (Inkeles and Smith 1974; Stinchcomb 1974).

5. Golembiewski and colleagues (1976) seem to suggest that evaluation of OD with fixed outcome standards is inappropriate. One must look for changes in the very nature of the system, including its goals, much as Argyris advocates double-loop learning.

6. Similarly, Ullrich (1972) suggests that workers may be motivated to "maintain the status quo."

7. See also Hage and Dewar (1973) on values for change and subsequent organizational change.

8. The first two seem to fall under the rubric of action systems, while the last seems to be one kind of understanding system. Task-oriented organizations may be either action or understanding systems.

9. In all, four types of organizational change agents were surveyed. Of these, the "outside pressure" type (Nader's Raiders, etc.) does not concern us since managers do not make use of such consultants. Another type, the "people change technology" consultants, had goals similar to the OD consultants' and seemed to fall between the OD and AFT groups in terms of background and the like—but they were concerned primarily with changing individuals rather than organizations.

10. In the same vein: "Too often consultants will prescribe the same form of OD to every organization without regard to its particular needs" (Strauss 1976, p. 651).

11. When the committee wished to ascertain hospital desires about continuing the project for another year, it called a general meeting of the hospital team members and simply excluded central team members.

12. Revans' General Electric Corporation Project seems to be closer to the individual end of the continuum, being an effort at "manager development . . . (and) slightly neglecting to focus on the actual changing of a company's behavior, embodied in and developing from the work done on the projects . . ." (Casey and Pearce 1977, p. 99).

13. Of the 30-point change from 85 percent to 115 percent of standard, 11 points were contributed by the training of supervisors in time-and-motion methods and their use in helping machine operators improve performance, and 5 points were contributed by "weeding out" poor operators. The psychological approach to change yielded 5 points in the form of sensitivity training and 3 points from the group discussion program. (The remaining 6 points were attributed to miscellaneous or combined change programs.)

    Furthermore, the evaluators (both psychologists) admit that this delimited evaluation of the changes is "unfair to the engineers" because the large-scale technical changes are better reflected in total system performance (e.g., costs per unit produced) than in terms of operator performance.

14. Not only is managerial action effective, it appears to be effective rather quickly. The effects of the structural changes showed up much more quickly in the action systems (surgical wards) than did the effects of the psychological changes in the understanding systems of the hospitals (medical wards). Figure 24-1 shows improvement in the surgical wards in the second year of the project, while the medical wards did not improve, on the average, till the fifth year after the project began (or two years after it ended). The psychological changes at top management levels took time to diffuse down the hierarchy. To achieve change in an understanding system, superiors facilitate and support psychological change in subordinates, and these changes then move down the hierarchy step by step (Franklin 1975). But managerial action need not wait the year or so apparently needed to transit each level. In one year, top managers can institute new structures that affect the functioning of all employees, even those at the bottom levels, in continual contact with patients. A year's time is enough to effect the relatively cognitive learning required for structural changes (see Chapter 8).

V

Summary and Implications

Introduction

This final section to the book provides an overview and summary of the main highlights of the readings (Chapter 26) and a short informal account of the implications for the practicing manager of action and understanding approaches to organizational change (Chapter 27).

26	Highlights and Overview of the Readings

George F. Wieland

The behavioral sciences, especially psychology, have been widely applied to the improvement of management, but relatively less so in hospitals or in other kinds of health care organizations. These are much more difficult settings than the typical organization. However, enormous pressures for improved management, and especially for more efficient patient care, have begun to incite a variety of innovative uses of behavioral science by health care managers, and that is what this book is about.

THE HOSPITAL ORGANIZATION

Part I takes a brief look at the nature of health care organizations and at the work of health care managers. Georgopoulos (Chapter 1) cites the enormous complexity of the hospital. A great variety of different, yet interdependent, specializations and skills are in frequent interaction. Authority and formal structures are used to minimize uncertainty and to ensure the continuity and uniformity of performance, especially required because of the critical nature of patient care. But the need to individualize and also personalize care means that formal structures cannot be applied across the board. There must be individual initiative and creativity, warm personal relations, and collaboration and cooperation among staff members. The problem of the autonomy of professionals and the additional lines of authority they provide also adds to the problems of coordinating the specialized and interdependent staff members.

All of this makes informal organizational coordination as important, if not more so, than formal modes of coordination. The bases of this informal coordination rest in a variety of social factors—complementary expectations and mutual understandings, informal norms of reciprocity, trust, and mutual helpfulness, as well as individual commitment, loyalty, and involvement. In general, "for hospitals, organizational effectiveness depends upon social efficiency more than it does upon technical-economic efficiency. . . ."

ROLE OF THE MANAGER

One of the first requisites of effective management in hospitals, according to Peter Drucker (Chapter 2) is the determination of how the manager actually spends his time. The practice of most managers, suggests Drucker, far from follows the strictures of textbooks advocating planning and other "rational" activities. As Mintzberg and colleagues (1976) showed in a study of a group of top executives (including one from a hospital), decision making is usually very complex, iterative, and subject to all kinds of interruptions. Drucker emphasizes how little control the hospital manager has over his or her time.

To start with, Drucker suggests, effective hospital managers must consider the contributions they can make in their work. Managers should:

> . . . not look down but, rather, up. In other words, they know that results do not exist inside an organization; only costs and efforts exist there. Results are with the patients . . . and the major hope of the patient is to get out of the hospital as fast as possible.

Allison and colleagues (Chapter 3) studied the activities of six "successful" chief executive officers in each of four types of health care organization, hospitals, long-term care facilities, multispecialty group practice clinics, and health maintenance organizations. A list of 46 different organizational activities was developed, and respondents indicated their extent of involvement in each and its importance to their role.

Using Katz and Kahn's typology of organizational subsystems, Allison and colleagues found that "adaptive" activities, such as market and product research and long-range planning, were "crucial" (i.e., entailing both high involvement and high importance to the role of the manager). "Supportive/ boundary" subsystem activities such as public relations, lobbying or influencing the rulings of government agencies, or establishing agreements with other health organizations were also "crucial." These days much of the work of the adaptive and supportive/boundary subsystems has to do with cost control.

One other interesting point from the study has to do with the way in which successful managers learned to become competent in performing some 46 basic activities in their managerial roles. They generally cited themselves as the source of their competence, that is, they saw their own on-the-job experience, self-instruction, and perhaps their basic common sense and personality as the most important sources of learning. They placed learning from discussions with others second. In last place, they put formal education, whether a specific workshop or institute, professional education, or general education.

MANAGERIAL ACTION TO IMPLEMENT COST-SAVING STRUCTURES

Part II provides readings on one of the two fundamental approaches to changing and improving the functioning of health care organizations. "Managerial action" refers to the traditional management strategy of changing work structures such as roles, routines, procedures, facilities, and other aspects of the organization that constrain the behavior of individuals. Management typically devises a solution to a problem, and then acts to implement that (structural) solution, paying attention to the psychological conditions that might help overcome resistance and ease its acceptance. Managerial and technical expertise take precedence in devising the solution to the problem, not the people involved in the problem, their feelings about what is wrong, and psychological elements.

Managerial action to change structures seems most appropriate to the traditional production organization, where routine technology and a mechanistic or bureaucratic structure predominate. Structural change is less important for organizations with nonroutine or individualized technologies and organic structures, or for organizations centered around professionals such as doctors. The psychological approach to change, described in Part III, seems more appropriate for dealing with these latter kinds of organizations.

The first reading (Chapter 4) in the section provides an introduction and overview of managerial action and structural change. Research by Hage and Aiken in seventeen health and welfare organizations shows that the two different kinds of organizations described above seem to vary systematically along a variety of dimensions. Most importantly, the organic organization, or one with many professionals, tends to be more dynamic and subject to creativity and change. The mechanistic organization tends to be more static. However, its managers can more easily innovate by making use of the organization's centralized power and authority. Innovation, or the successful implementation of a creative idea, is more feasible in the traditional mechanistic organization than in the more complicated professional and organic organization.

THE ADMINISTRATOR'S POWER TO IMPLEMENT

In Chapter 5, Allison describes structural change in the context of an experiment to control costs. Eleven hospitals voluntarily negotiated prospective reimbursement agreements with Blue Cross, agreements in which the hospital receives weekly payments of the expected reimbursement for the coming year.

According to Allison, one of the major factors facilitating the cost-containment subsequently observed in the experiment is the "administrator's power," his or her influence relative to the medical staff's influence, over areas with high cost-saving potential. Unfortunately the areas of highest rated cost-saving potential, such as patient length of stay or admissions or quality or care, are areas in which the administrator's power is rated low. Areas where the administrators rate their power as high, e.g., in making hospital investments in human and capital resources, have relatively low rated cost-saving potential. Allison concludes: "Those with formal authority to control hospital costs do not have enough power to control them." He estimates that, "at most, administrators control less than 25 percent of total hospital costs in the short run."

IMPLEMENTING STRUCTURES FOR COST CONTAINMENT

Chapters 7 to 10 describe an active program of structural change, or managerial action, for cost containment designed by John Griffith and colleagues at the University of Michigan. Two of the chapters report the implementation of an admissions scheduling program to enable the more optimal use of hospital staff and facilities. As one might expect, physician acceptance or rejection was a key determining element for the success in one hospital and the failure in the other.

But physician rejection did not come about in a vacuum. A whole host of other problems contributed to and interacted with the negative physician attitudes in the rejecting Able hospital. Technical, computer-caused delays in getting the experiment underway led to frustrations, as did early problems in learning how to use the new system. Some physicians reacted to frustrations by taking patients to another community hospital. Exaggeration and rumor amplified the difficulties flowing from technical problems in implementing the system. The doctors took more and more of an unsympathetic attitude; the new system inconvenienced them in too many ways. The nurses became caught in the middle of the administrative proponents and medical detractors, and they began to see negative aspects, such as possible job layoffs if the new scheduling system permitted reduced staffing levels. The final straw was some adverse publicity about the project, publicity that offended a doctor who happened also to be a hospital trustee.

The successful experiment at Baker hospital differed in a number of ways: in the technical nature of the system, in the hospital situation (e.g., the need at Baker to handle increased, not decreased occupancy levels), but, perhaps most significant, in the later start of the experiment, allowing the experimental team to use much of its experience from the earlier efforts at implementation. Frustration, conflict, and general problems of coordination occurred as in the earlier experiment. But with considerable learning and readjustment on the part of almost everybody, the system at Baker achieved a stable level of acceptance and showed positive effects on evaluation measures.

Munson and Hancock (Chapter 9) describe the dilemma of whether to give primacy to the technically correct solution or to the psychologically acceptable solution when implementing a structural or technological change. In general, they favor mastering the technical aspects of the change first, and then working on acceptance by organizational members.

Munson and Hancock suggest that success in implementing a change requires three factors. First, one must start with an innovation that is technically well devised, with a technically optimal solution, and then modify it for organizational feasibility. Second, the attitude toward the innovation of critical people should be favorable or at least neutral. Participation or, even better, negotiation, helps foster learning and positive attitudes. Third, those who are part of the innovation must not only know what to do, they must be able to behave differently (thus implying training of some kind).

They also suggest that managers and consultants think about implementation in terms of a negotiation process so as to avoid slipping into a manipulative attitude in dealing with members of the system requiring change. Negotiation allows (usually legitimate) objections to the innovation to be raised and the system members to make inputs based on their own expert knowledge of local conditions. Negotiation provides time for learning and attitude change on the part of the experts who wish to implement the change, as well as of those who resist.

In Chapter 10, Student details some of the psychological factors determining acceptance of an innovation: familiarizing staff members with the program, involving them in the implementation process, using top management authority and support to back up the change program, and also using (moderate) stress to motivate acceptance. These points overlap to some extent the points made in Chapter 4 on changing organizational structures. There it is suggested that management overcomes resistance to change by making sure the change is clearly and favorably perceived. This is done by providing considerable information, by providing psychological participation, and by building on past experiences in the organization in which changes were acceptable and created positive feelings.

IMPLEMENTING NEW STRUCTURES:
THE IMPORTANCE OF LEARNING

Another aspect of the managerial action approach to change is the concern for new kinds of formal organizational structures to enable more flexible, efficient performance. As the contingency theorists have indicated, organizations with complex tasks and dynamic environments function more effectively when they are differentiated and decentralized, with integration taking place at the lowest level feasible. These needs are especially evident where ambulatory and comprehensive care require the flexible integration of a whole host of specialists working with the patient (and often his or her family, too).

In the hospital, one move toward this kind of restructuring has been service unit management (SUM) (Chapters 11 and 12). Service units of several wards are created, with a manager assigned to take charge of such management activities as ordering supplies, scheduling maintenance services, supervising the ward clerks (who answer phones, greet visitors, schedule appointments, and maintain patient records), and coordinating requests for charts and records, and lab and x-ray information. One aim of SUM is to relieve nurses of administrative work (for which they may not be specially trained) and to allow them to do more nursing (for which they are trained). Cost savings are also expected.

Jelinek, Munson, and Smith conducted intensive studies of several hospitals implementing SUM, as well as surveys of larger numbers of hospitals, and found a variety of implementation problems. At the individual level there are problems such as the anxieties of the nurses regarding their new roles. At the unit level, the creation of the new unit manager role means that existing patterns of interaction and status will be disrupted and will have to be channeled appropriately. At the system level, there is the need to create new relationships between the unit manager (instead of the head nurse) and other units in the hospital.

Jelinek and colleagues emphasize the importance of unfreezing prior behavioral patterns and generating motivation for change through participation. Training in interpersonal skills, as well as technical competence, is very important, especially for the new unit manager, since the nurses otherwise are reluctant to relinquish their control to the newcomer. Training is also important for the head nurse, who must unlearn old behavior patterns as well as learn new patterns.

Griffith and colleagues (1973) similarly emphasize the importance of psychology and the great amount of learning needed to implement cost-saving structures such as an admission scheduling system:

Those involved in the process may well be obliged to learn new performance measures and control mechanisms. Mastery of the admissions scheduling system at Baker took six months, for example. Preliminary revisions of existing systems and thorough communication of plans took three months. Despite the lengthy preparation, the admitting, nursing, and medical staffs reacted strongly against the system when it went on line. The system was not completely turned over to departmental management until three months after start-up. It is obvious that the installation of such a system requires substantial time and continuous guidance by a representative of management (p. 138).

INVOLVING PHYSICIANS IN MANAGEMENT

One criticism of SUM is that it does not go far enough in restructuring, it does not make any direct effort to restructure the role of the physician. Physicians can help if they play a more active role in coordinating the various hospital staff members who provide care to each patient.

For the improvement of hospital management generally, perhaps the single most important task is to get the physicians to manage more, to facilitate coordination and to avoid waste, duplication, and inefficiency. A number of investigators indicate that physicians must be made to feel more a part of the hospital and they must work in ways that take the whole of the hospital into account, not just the physician-patient relationship.

Of course, there is a limit to the management role that physicians can play. They are busy people, and, after all, their primary training and interest is in patient care. Patients want and need them to play a direct and decisive role in the provision of their care. But as Allison and colleagues (Chapter 3) emphasize, there is a point of balance between the total lack of integration of the medical staff and integration to the extent that they actually run the hospital. "As one administrator put it, he must guide their [the medical staff's] use of power to a position of planned responsibility midway between the extremes of uninvolvement and assertion."

But why don't physicians manage? Probably the most important reason is their complete authority in the realm of patient care. Physicians are trained to expect to be individually responsible for the patient. They are the ones who have the most expertise, and who can claim that matters of life-and-death provide emergency powers. This enables the physician to exert a "professional dominance" over the other health care professions. In addition, as Weisbord indicates in Chapter 15, the training of the physician in autonomous, individualistic decision making is reinforced subsequently by the profession's emphasis on personal achievement and on improving one's own performance. Any diminution of autonomy thus is a direct threat to physicians' status, and a threat to their basic identity.

Physician independence could be addressed through the creation of structures which help to involve and integrate the medical staff into the management of the organization as a whole. Neuhauser (see Chapter 6) provides a vivid picture of how much patient care can be improved if physicians play a more influential role in running the organization and, especially, in structuring their own activities. Studying 30 Chicago-area hospitals, Neuhauser measured physician participation in terms of the percentage of medical membership on the board of trustees and also in terms of the frequency of meetings of the joint conference committee (in which the chiefs of the medical staff meet with the executive officers of the board). Such physician participation is positively associated with the quality of medical care as measured by outside expert evaluators, by the accreditation evaluation, and by the severity-adjusted death rate.

THE PSYCHOLOGICAL APPROACH TO IMPROVING ORGANIZATIONAL FUNCTIONING

It is fair to say that relatively few physicians have responded to invitations to become more involved in structures to improve the efficiency of their hospitals. Part III describes the second basic approach to organizational change, a psychological approach, which provides a way in which some hitherto uninterested physicians may become involved in management.

The psychological approach to change is especially suited to situations in which organizational members, usually professionals, must use a great array of knowledge and skills to respond to a highly complex work situation. Changing the work behavior of such professionals by means of structures is difficult. Because the work is dependent on their initiative, and their judgment, the implementation of new structures to provide constraints on professionals is usually inadequate to assure changed performance. The change must come from within individual professionals or groups of professionals. It is they who know the work problems first hand in all their complexity, and it is they who, with help, must develop the complex new behaviors and social organizations which are likely to provide the answers.

In the psychological approach to change, the organization development (OD) change agent first attempts to understand the needs, desires, attitudes, and feelings of the people involved in the problem. The change agent works with the existing social system and helps the individuals evolve new patterns of interpersonal and work behavior. By focusing on psychological and interpersonal factors, the change agent helps to unlock conflicts and release latent energies for new social patterns that better meet individual needs while also facilitating organizational efficiency and effectiveness. New structural or technological arrangements are not precluded (recall the accounts of flexi-time and other OD structural interventions in Chapter 14).

The psychological approach to change is not, by any means, a panacea, particularly when dealing with the great problem of physician autonomy and unwillingness to become involved. Weisbord, in Chapter 15, tells "Why Organization Development Hasn't Worked (So Far) in Medical Centers." He provides some concrete evidence on the freedom of physicians from organizational and managerial constraints. When medical center physicians were asked to whom they were responsible in dealing with patient care, 55 percent said "no one" or left the item blank. Organization development is meant to increase interdependency, so it is no wonder, as Weisbord says, that physicians see OD as a threat.

In addition, there are special features to the training of physicians which make their behavioral style inimical to OD and its emphasis on examining emotions. Physicians are trained to be rational and objective. To show feelings is an unprofessional retreat from reason. Similarly, the physician's emphasis on expert knowledge clashes with the OD approach that "process" rather than content (and "here-and-now," rather than theory) is important. Finally, physicians are socialized to be individualistic. Thus the emphasis in OD on interdependence and cooperation is similarly a threat to the physician.

But according to other accounts, OD has worked in some medical settings. By comparing these successes with the failures, one can learn about the apparent critical factors for success. A group of OD change agents, for example, report success in their work at the Martin Luther King, Jr. (MLK) Health Center (Chapter 16). The consultants focused on the multidisciplinary primary health care teams, composed of physicians, nurses, and family health workers. The fifteen hours of training for each team entailed many of the potent interventions of OD: diagnostic interviewing and feedback, with subsequent consultant facilitation of behavior changes especially in team meetings, and training in role negotiation, in feedback, and in sharing of feelings. The reaction of the teams was generally positive. The consultants observed "increased clarity of role expectations, greater flexibility in decision making, and more widely shared influence and participation. . . ." However, an attempt at training members of the bureaucratic central management for the MLK center was not successful.

The dimension of psychological "depth" (Chapter 14) helps explain why OD seems to work in the community health care team, but not in the medical center or in the bureaucratic structure of the health care center. Psychologically "shallow" interventions such as changes in managerial procedures (e.g., replacing an old report form with a new report form) are essentially cognitive, impersonal, "objective," and usually not objectionable in a personal way. On the other hand, OD is "deep" and involves emotions, changing attitudes and deeply felt convictions about trust, openness, and working with others in collaborative rather than authoritarian ways.

Individuals tend to resist deep interventions, but if a relatively powerful consultant is operating in the small training-group setting (where the clients have abdicated their structured roles), he or she can overcome the client's resistance. In terms of the classic OD paradigm, the consultant can use his or her power: (1) to "unfreeze" old behaviors, (2) to help the client model new behaviors ("change") and (3) to "refreeze" or reinforce new, more appropriate behaviors.

In short, to intervene at a deep level, as in OD, the consultant must have power over the client. In the medical center, physicians are very powerful; their expertise, needed by the organization, makes them independent of others. If need be, the physician may even enlist the collective power of the medical staff to resist any OD efforts. In contrast, in the community care setting, the physician is rather dependent on other team members and their expertise. The physician is only one part of an interdependent team with the goal of providing comprehensive care and needs the help of the others on the team.

LESS DEEP OD INTERVENTIONS

An apparently successful OD intervention in another kind of health care setting, a health maintenance organization, seems to confirm the value of viewing settings in terms of the power available to physicians to resist deep OD interventions. Margulies (Chapter 18) describes survey feedback at Kaiser-Permanente, a large bureaucratically structured organization in which physicians are employees and work with other staff to provide care to those covered by the health insurance program.

A survey conducted by means of a questionnaire on organizational climate was followed by data feedback, extensive discussion of problems, and then the designing and implementation of concrete operational improvements. Areas of focus were freer communications, improved relationships between those from the "hospital culture" and those from the "clinic culture," better relationships between physicians and managers (especially providing the physicians with more of a managerial orientation), better interdepartmental cooperation, more clarity on responsibilities and authority, more opportunities for employee "growth" and advancement, and the development of more concern for patient education.

This OD effort apparently achieved success in part because the physicians are less powerful than those in the medical center. The physicians at Kaiser probably have more power to resist than do those in community health care teams, because they are in relatively familiar hospital or clinic settings and they have colleagues for support. But they have less power than those in the medical center or usual hospital setting because they are employees with a contractual and integrated relationship with their organization, not permitting the autonomous behavior more common in the medical center or hospital.

In addition, the project by Margulies was apparently successful because it was a relatively shallow intervention, an effort which would not arouse much resistance from physicians or other organizational members. (This may be true not only of the survey feedback but also of management by objectives, the technique described in Chapter 19.) Physicians were less likely to use whatever power they had, because the intervention was not as deep or as threatening as most OD efforts involving emotional issues in small-group settings. In part, this was because the interventions were by means of relatively impersonal questionnaires and feedback reports. Even more important, however, is the fact that a great emphasis was apparently placed on what Margulies terms "concrete operational improvements," structural matters such as reassignment of staff or procedural changes such as new kinds of reports to patients or a new orientation program on the role and function of other departments. Such a relatively shallow focus on managerial problems, rather than deeper interpersonal or individual problems, is not so likely to arouse the power of physicians to resist (the "systems" intervention in Chapter 13 used a similar, relatively shallow approach to change).

Weisbord's analysis of OD in the medical center setting supports this point about the importance of using relatively shallow interventions where the clients have considerable power to resist deep interventions. Weisbord suggests that OD consultants and managers should work with physicians on matters such as budgeting procedures, clarifying goals, planning resource management—and generally involving physicians in managerial activities. Similar shallow interventions were also used by Stoelwinder and Clayton, as described in Chapter 20.

CLIENT-DIRECTED CHANGE LEADING TO A VARIETY OF CHANGE EFFORTS

Perhaps the strongest evidence for the role of intervention depth and relative client power comes from the evaluation of the Hospital Internal Communications (HIC) Project described in Part IV (Chapters 22 to 25). In this project, the most senior administrators, nurses, and doctors from each of ten hospitals studied their own organizations, often with the help of a small group of student assistants and change facilitators. A variety of studies, usually involving the collection of survey, observational, or records data was made, and various actions and changes were undertaken, culminating in reduced length of stay compared to other hospitals in the same regions.

The project was successful, despite the physician's potentially high power in the hospital setting, apparently because hospital staff members, including physicians, were invited to take direct charge of the interventions. They did not merely "participate"; they themselves directed the teams of college students who gathered a variety of data in the hospitals. Because the change program was truly nondirective, some of the hospital staff and teams of helpers undertook relatively deep psychological interventions (e.g., group meetings and discussions and sensitivity training) while others commissioned shallow, structural interventions (e.g., operations research studies of the scheduling in the surgical theaters or the flow of medical records). The clients, in other words, were able to select the particular depth of intervention which they wished to experience. This was in contrast to the usual circumstance in which an outside management or OD consultant tends to prescribe the same kinds of solutions for a variety of different organizational situations.*

Two Separate Processes for Structural and Psychological Change

Further insight comes from the data analyses showing that hospital teams used two separate processes of change, leading to two different forms of improved organizational efficiency. One change process was closely akin to that observed in much of organization development. Psychological and social change, learning in individuals, and improved interpersonal relations were emphasized. In contrast, the second change process did not emphasize people, but rather structure and technology. In a process more akin to everyday management or traditional management consultancy, there was a focus on management problems, coming up with a solution, and then setting matters right by means of administrative action.

Correlational analyses showed that the latter, traditional management approach to change occurred in those organizations which were well

---

*Perhaps the success of self-help and learning by doing in this project also lends some support to the finding by Allison and colleagues (Chapter 3) that successful top health care managers learn more from their own experience than from the experience of others or from training which attempts to simulate real work problems.

organized and well structured for change. These organizations were responsive to internally instituted changes, had strong, influential hierarchies, and were well integrated (with agreement among different groups and levels about priorities and awareness of each other's problems). Teams in these hospitals took a direct and authoritative approach to change. They emphasized the solving of problems, about which they tried to get clear data so they could take administrative action (instituting new procedures, routines, or structures or altering technological arrangements). In the hospitals, this kind of project approach yielded a high degree of problem solving and significant reductions in surgical length of stay over the subsequent years.

In contrast, the psychological or OD approach to change occurred in those hospitals which had teams which were suffering some distress: the team members were rated as being poor communicators, and the organization as a whole was poorly integrated. Over time, the most senior team members in these hospitals became emotionally committed, active, and influential in the project, and they provided psychological support for the junior, operational members of the hospital teams.

These teams of managers with a psychological or OD orientation generally took a critical approach to the project. They saw many psychological and interpersonal problems in their organizations, and they were intellectually critical about the nature of the project data they collected, too. (Those taking the first approach, in contrast, were more closed minded and authoritarian in attitude and were not interested in discussing matters, learning about the views of others, or meeting with facilitators to get help.)

The result of this second, OD approach to change was acquisition of significant new information and changes in the patterning of team member (and close associate) work behavior. Hospital team members were also subsequently rated by facilitators as showing desirable psychological changes (becoming more open). Finally, and most importantly, these teams' hospitals showed, over the subsequent years, an improvement in length of stay for internal medicine patients, but not for surgical patients.

The implications of these two separate change processes become clearer when one recognizes the very different nature of surgical and medical ward organization. Surgery is a mechanistic and relatively routine system, with relatively simple tasks requiring low amounts of information processing, and with an external management control system emphasizing formal organizational structures and hierarchical controls. Internal medicine is a complex, "organic" system characterized by complex tasks and by the more internal controls possessed by professionals. Informal relations and other interpersonal and psychological characteristics are very important for diagnosing patient illness, and for instituting effective therapies.

A CONTINGENCY APPROACH TO CHANGE:
ACTION AND UNDERSTANDING SYSTEMS

In more general terms, surgery is an "action" system, internal medicine, an "understanding" system. The nature of action and understanding systems, as detailed in Chapter 25, is outlined in Table 26-1.

It seems that different kinds of organizational systems, when given a free rein and resources in a self-help change project, will choose different approaches to change and will emphasize different kinds of improvements. The approach is contingent on the nature of the system to be changed. Those organizations operating more nearly as action systems will take a quick, direct approach to changing structures and technologies. These organizational elements are the critical ones and the ones which, when changed, will lead to improved functioning. The understanding systems will take a slower OD approach to change, so as to improve the "people" element of the organization. The psychological forms of help allow individuals to develop new ways of thinking and feeling. Groups of individuals collaborating in the changes can exchange views and share information, and they can build up commitments to new ways of working that enhance the informal relations that are so critical in understanding systems.

If one is to improve the efficiency of hospitals and other health care facilities, one must look closely at the nature of the organizational systems and subsystems involved. Do the structures, technologies, people, and, most of all, the goals, more nearly make up an action system or an understanding system? Do the managers, for example, prefer a strict regimen with clear objectives, close controls, and a routine, relatively simple and straightforward technology? Or is there more learning in the system, with attempts to explore and improve patient care quality, and with egalitarian input in decision making because there are no simple answers, no simple techniques? These are the kinds of questions that have to be asked, if change techniques are to be tailored to the system needing improvement.

Psychological (i.e., relatively deep) approaches to change will be the method of choice in an understanding system, while structural and technological approaches will have the most direct impact for improving the functioning of an action system. The psychological approaches get inside of people's heads, so to speak; they get at the internal and interpersonal control systems that Georgopoulos has highlighted as key elements in the functioning of professionals in hospitals. The psychological approaches focus on the mutual awareness, the complementarity of expectations, and the informal norms of trust and cooperation which are especially important in the functioning of internal medicine wards.

TABLE 26-1
SUMMARY OF IMPORTANT DIFFERENCES BETWEEN
ACTION AND UNDERSTANDING SYSTEMS

Action	Understanding
Management Process	
Dealing with problems (discrepancies)	Intellectual and emotional understanding
Problem discernment	Clarifying, understanding the task
Action toward goal	Emotional commitment to a solution
Evaluation	Implementation
Critical task: perfecting an action	Critical task: perfecting a commitment
Tasks	
Simple, little information needed	Complex, much information needed
Task Organization	
Specialized, with centralized direction	Generalists, organized as professional peers
Control System	
External or programmed coordination	Internal (professional) or coordination by feedback
Structural Organization	
Mechanistic	Organic
Individuals (Personalities)	
Doers, value results, practice perfecting action, are closed to new knowledge, act on external environment in terms of self-fulfilling prophecies, "authoritarian"	Knowers, value (breadth of) knowledge as an end, sensitive to the psychological and the subjective, doubting and uncertain, egalitarian in attitude toward others

Psychology is not nearly so important in the functioning of other systems. In fact, in order to obtain quick and error-free functioning, the operating room and emergency department, for example, rely on structures external to people, structures that do not allow people to question, doubt, criticize, and then synthesize better solutions to problems.

In other sectors of the hospital, the high reliance on routines enhances the efficient production of large quantities of goods and services. Much of the work in the laundry, dietetics, and admissions departments can be routinized, and when there are problems, they can usually be solved by examining these routines, procedures, and systems. Therefore, a structural or an action orientation to change is here the method of choice. Of course, no system can operate without people, and the psychology of implementing better structures and systems (Chapter 4) is also relevant, as was seen in the Michigan experiments conducted by Griffith and colleagues (Chapters 7 to 10) and in the reviews of factors important in implementing SUM (Chapters 11 and 12). But it should be remembered that the key elements in those changes of action systems were the structural elements, not the psychological elements. As Munson and Hancock (Chapter 9) suggest, one probably should try to get the technical solution right first, and then worry about the human elements of implementation.

What happens if an incongruent change approach is used? What happens if a psychological approach to change is used in an action system? Roberts and colleagues (Chapter 21) describe an excellently evaluated (control-groups and before-and-after design) attempt at improving communications in an emergency room. Patients complained about impersonal staff attitudes, while staff were dissatisfied with their level of influence on the organization and often failed to understand what was expected of them. Training facilitators held ten hours of sessions which featured "learning to listen, providing feedback and accurate information, building trust and teamwork . . . , [and] increasing self-esteem. . . ." An evaluation questionnaire showed that after the training, staff had more positive attitudes in a number of areas. However, their ratings of actual communications behavior in the emergency room showed no change. The system still behaved as before, presumably because the control structures, procedures, etc., were not changed through managerial action aimed at improving an action system such as an emergency department.

EVALUATION RESEARCH ON ORGANIZATIONAL CHANGE EFFORTS

Unfortunately, much of the analysis in this book is inferential, because systematic evaluation research is lacking in most of the studies that have been reviewed here. The study by Roberts and colleagues is one of the few exceptions. A special plea for better evaluation research on OD and organization change is in order. While the evaluation of the HIC Project (Chapter 24) is no model of perfection, it does provide some suggestions for improvement.

A systematic evaluation study should assess the ultimate outcomes of an intervention. OD interventions, for example, are commonly expected to improve the degree of trust, openness, and cooperation in the organization, with the assumption that these psychological characteristics will in turn improve organizational productivity and efficiency. As Suchman (1967) indicates, this kind of assumption about results is often open to question.

When ultimate outcomes as well as more immediate outcomes are evaluated, the ineffective nature of many interventions is discovered. Participants in a traditional lecture-type training course, for example, may be attentive and may like the course, but they may fail to apply the material to their work situation (Wolfe and Moe 1973). Implementation of a management-by-objectives program may lead to expressions of satisfaction but no changes in actual behavior (Sloan and Schrieber 1971) or may lead to temporary changes that disappear after a year or so (Ivancevich 1972).

In general, then, an evaluation of social interventions must trace their impact until the effects reach a value in and of itself, without depending on an assumption of subsequent consequences of value. Thus, in the hospital, the intervention must be shown to affect patient care. To demonstrate these effects, the evaluator must make use of one or more experimental and quasi-experimental designs which will eliminate extraneous explanations for the desired outcomes (Campbell and Stanley 1963; Cook and Campbell 1976).

However, having demonstrated valued outcomes as resulting from the intervention, the evaluator is not done. The various more-or-less separable processes in the intervention must be assessed in order to determine what in the usually complex intervention was of value and what was not. This can be done by means of a survey-correlational design (Wieland 1969). Surveys can be used to provide cross-sectional assessments of the intervention and immediate outcomes at several points in time. These data can then be correlated with the above described criterion measures for immediate and ultimate valued outcomes.

Because real-life interventions risk the reputation of the change agent and the participating managers, interventions are usually complex, with many components utilized to help ensure success. A correlational evaluation can show that certain aspects of the intervention may have been relatively valueless, i.e., having no impact on ultimate criteria (or perhaps even having a detrimental effect). For example, the evaluation of the HIC Project shows that the degree of participation by top hospital staff in the survey work (e.g., administration of instruments, analysis of data, writing reports) in their own hospitals was of relatively little ultimate value. The students could have done all of this work, saving an enormous amount of valuable top management time.

A correlational design also helps differentiate interventions according to differently valued outcomes. In the HIC evaluation, hospital projects which took an action orientation (e.g., surveys focusing on management problems) triggered a process which eventuated in improved efficiency in the care of surgical patients, while hospital projects or surveys with an understanding orientation (e.g., using surveys and discussion groups for better interpersonal undertanding) triggered a process which ultimately led to improved efficiency in the care of internal medicine patients. By studying the process of change, then, one learns which inputs to emphasize in order to obtain the particular results desired. In conclusion, attempts at improving management and organizational functioning are likely to have relatively little value beyond the specific hospital setting unless they are accompanied by evaluation research which allows one to generalize about valued outcomes and the processes leading to such outcomes.

REFERENCES

Campbell, Donald T., and Stanley, J. Experimental and quasi-experimental designs for research on teaching. In N. L. Gage (Ed.) *Handbook of research on teaching.* Chicago: Rand McNally, 1963.

Cook, Thomas D., and Campbell, Donald T. The design and conduct of quasi-experiments and time experiments in field settings. In Marvin D. Dunnette (Ed.) *Handbook of industrial and organizational psychology.* Chicago: Rand McNally, 1976. Pp. 223–326.

Griffith, John R., Hancock, Walton M., and Munson, Fred C. Practical ways to contain hospital costs. *Harvard Business Review,* 1973, *51,* 6 (November–December), 131–139.

Ivancevich, John M. A longitudinal assessment of management by objectives. *Administrative Science Quarterly,* 1972, *17,* 126–138.

Sloan, Stanley, and Schrieber, David E. *Hospital management . . . an evaluation. Bureau of Business Research and Service Monograph No. 4.* Madison, Wisc.: Graduate School of Business, University of Wisconsin, 1971.

Suchman, Edward A. *Evaluation research: principles and practice in public service and social action programs.* New York: Russell Sage Foundation, 1967.

Wieland, George F. Evaluating the Hospital Internal Communications Project: The use of survey methods in evaluation. *International Nursing Review,* 1969, *16,* 106–114.

Wolfe, Joseph, and Moe, Barbara L. An experimental evaluation of a hospital supervisory training program. *Hospital Administration,* 1973, *18,* 4(Fall), 65–77.

27 | # Action and Understanding: Some Implications for Practicing Managers

George F. Wieland

"Action" and "understanding" are two fundamental approaches to using behavioral science techniques for improving management and organizational functioning. One might think of managers who emphasize the action approach as "doers," and those who emphasize understanding as "talkers." Systematic research shows that both approaches are effective, if used in their proper places.

The action approach to change uses the style of the traditional management consultant. Improvement studies focus on the structure or technology of the hospital, on its skeleton or mechanics of functioning, so to speak. Hospital staff are viewed from "outside," as objects to be changed by means of altered procedures, policies, roles, or technological arrangements. An action-oriented study usually focuses on a specific problem, gathers data on that problem, and quickly moves to some sort of administrative action to deal with the problem.

The understanding approach to change follows a more psychological, people-oriented tack, one commonly used by organization development (OD) consultants. These studies focus on the nervous system of the hospital. The attempt is to change people from the "inside," to change what they think and feel. Discussion groups of one form or another are the primary vehicle of change.

Adapted, by permission of the publisher, from HEALTH SERVICES MANAGER, February 1980, © 1980 by AMACOM, a division of the American Management Association. All rights reserved.

An understanding-oriented study typically emphasizes the gathering of a great breadth of data, often by means of open-ended interviews. Group meetings and discussion of data may raise fundamental questions, such as "What is the goal of this hospital to be?" and they may develop into the sensitivity-training and team-building efforts often used in organization development. The discussions lead to the learning of much information, to changes in attitudes, and to improved interpersonal relations, and these eventually affect the work of the hospital.

These two approaches to improving management seem to arise from the fundamental ways in which we look at the world—from our assumptions about human nature and what is important in life. Most people tend to prefer one approach to the other and find it hard to appreciate the opposite approach, yet both are effective when used appropriately. The following statements provide some illustrations and ideas for diagnosing whether colleagues or management consultants favor one approach over the other:

The Understanding Approach

1. An administrator: "All knowledge is good knowledge; the project gave me a greater understanding of people and the organization of people."
2. A nurse: "You have to hurt, before you can get better."
3. A change consultant: It's a question of getting people to want to do the right things . . . ; if they don't feel it in their hearts, they won't do it effectively and it won't be productive at all."
4. A nurse: "Differences of ideas and conflicting opinions are usually more of an asset than a liability."

The Action Approach

1. A change consultant: "I think the reason why a number of hospital staff did . . . change was that, for almost the first time, they were given a certain direction in which change was recommended."
2. A change consultant: "There are occasions when manipulative action is appropriate."
3. A nurse: "Usually there is only one right and simple way to do a job."
4. An administrator: ". . . by continuing to examine the problems on a narrow front and dealing with one matter at a time, we shall make positive progress. . . ."
5. An administrator (reporting that he changed the way he works, as a result of the project): "I can be clearer in what I am trying to accomplish and be more specific in my discussion with other people as to what I'm after."
6. An administrator: "Too much communicating of the wrong sort. Wads and

wads of paper which no one reads. . . . People get bored and irritated by projects which don't seem to be heading anywhere."

What are the implications of differentiating between the action and understanding approaches to change?

1. You can diagnose management problems and sites for change in terms of whether they are part of action or understanding systems, calling for one or the other approach to change. If the people involved tend to agree with this ("the best way to solve a work problem is to call everyone together for a discussion"), then you have at least one element of an understanding system. On the other hand, if you notice a department or even a whole hospital run as a "tight ship," with managers displaying no-nonsense attitudes, and little evidence of informal discussion in the corridors, then you are dealing with an action system.

In the same way, you can look at the structures and technologies at a site for change. Is there a reliance on formal controls or, instead, on informal psychological approaches to management? The more bureaucratic the organization, the more it is an action system. Are the tasks and technologies complex, requiring considerable information and time to think through the work problems? These point to an understanding system.

2. Choose your change tactics according to the nature of the system involved. Studies using an understanding approach tend to be more effective in improving work on the medical wards. Surveys, for example, can deal with psychological matters such as patient anxieties, interpersonal conflicts between nursing and domestic staff, and problems of staff morale. The surveys can be used as an organization development tool. The findings can be widely discussed and there can be considerable feedback to respondents, facilitating changes in attitude and behavior. Similar kinds of studies seem to be effective in dealing with feelings of pressure and a high drop-out rate among student nurses, poor interpersonal relations between different levels in the nursing hierarchy, inadequate motivation and skill development among junior administrators, and problems of communication between top nursing, administrative, and medical staff members.

Studies with an action approach tend to be more effective in improving the work on surgical wards. These studies can focus on a specific problem and look for administrative actions to deal with that problem. Missing lab and x-ray reports can be traced and new procedures instituted for their safe transmittal. Operating room records can be studied and more efficient schedules set up. The same kinds of studies seemed to be effective in dealing with medical records departments, emergency departments, messenger services, admissions and discharge procedures, and dietetics departments.

3. Give some thought to your own management style. Does it fit the predominant emphasis of your organizational system? Furthermore, if you tend

toward an extreme in either action or understanding, it might be useful to ensure that your management team includes staff with complementary propensities and skills. Most complex organizational systems include both action and undertanding subsystems, medical *and* surgical departments, emergency departments *and* interdisciplinary community care teams, etc.

4. Look at management consultants in terms of action and understanding approaches and their appropriateness to your needs and problems. Obviously, operations research is more suited to an action system, while organization development is suited for an understanding system. But often the label a consultant uses doesn't tell you the whole story, so you have to diagnose his or her basic approach to change. Management by objectives (MBO) can be an action approach to change, emphasizing paper work and procedures as a way of getting clearer links between overall organizational goals and the subgoals that direct the efforts of lower-level staff. On the other hand, a consultant may use MBO as a vehicle for increasing discussion of goals between superiors and subordinates and as a means of engendering greater motivation on the part of those subordinates. You have to look beyond the label, beyond the technique, to get at the basic "chemistry" of the consultant's approach.

5. Finally, the action and understanding distinction is really crucial when dealing with organizational matters over which doctors have some control (75 percent of all hospital costs, according to many observers). To improve organizational functioning successfully, an appropriate approach to doctors will tailor the change tactics very closely to their preferences. In the ten-hospital project that the author observed, this was done by letting doctors themselves decide on the major problems to be studied, and then letting them direct the student help in the appropriate action or understanding kind of study, as the doctors themselves preferred. If an administrator or an outside consultant had offered only a one-sided approach to change and improvement, many doctors would have undoubtedly dropped out. The key seems to be to offer both approaches to change and let them select and devise change efforts that are most compatible with their own personality and work requirements.

Bibliography

The following is a list of articles and books about organization change and organization development in health care organizations. Research studies from the behavioral sciences are emphasized, although some practical, how-to-do-it articles and books are included, too.

To conserve space, multiple chapters from an edited collection are provided with a citation consisting of the editor's name and the date of the volume. The full citation, giving the title and other details of the edited volume, will be found in the list under the editor's name.

Abernathy, William J., and Prahalad, Coimbatore K. "Technology and Productivity in Health Organizations." In Abernathy et al., 1975, pp. 189–203.

Abernathy, William J.; Sheldon, Alan; and Prahalad, Coimbatore K., eds. *The Management of Health Care.* Cambridge, Mass.: Ballinger, 1975.

Alford, Robert R., *Health Care Politics: Ideological and Interest Group Barriers to Reform.* Chicago: University of Chicago Press, 1975.

Allison, Robert F. "Administrative Responses to Prospective Reimbursement." *Topics in Health Care Financing* 3, no.2(Winter 1976):97–111.

Allison, Robert F.; Dowling, William L.; and Munson, Fred C. "The Role of the Health Services Administrator and Implications for Education." *Education for Health Administration,* Vol. 2. Ann Arbor, Mich.: Health Administration Press, 1975, pp. 147–82.

Alpander, Guvene G. "Role Clarity and Performance Effectiveness." *Hospital & Health Services Administration* 24 no.1(Winter 1979):11–24.

American Hospital Association. Research capsule no.15: "Hospital Use of Industrial Engineers." *Hospitals, J.A.H.A.* 49, no.5(1 February 1975): 186–88.

Anderson, Ronald. "Social Factors Influencing Administrators' Use of Research Results." *Inquiry* 12(1975):235–38.

Anthony, Robert N., and Herzlinger, Regina. *Management Control in Nonprofit Organizations.* Homewood, Ill.: Richard D. Irwin, 1975.

Appelbaum, Steven H. "A Profile of Leadership and Motivation within a Closed Hospital Climate." *Health Care Management Review* 3(Winter 1978):77–85.

Arthur, David M. *Organization Development: Behavioral Science Strategies for Increasing Hospital Effectiveness in a Changing Environment.* Iowa City: University of Iowa, 1977.

Balint, M.; Balint, E.; Gosling, R.; and Hildebrand, P. *A Study of Doctors: Mutual Selection and the Evaluation of Results in a Training Programme for Family Doctors.* Philadelphia: Lippincott, 1966.

Banta, H. D., and Fox, R. "Role Strain of a Health Care Team in a Poverty Community." *Social Science and Medicine* 6(1972):692–722.

Bartee, Edwin M., and Cheyunski, Fred. "A Methodology for Process-oriented Organizational Diagnosis." *Journal of Applied Behavioral Science* 13(1977):53–68.

Bartscht, Karl G., and Coffey, Richard J. "Management Engineering—a Method to Improve Productivity." *Topics in Health Care Financing* 3, no.3(Spring 1977):39–67.

Battistella, Roger M., and Chester, Theodore E. "Reorganization of the National Health Service: Background and Issues in England's Quest for a Comprehensive-Integrated Planning and Delivery System." *Milbank Memorial Fund Quarterly: Health and Society* 51(1973):489–530.

Bauerschmidt, Alan D., and Brunson, Richard W. "Organization Development: Part one: Definition, Origin, Methods, and Modes of Delivery. Part two: Applications in a Hospital Setting." *Hospital Progress* 54, no.9 (September 1973):62–68, and no.10(October 1973):44–52.

Becker, Selwyn W., and Neuhauser, Duncan. *The Efficient Organization.* New York: Elsevier, 1975.

Beckhard, Richard. "Organizational Implications of Team Building: The Larger Picture." In Wise et al., 1975, pp. 69–98.

Beckhard, Richard. "ABS in Health Care Systems: Who Needs It?" *Journal of Applied Behavioral Science* 10(1974):93–106.

Beer, H. R. "Problems Encountered in Introducing Management by Objectives." *Hospital and Health Services Review* 68(1972):353–58.

Bennett, Addison C. "Managing Change in the Hospital." Pt.1. *Hospital Topics* 50, no.6(June 1972):53–56. Pt.2. *Hospital Topics* 50, no.7(July 1972):22–26.

Bennett, Wallace F. "Education Is PSRO Goal." *Hospitals, J.A.H.A.* 48, no.5(1 March 1974):53–62+.

Blum, Henrik L. *Planning for Health: Development and Application of Social Change Theory.* New York: Human Sciences Press, 1974.

Berlin, Victor. "Organizational Structure and Effectiveness: an Administrative Experiment in an Urban Health Department." *IEEE Transactions on Engineering Management,* May 1974, pp. 57–72.

Brady, Rodney H. "MBO Goes to Work in the Public Sector." *Harvard Business Review* 51, no.2(March–April 1973):65–74.

Bragg, J. E., and Andrews, I. R. "Participative Decision Making: an Experimental Study in a Hospital." *Journal of Applied Behavioral Science* 9(1973):727–35.

Bucher, Rue, and Stelling, Joan. "Characteristics of Professional Organizations." *Journal of Health and Human Behavior* 10(1969):3–15.

Burling, Temple; Lenz, Edith; and Wilson, Robert. *The Give and Take in Hospitals.* New York: G.P. Putnam's Sons, 1956.

Cain, Cindy, and Luchsinger, Vince. "Management by Objectives: Applications to Nursing." *Journal of Nursing Administration* 8, no.1(January 1978):35–38.

Carithers, Robert W. "What to Expect from an Outside Consultant and How to Get It." *Health Care Management Review* 2, no.3(Summer 1977):43–46.

Cartwright, Ann. *Human Relations and Hospital Care.* London: Routledge and Kegan Paul, 1964.

Charnes, Martin P. "Breaking the Tradition Barrier: Managing Integration in Health Care Facilities." *Health Care Management Review* 1, no.4 (Winter 1976):55–67.

Chaska, Norma L. "The 'Cooling Out' Process in a Complex Organization." *Journal of Nursing Administration* 9, no.1(January 1979):22–28.

Clarke, Roberta N. "Marketing Health Care: Problems in Implementation." *Health Care Management Review* 3, no.1(Winter 1978):21–27.

Coe, Rodney M., ed. *Planned Change in the Hospital: Case Studies of Organizational Innovations.* New York: Praeger, 1970.

Coghill, Nelson F. "Change and Growth in Hospitals." *Lancet* 2, no.7629 (November 15, 1969):1058–61.

Colarelli, Nick J., and Siegal, Saul M. *Ward H: An Adventure in Innovation.* Princeton: Van Nostrand, 1966.

Coleman, James S.; Katz, Elihu; and Menzel, Herbert. *Medical Innovation: A Diffusion Study.* Indianapolis: Bobbs-Merrill, 1966.

Collen, Morris F. "Planning and Implementing Large Medical Information Systems." In Abernathy et al., 1975, pp. 127–39.

Cornish, John B. "Research and the Management of Hospitals." In *Portfolio for Health,* edited by G. McLachlan, pp. 169–75. London: Oxford University Press, 1971.

Coser, Rose Laub. "Authority and Decision-making in a Hospital." *American Sociological Review* 23(1958):56–63.

Coser, Rose Laub. "Alienation and the Social Structure: Case Analysis of a Hospital." In *The Hospital in Modern Society,* edited by Eliot Freidson, pp. 231–65. New York: Free Press, 1963.

Corwin, Ronald G. "The Professional Employee: A Study of Conflict in Nursing Roles." *American Journal of Sociology* 66(1961):604–15.

Crichton, Ann. "Research and Hospital Management." *Hospital (London)* 62(1966):66–68.

Davies, Celia. "Professionals in Organizations: Some Preliminary Observations on Hospital Consultants." *Sociological Review* 20(1972):553-67.

Deegan, Arthur X., II. *Management by Objectives for Hospitals.* Germantown, Md.: Aspen Systems, 1977.

Demone, Harold W., Jr., and Harshberger, Dwight. *The Planning and Administration of Human Services.* New York: Behavioral Publications, 1973.

Department of Health and Social Security, United Kingdom. *Guide to Good Practices in Hospital Administration.* London: Her Majesty's Stationery Office, 1970.

Dobson, Allen, et al. "PSROs: Their Current Status and Their Impact to Date." *Inquiry* 15, no.2(June 1978):113-28.

Donabedian, Avedis. *Aspects of Medical Care Administration: Specifying Requirements for Health Care.* Cambridge, Mass.: Harvard University Press, 1973.

Dornbusch, Sanford M., and Scott, W. Richard. *Evaluation and the Exercise of Authority.* San Francisco: Jossey-Bass, 1975.

Draper, Peter, and Smart, Tony. "Social Science and Health Policy in the United Kingdom: Some Contributions of the Social Sciences to the Bureaucratization of the National Health Services." *International Journal of Health Services* 14, no.3(Summer 1974):453-70.

Duff, Raymond S., and Hollingshead, August B. *Sickness and Society.* New York: Harper and Row, 1968.

Dykens, James W.; Hyde, Robert W.; Orzack, Louis H.; and York, Richard H. *Strategies of Mental Hospital Change.* Boston: Department of Mental Health, 1964.

Eisenberg, John M. "An Educational Program to Modify Laboratory Use by House Staff." *Journal of Medical Education* 52(1977):578-81.

Engel, Gloria V. "The Effect of Bureaucracy on the Professional Autonomy of the Physician." *Journal of Health and Social Behavior* 10(1969):30-41.

Ermann, M. David. "Long-Term Responses to Control Systems." In Griffith et al., 1976, pp. 317-26.

Falck, Hans S. "The Consultant As Insider and Change Agent: The Problem of Boundaries in Social Systems." *Administration in Mental Health* 5, no.1(Fall-Winter 1977):55-67.

Farlee, Coralie, "The Computer As a Focus of Organizational Change in the Hospital." *Journal of Nursing Administration* 8, no.2(February 1978): 20-26.

Findley, Wilfred J. "Management by Objectives." *Dimensions in Health Service (Canadian Hospital Journal)* 51, no.7(July 1974):17-18.

Franklin, Jack L., and Kittredge, Lee D. "Organizational Problems in Community Mental Health Centers." *Administration in Mental Health*, Spring 1975, pp. 60-65.

Fredrickson, James W. "Organizing for Better Medical School Management." *Health Care Management Review* 2, no.2(Spring 1977):71–76.

Freedman, Arthur M. "Organization Development in a State Mental Health Setting." In *Current Perspectives in Organization Development,* edited by J. Jennings Partin, pp. 195–210. Reading Mass.: Addison-Wesley, 1973.

Freeman, Howard; Levine, Sol; and Reeder, Leo G., eds. *Handbook for Medical Sociology.* 2d ed. Englewood Cliffs: Prentice-Hall, 1972.

Freidson, Eliot. "Dominant Professions, Bureaucracy and Client Services." In *Organizations and Clients,* edited by W. R. Rosengren and M. Lefton, pp. 71–92. Columbus: Charles E. Merrill, 1970.

Freidson, Eliot. *Professional Dominance: the Social Structure of Medical Care.* New York: Atherton Press, 1970.

Freidson, Eliot. *Profession of Medicine: a Study of the Sociology of Applied Knowledge.* New York: Dodd, Mead, 1970.

Freidson, Eliot, and Lorber, Judith, eds. *Medical Men and Their Work.* Chicago: Aldine-Atherton, 1972.

Freidson, Eliot, and Rhea, Buford. "Processes of Control in a Company of Equals." *Social Problems* 2(1963):119–31.

Fry, Ronald E.; Lech, Bernard A.; and Rubin, Irwin. "Working with the Primary Care Team: the First Intervention." In Wise, et al., 1975, pp. 27–67.

Ganong, Warren L., and Ganong, Joan Mary. "Reducing Organizational Conflict through Working Committees." *Journal of Nursing Administration* 2, no.1 (January-February 1972):12–19.

Garrison, John E., and Raynes, Anthony E. "Results of a Pilot Management-by-Objectives Program for a Community Mental Health Outpatient Service." *Community Mental Health Journal* 16(1980):121–129.

Geiger, H. F. "Hidden Professional Roles: The Physician as Reactionary, Reformer, Revolutionary." *Social Policy* 1(1971):24–33.

Georgopoulos, Basil S. "The Hospital As an Organization and Problem-solving System." In Georgopoulos, 1972, pp. 9–48.

Georgopoulos, Basil S. *Hospital Organization Research: Review and Source Book.* Philadelphia: W. B. Saunders, 1975.

Georgopoulos, Basil S., ed. *Organization Research on Health Institutions.* Ann Arbor: Institute for Social Research, 1972.

Georgopoulos, Basil S., and Mann, Floyd, C. *The Community General Hospital.* New York: Macmillan, 1962.

Georgopoulos, Basil S., and Matejko, Alexander. "The American General Hospital As a Complex Social System." *Health Services Research* 2(1967): 76–112.

Georgopoulos, Basil S., and Wieland, George F. *Nationwide Study of Coordination and Patient Care in Voluntary Hospitals.* Ann Arbor: Institute for Social Research, 1968.

Gerstenfield, Arthur. "Innovation and Health Care Management." *Hospital*

& *Health Services Administration* 23, no.2(Spring 1978):38–50.

Gerstenfield, Arthur. "MBO Revisited: Focus on Health Systems." *Health Care Management Review* 2, no.4(Fall 1978):51–57.

Gilbert, G. Ronald. "Evaluation for Institutional Learning: A Behavioral Perspective." *Journal of Health and Human Resources Administration* 1(1979):307–16.

Gilbert, G. Ronald. Introduction to Symposium—"Evaluation Management: Can We Improve Organizational Learning?" *Journal of Health and Human Resources Administration* 1(1979):274–77.

Glaser, Edward M. and Backer, Thomas E. "Durability of Innovations: How Goal Attainment Scaling Programs Fare Over Time." *Community Mental Health Journal* 16(1980):130–142.

Goffman, Erving. *Asylums: Essays on the Social Situation of Mental Patients and Other Inmates.* Garden City: Doubleday Anchor, 1961.

Goldstein, S. G. "A Structure for Change." *Human Relations* 31(1978): 957-83.

Golightly, Cecilia. "MBO and Performance Appraisal." *Journal of Nursing Administration* 9, no.9(September 1979):11–20.

Gordon, Gerald; Tanon, Christian P.; and Morse, Edward V. "Decision-making Criteria and Organizational Performance." In Shortell and Brown, 1976, pp. 62–71.

Goss, Mary E. W. "Influence and Authority among Physicians." *American Sociological Review* 26(1961):39–50.

Goss, Mary E. W. "Patterns of Bureaucracy among Hospital Staff Physicians." In *The Hospital in Modern Society*, edited by Eliot Freidson, pp. 170–94. New York: Free Press, 1963.

Goss, Mary E. W. "Organizational Goals and Quality of Medical Care: Evidence from Comparative Research in Hospitals." *Journal of Health and Social Behavior* 11(1970):225–68.

Gray, A. F. "Management Consultants in the Hospital Service: an Assessment." *Hospital (London)* 64, no.1(January 1968):11–13.

Green, Stephen. "Professional/Bureaucratic Conflict: the Case of the Medical Profession in the National Health Service." *Sociological Review* 23(1975):121–41.

Griffith, John R. "An Analysis of the Results at Baker Hospital." In Griffith et al., 1976, pp. 387–435.

Griffith, John R.; Hancock, Walton M.; and Munson, Fred C. "Practical Ways to Contain Hospital Costs." *Harvard Business Review* 51, no.6 (November-December 1973):131–39.

Griffith, John R.; Hancock, Walton M.; and Munson, Fred C., eds. *Cost Control in Hospitals.* Ann Arbor: Health Administration Press, 1976.

Groner, Pat N. *Cost Containment through Employee Incentive Programs.* Germantown, Md.: Aspen, 1977.

Grossman, Jerome H. "Shifting Patterns in the Nature of Technological Innovations in Health Care Delivery." In Abernathy et al., 1975, pp. 63–66.

Gue, Ronald L. "Operations Research in Health and Hospital Administration." *Hospital Administration* 10, no.4(Fall 1975):6–25.

Guest, Robert H. "The Role of the Doctor in Institutional Management." In Georgopoulos, 1972, pp. 283–300.

Hage, Jerald. *Communication and Organizational Control: Cybernetics in Health and Welfare Settings.* New York: John Wiley, 1964.

Hage, Jerald, and Aiken, Michael. "Program Change and Organizational Properties." *American Journal of Sociology* 72(1967):503–19.

Hage, Jerald, and Aiken, Michael. "Routine Technology, Social Structure, and Organizational Goals." *Administrative Science Quarterly* 14(1969): 366–77.

Hage, Jerald, and Aiken, Michael. *Social Change in Complex Organizations.* New York: Random House, 1970.

Hage, Jerald, and Dewar, Robert. "Elite Values Versus Organization Structure in Predicting Innovation." *Administrative Science Quarterly* 18(1973): 279–90.

Halachmi, Arie. "Dealing with the Conflict of Loyalties: The Continuing Seminar and Action Research." *Journal of Health and Human Resources Administration* 2(1980):505–31.

Hall, David J. "Problems of Innovation in a Hospital Setting: The Example of Playleaders." *Sociology of Work and Occupations* 4(1977):63–86.

Halperin, William, and Neuhauser, Duncan. "MEU: Measuring Efficient Utilization of Hospital Services." *Health Care Management Review* 1, no.2(Spring 1976):63–70.

Hand, Herbert H., and Hollingsworth, A. Thomas. "Tailoring MBO to Hospitals." *Business Horizons* 18, no.1(February 1975):45–52.

Harris, Reuben T. "Improving Patient Satisfaction through Action Research." *Journal of Applied Behavioral Science* 14(1978):382–99.

Harris, Ruth J. "Facilitating Change to the Problem-oriented Medical Record System." *Journal of Nursing Administration* 8, no.8(August 1978): 35–38.

Haussmann, Dieter. "Implementing Technology-based Management Systems in Health Organizations." In Abernathy et al., 1975, pp. 141–49.

Haveliwala, Yoosuf A. "Changing a Mental Hospital." *Administration in Mental Health* 7(1979):112–19.

Hersch, Charles. "The Process of Collaboration: A Case Study." *Community Mental Health Journal* 3(1967):254–58.

Hersch, Charles. "The Process of Collaboration II: Implementation and Its Discontents or You Don't Learn That in School." *Community Mental Health Journal* 6(1970):300–12.

Herzlinger, Regina E. "Fiscal Management in Health Organizations." *Health*

Care Management Review 2, no.3(Summer 1977):37–42.

Herzlinger, Regina E., Moore, Gorton T., and Hall, Elizabeth A. "Management Control Systems in Health Care." *Medical Care* 11(1973):416–29.

Heydebrand, Wolf V. *Hospital Bureaucracy: A Comparative Study of Organizations.* New York: Dunellen, 1973.

Highman, Arthur, and Davidson, Leth. "Survey Shows How Management Technics Change." *Modern Hospital* 117, no.6(December 1971):60–62.

Hollister, Robert M.; Kramer, Bernard M.; and Bellin, Seymour S., eds. *Neighborhood Health Centers.* Lexington, Mass.: D. C. Heath, 1974.

Holloway, Robert G. "Management Can Reverse Declining Employees Work Attitudes." *Hospitals* 50, no.20(16 October 1976):71–77.

Holloway, Robert G., and Lonergan, Wallace G. "A Survey Program for Management and Organizational Development." *Hospitals J.A.H.A.* 42(16 August 1968):59–65.

Houghton, Hazel. "Problems of Hospital Communication: An Experimental Study." In *Problems and Progress in Medical Care: Essays on Current Research.* 3d. ser., edited by Gordon McLachlan. London: Oxford University Press, 1968.

Hughes, Shirley J. "Installing a Computer-Based Patient Information System." *Journal of Nursing Administration* 10, no.5(May 1980):7–10.

Hulka, et al. "Peer Review in Ambulatory Care: Use of Explicit Criteria and Implicit Judgments." *Medical Care* 13, no.3(1975), Supplement.

Jaco, E. Gartly. "Ecological Aspects of Patient Care and Hospital Organization." In Georgopoulos, 1972, pp. 223–70.

Johnson, Nancy D. "The Professional-Bureaucratic Conflict." *Journal of Nursing Administration* 1, no.3(May-June 1971):31–39.

Jelinek, Richard C.; Munson, Fred; and Smith, Robert L. *SUM (Service Unit Management): An Organizational Approach to Improved Patient Care.* Battle Creek, Mich.: W. K. Kellogg Foundation, 1971.

Johnson, Richard L. "The Power Broker—Prototype of the Hospital Chief Executive?" *Health Care Management Review* 3, no.4(Fall 1978):67–73.

Kalish, Beatrice J., and Kalish, Philip A. "An Analysis of the Sources of Physician-Nurse Conflict." *Journal of Nursing Administration* 7, no.1 (January 1977):51–57.

Kaluzny, Arnold D. "Innovation in the Health System: A Selective Review of System Characteristics and Empirical Research." *Health Services Research* 9, no.2(Summer 1974):101–20.

Kaluzny, Arnold D.; Glasser, Jay H.; Gentry, John T.; and Sprague, Jane. "Diffusion of Innovative Health Care Services in the United States: A Study of Hospitals." *Medical Care* 8(1970):474–87.

Kaluzny, Arnold D., and Veney, James E. "Who Influences Decisions in the Hospital? Not Even the Administrator Really Knows." *Modern Hospital* 119, no.6(December 1972):52–53.

Kaluzny, Arnold D., and Veney, James E. "Attributes of Health Services As Factors in Implementation." *Journal of Health and Social Behavior* 14(1973):124–33.

Kaluzny, Arnold D.; Veney, James E.; and Gentry, John T. "Innovation of Health Services: A Comparative Study of Hospitals and Health Departments." *Milbank Memorial Fund Quarterly: Health and Society* 52, no.1(Winter 1974):51–82.

Kaluzny, Arnold D.; Veney, James E.; Smith, David B.; and Elliot, William. "Predicting Two Types of Hospital Innovation." *Hospital and Health Services Administration* 21, no.2(Spring 1976):24–43.

Kaplan, Howard B. "Implementation of Program Change in Community Agencies." *Milbank Memorial Fund Quarterly* 45(July 1967):321–31.

Kendall, Patricia L. "The Learning Environments of Hospitals." In *The Hospital in Modern Society*, edited by Eliot Freidson, pp. 195–230. New York: Free Press, 1963.

Kennedy, Rose, and Vose, Ann B. "Preparing the Nurse Manager to Assume New Accountabilities." *Hospitals, J.A.H.A.* 52, no.2(1 January 1978): 66–69.

Kimberly, John R. "Hospital Adoption of Innovation: The Role of Integration into External Informational Environments." *Journal of Health and Social Behavior* 19(1978):361–73.

Klein, Rudolf. "Reorganisation: What Went Wrong." *New Society* 41, no.781 September 1977):592–93.

Kopelke, Charlotte E. "The Nominal Group Approach As an Evaluation Tool." *Journal of Nursing Administration* 6, no.10(December 1976): 32–34.

Kovner, Anthony R. "The Hospital Administrator and Organizational Effectiveness." In *Organization Research on Health Institutions*, edited by Basil S. Georgopoulos. Ann Arbor: Institute for Social Research, 1972.

Kovner, Anthony R.; Katz, Gerald; Kahane, Stanley B.; and Sheps, Cecil G. "Relating a Neighborhood Health Center to a General Hospital: A Case Study." *Medical Care* 7(1969):118–23.

Kovner, Anthony R., and Neuhauser, Duncan, eds. *Health Services Management: Readings and Commentary*. Ann Arbor: Health Administration Press, 1978.

Kramer, Marlene, and Schmalenberg, Claudia E. "Conflict: the Cutting Edge of Growth." *Journal of Nursing Administration* 6, no.8(October 1976): 19–25.

Kyte, Arleen L. "Creating a Self-Renewing Capability: An OD Odyssey." In Wise et al., 1974, pp. 101–46.

Lammert, Marilyn H. "Power, Authority, and Status in Health Systems: A Marxian-based Conflict Analysis," *Journal of Applied Behavioral Science* 14(1978):321–33.

Landay, Merwyn A. "Organization Development in a School of Dentistry: A Client Reflects on Theory and Practice." *Journal of Applied Behavioral Science* 14(1978):415–30.

Lawrence, Robert S. "The Role of Physician Education in Cost Containment." *Journal of Medical Education* 54(1979):841–47.

Lehman, Edward W. *Coordinating Health Care: Explorations in Interorganizational Relations.* Sage Library of Social Research, Vol. 17. Beverly Hills: Sage Publications, 1975.

Leigh, Hilary; Wieland, George F.; and Anderson, John A. D. "The Hospital Internal Communication Project." *Lancet* 1, no.7707(15 May 1971): 1005–1009.

Levenstein, Aaron. "Effective Change Requires Change Agent." *Hospitals, J.A.H.A.* 50, no.24(16 December 1976):71–74.

Levey, Samuel. "Sources of Medical-Administrative Conflict: A Survey Report." *Hospitals, J.A.H.A.* 36, no.14(16 July 1962):60–66.

Levey, Samuel, and Loomba, N. Paul. *Health Care Administration: A Managerial Perspective.* Philadelphia: J. B. Lippincott, 1973.

Levinson, Harry. "The Changing Role of the Hospital Administrator." *Health Care Management Review* 1, no.1(Winter 1976):79–89.

Lewis, Joyce H. "Conflict Management." *Journal of Nursing Administration* 6, no.10(December 1976):18–22.

Lindner, Joseph, Jr. "Point of View: Better Management Not Just More Money: Physician Involvement." *Health Care Management Review* 2, no.3(Summer 1977):47–50.

Lippitt, Gordon L. "Hospital Organization in the Post Industrial Society." *Hospital Progress* 54, no.6(June 1973):55–64.

Litman, Theodore J. *The Sociology of Medicine and Health Care: A Research Bibliography.* San Francisco: Body and Fraser, 1976.

Longest, Beaufort B., Jr. "Productivity in the Provision of Hospital Services: A Challenge to the Management Community." *Academy of Management Review* 2(1977):475–83.

Longest, Beaufort B., Jr. "The Contemporary Hospital Chief Executive Officer." *Health Care Management Review* 3, no.2(Spring 1978):43–53.

Ludwig, Patric E. *Dollars and Sense: An Approach Toward Hospital, Cost Containment and Quality Improvement through Management Engineering Programs.* Battle Creek, Mich.: W. K. Kellogg Foundation, 1971.

Lundstedt, Sven, and Lillibridge, John. "Effects of Increased Staff Participation on Patient Care and Staff Attitudes." *Mental Hygiene* 50(1966): 432–38.

Lyle, Carl B. Jr.; Bianchi, Raymond F.; Harris, Judith H.; and Wood, Zoe L. "Teaching Cost Containment to House Officers at Charlotte Memorial Hospital." *Journal of Medical Education* 54(1979):856–62.

McConkey, Dale D. *MBO (Management by Objectives) for Nonprofit*

Organizations. New York: American Management Association, 1975.

McLaughlin, Curtis P. "Productivity and Human Services." *Health Care Management Review* 1, no.4(Fall 1976):47–60.

Margulies, Newton. "Managing Change in Health Care Organizations." *Medical Care* 15(1977):693–704.

Marsden, Lorna R. "Power within a Profession: Medicine in Ontario." *Sociology of Work and Occupations* 4(1977):3–24.

Mazade, Noel A. "Consultation and Education Practice and Organizational Structure in Ten Community Mental Health Centers." *Hospital & Community Psychiatry* 25(1974):673–75.

Menzel, Herbert. Innovation, Integration, and Marginality: A Survey of Physicians." *American Sociological Review* 25(1960):704–13.

Menzies, Isabel E. P. "A Case-Study in the Functioning of Social Systems As a Defense Against Anxiety." *Human Relations* 13(1960):95–121.

Milch, Robert Austin. "Product-Market Differentiation: A Strategic Planning Model for Community Hospitals." *Health Care Management Review* 5, no.2(Spring 1980):7–16.

Milio, Nancy. "Health Care Organizations and Innovation." *Journal of Health and Social Behavior* 12(1971):163–73.

Mill, Cyril R. "Short-term Consultation in Organization Development for Mental Health Agencies." *Hospital & Community Psychiatry* 25(1974): 726–29.

Millman, Marcia. *The Unkindest Cut: Life in the Backrooms of Medicine.* New York: William Morrow, 1977.

Moore, Terence F., and Lorimer, Bernard E. "The Matrix Organization in Business and Health Care Institutions: A Comparison." *Hospital & Health Services Administration* 21, no.4(Fall 1976):26–34.

Moore, T., et al. "Power and the Hospital Executive." *Hospital & Health Services Administration* 24, no.2(Spring 1979):30–41.

Morrell, Joan; Podlone, Michael; and Cohen, Stanley N. "Receptivity of Physicians in a Teaching Hospital to a Computerized Drug Interaction Monitoring and Reporting System." *Medical Care* 15(1977):68–78.

Morse, Edward V.; Gordon, Gerald; and Moch, Michael. "Hospital Costs and Quality of Care: An Organizational Perspective." *Milbank Memorial Fund Quarterly* 52(1974):315–46.

Mosely, S. Kelley, and Grimes, Richard M. "The Organization of Effective Hospitals." *Health Care Management Review* 1, no.3(Spring 1976):13–23.

Moss, Arthur B.; Broehl, Wayne G., Jr.; Guest, Robert H.; and Hennessey, John W., Jr. *Hospital Policy Decisions: Process and Action.* New York: Putnam, 1966.

Mott, Paul E. *The Characteristics of Effective Organizations.* New York: Harper & Row, 1972.

Mumford, Emily, and Skipper, James K., Jr. *Sociology in Hospital Care.*

New York: Harper & Row, 1967.

Munson, Fred C. "Crisis Points in Unit Management Programs." *Hospitals, J.A.H.A.* 47, no.14(16 July 1973):122+.

Munson, Fred C., and Hancock, Walton M. "Implementation of Hospital Control Systems." In Griffith et al., 1976, pp. 297–316.

Musschoot, Frederik, and Van Oyen, M. "Optimal Patient Care through Action Learning." *Acta Hospitalia* 18(1978):335–56.

Nadler, David A. "Hospitals, Organized Labor and Quality of Work: An Intervention Case Study." *Journal of Applied Behavioral Science* 14(1978): 366–81.

Nathanson, Constance A., and Becker, Marshall H. "Control Structure and Conflict in Outpatient Clinics." *Journal of Health and Social Behavior* 13(1972):251–62.

Nathanson, Constance A., and Morlock, Laura L. "Control Structure, Values, and Innovation: A Comparative Study of Hospitals." Paper presented at American Sociological Meetings, September 1978, San Francisco, California.

Neilsen, Eric H. "Physicians and Organization Development." *Proceedings of the Academy of Management*, 8–11 August, 1979. Atlanta, Ga.

Neuhauser, Duncan. *The Relationship between Administrative Activities and Hospital Performance.* Chicago: Center for Health Administration, University of Chicago, 1971.

Neuhauser, Duncan. "The Hospital As a Matrix Organization." *Hospital Administration* 4(Fall 1972):8–23.

Neuhauser, Duncan. "Information Systems for Hospitals: An Organizational Approach." In Kovner and Neuhauser, 1978, pp. 206–12.

O'Donovan, Thomas R. "Management by Objectives." *Hospital Topics* 49, no.2(February 1971):34–37, 42.

Palmer, Jeanne. "Management by Objectives." *Journal of Nursing Administration* 1, no.1(January 1971):17–23.

Pantall, John, and Elliot, James. "Can Research Aid Hospital Management?" Hospital Centre Reprint 234: London: King's Fund Hospital Centre, 1968.

Pellegrino, Edmund D. "The Changing Matrix of Clinical Decision-making in the Hospital." In Georgopoulos, 1972, pp. 301–28.

Penchansky, Roy, ed. *Health Services Administration: Policy Cases and the Case Method.* Cambridge, Mass.: Harvard University Press, 1968.

Perrow, Charles. "Organizational Prestige." *American Journal of Sociology* 66(1961):335–41.

Perrow, Charles. "Goals and Power Structures—a Historical Case Study." In *The Hospital in Modern Society*, edited by Eliot Freidson, pp. 112–46. New York: Free Press, 1963.

Perrow, Charles. "Hospitals: Technology, Structure, and Goals." In *Handbook of Organizations*, edited by James G. March, pp. 910–71. Chicago: Rand McNally, 1965.

Peterson, Grace G. "Power: A Perspective for the Nurse Administrator." *Journal of Nursing Administration* 9, no.7(July 1979):7–10.

Peterson, Ronald R. "Cost Improvement Program Generates Major Savings." *Hospitals, J.A.H.A.* 52, no.13(1 July 1978):83–90.

Pfeffer, Jeffrey. "Size, Composition, and Function of Hospital Boards of Directors: A Study of Organization-Environment Linkage." *Administrative Science Quarterly* 18(1973):349–64.

Plog, Stanley C., and Ahmed, Paul I., eds. *Principles and Techniques of Mental Health Consultation.* New York: Plenum, 1977.

Plovnick, Mark S.; Fry, Ronald E.; and Rubin, Irwin M. "Re-thinking the 'What' and 'How' of Management Education for Health Professionals." *Journal of Applied Behavioral Science* 14(1978):348–63.

Plovnick, Mark S.; Rubin, Irwin M.; and Fry, Ronald E. "Design and Evaluation of an Applied Behavioral Science Course for Health Administration Students." *Association of University Programs in Health Administration Program Notes.* No.73(February 1977):37–50.

Pozen, Michael W., and Bonnet, Philip D. "Effectiveness of Educational and Administrative Interventions in Medical Outpatient Clinics." *American Journal of Public Health* 66, no. 2(February 1976):151–55.

Pozen, Michael W., and Gloger, Hershel. "The Impact on House Officers of Educational and Administrative Intervention in an Outpatient Department." *Social Science and Medicine* 10(1976):491–95.

Prahalad, Coimbatore K. "Toward a Healthier Hospital—Balancing Technology and Organizational Goals." In Abernathy et al., 1975, pp. 215–27.

Prahalad, Coimbatore K., and Abernathy, William J. "A Strategy Approach to the Management of Technology in the Health System." In Abernathy et al., 1975, pp. 89–104.

Prussin, Jeffry A. "The Use of Role Studies for Improvement of Health Administration Training: A Conceptual Framework." *Journal of Mental Health Administration* 4, no.2(Winter 1975–76):18–35.

Rakich, Jonathon S.; Longest, Beaufort B.; and O'Donovan, Thomas R. *Managing Health Care Organizations.* Philadelphia: W. B. Saunders, 1977.

Reddin, W. J. "Managing Organizational Change." *Hospital Administration* 15, no.1(Winter 1970):79–86.

Resnick, H. "Effecting Internal Change in Human Service Organizations." *Social Casework* 58, no.9(1977):546–53.

Revans, Reginald W. *Standards for Morale: Cause and Effect in Hospitals.* London: Oxford University Press, 1964.

Revans, Reginald W. "Research into Hospital Management and Organization." *Milbank Memorial Fund Quarterly* 44, no.3, pt. 2(1966):207–45.

Revans, Reginald W., ed. *Hospitals: Communication, Choice and Change.* London: Tavistock, 1972.

Revans, Reginald W. *Action Learning in Hospitals: Diagnosis and Therapy.* London: McGraw-Hill, 1976.

Rhee, Sang-o. "Factors Determining the Quality of Physician Performance in Patient Care." *Medical Care* 14(1977):733–50.

Rhenman, Eric. *Managing the Community Hospital: a Systems Analysis.* Lexington, Mass.: Saxon House-Lexington, 1973.

Ritvo, Roger A. "Adaptation to Environmental Change: The Board's Role." *Hospital & Health Services Administration* 25, no.1(Winter 1980):23–37.

Robbins, Alan S.; Kauss, David R.; Heinrich, Richard; Abrass, Itamar; Dreyer, Jerrold; and Clyman, Basil. "Interpersonal Skills Training: Evaluation in an Internal Medicine Residency." *Journal of Medical Education* 54(1979):885–94.

Roberts, Karlene H.; Cerruti, Nannette L.; and O'Reilly, Charles A., III. "Changing Perceptions of Organizational Communication: Can Short-Term Intervention Help?" *Nursing Research* 25, no.3(May-June 1976): 197–200.

Rockart, J. F. "On the Implementation of Information Systems." In Abernathy et al., 1975, pp. 175–86.

Roemer, Milton I., and Friedman, Jay W. *Doctors in Hospitals: Medical Staff Organization and Hospital Performance.* Baltimore: Johns Hopkins Press, 1971.

Rosengren, William R., and DeVault, Spencer. "The Sociology of Time and Space in an Obstetrical Hospital." In *The Hospital in Modern Society*, edited by Eliot Freidson, pp. 266–92. New York: Free Press, 1963.

Rosner, Marvin M., "Administrative Controls and Innovation." *Behavioral Science* 13(1968):36–43.

Rosner, Marvin M. "Economic Determinants of Organizational Innovation." *Administrative Science Quarterly* 12(1968):614–25.

Rossman, Betty B.; Hober, Diane I.; and Ciarlo, James A. "Awareness, Use, and Consequences of Evaluation Data in a Community Mental Health Center." *Community Mental Health Journal* 15(1979):7–16.

Roth, Julius A. "Information and Control of Treatment in Tuberculosis Hospitals." In *The Hospital in Modern Society*, edited by Eliot Freidson, pp. 293–318. New York: Free Press, 1963.

Rothman, Jack; Erlich, John L.; and Teresa, Joseph G. *Promoting Innovation and Change in Organizations and Communities: A Planning Manual.* New York: John Wiley, 1976.

Rowbottom, Ralph, et al., *Hospital Organization.* London: Heinemann, 1973.

Rubenstein, Albert H.; Rath, Gustave J.; O'Keefe, Robert D.; Kernaghan, John A.; Moore, Evelyn A.; Moor, William C.; and Werner, David J. "Behavioral Factors Influencing the Adoption of an Experimental Information System." *Hospital Administration* 18, no.4(Fall 1973):27–43.

Rubin, Irwin, and Beckhard, Richard. "Factors Influencing the Effectiveness of Health Teams." *Milbank Memorial Fund Quarterly* 2(July 1972): 327–35.

Rubin, Irwin M.; Fry, Ronald E.; and Plovnick, Mark S. *Managing Human Resources in Health Care Organizations: an Applied Approach.* Reston, Va.: Reston Publishing Co., 1978.

Rubin, Irwin; Fry, Ronald; Plovnick, Mark; and Stearns, Norman. "Improving the Coordination of Care: An Educational Program. *Hospital & Health Services Administration* 22(Spring 1977):57–70.

Rubin, Irwin; Plovnick, Mark; and Fry, Ronald. "Initiating Planned Change in Health Care Systems." *Journal of Applied Behavioral Science* 10(1974): 107–24.

Rubin, Irwin; Plovnick, Mark; and Fry, Ronald. "The Role of the Consultant in Initiating Planned Change: A Case Study in Health Care Systems." In *Current Issues in Organization Development*, edited by W. Warner Burke, pp. 324–60. New York: Human Sciences Press, 1977.

Russell, A. Yvonne; Zimmerman, Shirley; and Bruce, Ray. "Organization Development at Work in a Medical Center." *Health Care Management Review* 4, no.3(Fall 1978):59–66.

Saxl, Joseph. "Evaluation's Evaluation: The Public Sector." *Hospital Administration* 20, no.4(Fall 1975):33–43.

Schermerhorn, John R., Jr. "The Health Care Manager's Role in Promoting Change." *Health Care Management Review* 4, no.1(Winter 1979):71–79.

Schoonhoven, Claudia Bird. "Computerized Planning Systems: A Professional Tool or an Administrative Control Device." Paper presented at the Academy of Management meetings, August 1979, Atlanta, Georgia.

Schroeder, Steven A.; Kenders, Kathryn; Cooper, James K.; and Piemme, Thomas E. "Use of Laboratory Tests and Pharmaceuticals: Variation among Physicians and Effect of Cost Audit on Subsequent Use." *JAMA, Journal of the American Medical Association* 225(1973):969–73.

Schulman, John *Re-making an Organization.* Albany: State University of New York Press, 1969.

Schultz, Rockwell. "Does Staff Participation Equal Active Participation?" *Hospitals, J.A.H.A.* 46, no.24(16 December 1972):51–55.

Schulz, Rockwell. "How to Get Doctors Involved in Governance, Management." *Trustee* 29, no.6(June 1976):34–37.

Schulz, Rockwell, and Johnson, Alton C. "Conflict in Hospitals." *Hospital Administration* 16(Summer 1971):36–49.

Schulz, Rockwell, and Johnson, Alton C. *Management of Hospitals.* New York: McGraw-Hill, 1976.

Schulz, Rockwell I., and Rose, Jerry. "Can Hospitals Be Expected to Control Costs?" *Inquiry* 10, no.2(June 1973):3–8.

Scott, W. Richard. "Professionals in Hospitals: Technology and the Organization of Work." In Georgopoulos, 1972, pp. 139–58.

Scott, W. Richard, and Volkart, Edmund H., eds. *Medical Care: Readings in the Sociology of Medical Institutions.* New York: John Wiley & Sons, 1966.

Scott, W. Richard; Flood, Ann Barry; and Ewy, Wayne. "Organizational Determinants of Services, Quality and Cost of Care in Hospitals." *Milbank Memorial Fund Quarterly: Health and Society,* in press.

Sheldon, Alan. *Managing Change and Collaboration in the Health System: The Paradigm Approach.* Cambridge, Mass.: Oelgeschlager, Gunn and Hain, 1979.

Sheldon, Alan. "On Consulting to New, Changing, or Innovative Organizations." *Community Mental Health Journal* 7(1971):62–71.

Sheldon, Alan. *Organizational Issues in Health Care Management.* New York: Spectrum Publications, 1975.

Sheldon, Alan, and Barrett, Diana. "The Janus Principle." *Health Care Management Review* 2, no.2(Spring 1977):77–99.

Sherman, Herbert. "Research, Development and Innovation in Health Care Organizations." In Abernathy, et al., 1975, pp. 105–24.

Shortell, Stephen M., and Richardson, William C. *Health Program Evaluation.* St. Louis: Mosby, 1968.

Shortell, Stephen M.; Becker, Selwyn W.; and Neuhauser, Duncan. "The Effects of Management Practices on Hospital Efficiency and Quality of Care." In Shortell and Brown, 1976, pp. 90–107.

Shortell, S. M., and Brown, Montague., eds. *Organizational Research in Hospitals.* Chicago: Blue Cross Association, 1976.

Sigmond, Robert M. "Changing Hospital Goals." *Journal of the Albert Einstein Medical Center* 17(Spring 1969):6–16.

Simon, James K. "Marketing the Community Hospital: A Tool for the Beleaguered Administrator." *Health Care Management Review* 3, no.2 (Spring 1978):11–23.

Sloan, Stanley, and Schrieber, David E. *Hospital Management . . . an Evaluation.* Bureau of Business Research and Service Monograph No. 4. Madison: Graduate School of Business, University of Wisconsin, 1971.

Smalley, Harold E., and Freeman, John R. *Hospital Industrial Engineering: A Guide to the Improvement of Hospital Management Systems.* New York: Reinhold, 1966.

Smith, Claggett. "A Comparative Analysis of Some Conditions and Consequences of Intraorganizational Conflict." *Administrative Science Quarterly* 10(1966):504-29.

Smith, David B., and Kaluzny, Arnold D. *The White Labyrinth: Understanding the Organization of Health Care.* Berkeley: McCutchan, 1975.

Smith, Robert L. "Management of Change." In Jelinek, et al., 1971, pp. 57-78.

Sofer, Cyril. "Reactions to Administrative Change, Study of Staff Relations in Three British Hospitals." *Human Relations* 8(1955):291-316.

Solomon, Stephen. "How One Hospital Broke Its Inflation Fever." *Fortune* 99, no.12(18 June 1979):148-54.

Sommer, Robert, and Dewar, Robert. "The Physical Environment of the Ward." In *The Hospital in Modern Society*, edited by Eliot Freidson, pp. 319-42. New York: Free Press, 1963.

Southard, Samuel. "A Case Study of Planning for Program Change." *Administration in Mental Health*, Spring 1975, pp. 71-80.

Stanton, Alfred H., and Schwartz, Morris S. *The Mental Hospital.* New York: Basic Books, 1954.

Stearns, Norman S.; Bergan, Thomas A.; Roberts, Edward B.; and Cavazos, Lauro F. "A Systems Intervention for Improving Medical-School-Hospital Interrelationships." *Journal of Medical Education* 53(1978):464-72.

Stearns, Norman S.; Bergan, Thomas A.; Roberts, Edward B.; and Quigley, John L. "Systems Integration: New Help for Hospitals." *Health Care Management Review* 1, no.4(Fall 1976):9-18.

Stewart, Rosemary, and Sleeman, J. *Continuously under Review.* Occasional Papers in Social Administration, No. 20. London: Bell, 1967.

Stoelwinder, Johannes U., and Clayton, Peter S. "Hospital Organization Development: Changing the Focus from 'Better Management' to 'Better Patient Care.'" *Journal of Applied Behavioral Science* 14(1978):400-414.

Strauss, Anselm. "Healing by Negotiation: Specialty of the House." *Transaction* 1, no.6(1964):13-15.

Strauss, Anselm; Schatzman, Leonard; Ehrlich, Danuta; Bucher, Rue; and Sabshin, Melvin. "The Hospital and Its Negotiated Order." In *The Hospital in Modern Society*, edited by Eliot Freidson, pp. 147-69. New York: Free Press, 1963.

Student, Kurt R. "Understanding the Implementation of Change." *Hospital Progress* 55, no.6(June 1974):54-59.

Student, Kurt R. "The Failure of Admission Scheduling at Able Hospital." In Griffith et al., 1976, pp. 327-341.

Student, Kurt R. "The Success of Admission Scheduling at Baker Hospital." In Griffith et al., 1976, pp. 342-56.

Student, Kurt R. "Understanding Change in the Hospital." In Griffith et al., 1976, pp. 372-384.

Suchman, Edward A. *Evaluative Research.* New York: Russell Sage, 1967.
Taylor, Carol. *In Horizontal Orbit: Hospitals and the Cult of Efficiency.*
    New York: Holt, Rinehart and Winston, 1970.
Teulings, Ad. W. M.; Jansen, Louis Ch. O.; and Verhoeven, William G.
    "Growth, Power Structure and Leadership Functions in the Hospital
    Organization." *British Journal of Sociology* 24(1973):490–505.
Thurkettle, Mary Ann, and Jones, Susan L. "Conflict As a Systems Pro-
    cess." *Journal of Nursing Administration* 8, no.1(January 1978):39–43.
Tichy, Monique K. *Behavioral Science Techniques: An Annotated Bibliog-
    raphy for Health Professionals.* New York: Praeger, 1975.
Tichy, Monique K. *Health Care Teams: An Annotated Bibliography.* New
    York: Praeger, 1974.
Tichy, Noel M. *Organization Design for Primary Health Care: The Case of
    the Dr. Martin Luther King, Jr. Health Center.* New York: Praeger, 1977.
Tichy, Noel M. "Diagnosis for Complex Health Care Delivery Systems: A
    Model and Case Study." *Journal of Applied Behavioral Science* 14(1978):
    305–20.
Topliss, E. P. "Organizational Change As Illustrated by a Case-Study of a
    Geriatric Hospital." *British Journal of Sociology* 25(1974):356–66.
Torrens, Paul R. "Administrative Problems of Neighborhood Health Cen-
    ters." *Medical Care* 9(1971):487–97.
Tuller, Edwin H. "The Baker Hospital Nursing Department Accommodates
    to Change." In Griffith et al., 1976, pp. 357–71.
United Hospital Fund of New York. *Analyzing and Reducing Employee
    Turnover in Hospitals: A Special Study in Management Practices and
    Problems.* New York: United Hospital Fund, 1968.
Varney, Glenn H., and Scott, W. Sherwood. "Initiating Hospital-wide Goal
    Setting for Organizational Improvement." Paper presented at Academy of
    Management meetings, August 1979, Atlanta, Georgia.
Veninga, Robert. "The Management of Conflict." *Journal of Nursing Admin-
    istration* 3, no.4(July-August 1973):12–16.
Veninga, Robert. "The Management of Organizational Change in Health
    Agencies." *Public Health Reports* 90, no.2(March-April 1975):149–53.
Veninga, Robert. "The Management of Disruptive Conflicts." *Hospital &
    Health Services Administration* 24, no.2(Spring 1979):8–29.
Viguers, Richard T. "The Politics of Power in a Hospital." *Modern Hos-
    pital* 96, no.5(May 1961):89–94.
Vraciu, Robert A., and Griffith, John R. "Cost Control Challenges for
    Hospitals." *Health Care Management Review* 4, no.2(Spring 1979):63–73.
Weaver, Jerry L. *Conflict and Control in Health Care Administration.* Sage
    Library of Social Research, Vol.14. Beverly Hills: Sage Publications, 1974.
Weaver, Jerry L. "Answering the Challenges to Effective Health Care

Administration." *Journal of Health and Human Resources Administration* 1, no.2(November 1978):231-47.

Weisbord, Marvin R. "Why Organization Development Hasn't Worked (So Far) in Medical Centers." *Health Care Management Review* 1, no.2(Spring 1976):17-28.

Weisbord, Marvin R. "A Mixed Model for Medical Centers: Changing Structure and Behavior." In *New Technologies in Organization Development,* edited by J. D. Adams, pp. 211-54. La Jolla: University Associates, 1975.

Weisbord, Marvin R., and Goodstein, Leonard D., eds. "Towards Healthier Medical Systems: Can We Learn from Experience?" *Journal of Applied Behavioral Science* 14, no.3(July 1978):whole issue.

Weisbord, Marvin R.; Lawrence, Paul R.; and Charns, Martin P. "Three Dilemmas of Academic Medical Centers." *Journal of Applied Behavioral Science* 14(1978):284-304.

Weisbord, Marvin R., and Stoelwinder, Johannes U. "Linking Physicians, Hospital Management, Cost Containment and Better Medical Care." *Health Care Management Review* 4, no.2(Spring 1979):7-13.

Westphal, Milton; Frazier, Emma; and Miller, M. Clinton. "Changes in Average Length of Stay and Average Charges Generated Following Institution of PSRO Review." *Health Services Research* 14(1979):253-65.

White, Rodney F. "Contributions of Social Science to Hospital Administration." *Hospital Administration* 6(1961):6-25.

Wieland, George F. "Evaluating the Hospital Internal Communications Project: The Use of Survey Methods in Evaluation." *International Nursing Review* 16(1969):106-14.

Wieland, George F. "Hospitals and Social Research: A Review of Research Relevant to Management." *World Hospitals* 4(1969):201-205.

Wieland, George F. "Manager-directed Surveys for Organizational Improvement." *Journal of Nursing Administration* 6(November-December 1972): 42-47.

Wieland, George F. "Two Ways of Using Behavioral Science to Improve Management." *Health Services Manager* (February, 1980):1-4.

Wieland, George F., and Leigh, Hilary, eds. *Changing Hospitals: A Report on the Hospital Internal Communications Project.* London: Tavistock, 1971.

Wilkie, Roy. "Coping with Organizational Change." *Hospital and Health Services* 75(1979):353-56.

Wilkinson, Gregg S. "Interaction Patterns and Staff Response to Psychiatric Innovations." *Journal of Health and Social Behavior* 14(1973):323-29.

Wilson, Robert N. "Teamwork in the Operating Room." *Human Organization* 12(1954):9-14.

Wise, Harold; Beckhard, Richard; Rubin, Irwin; and Kyte, Aileen I. *Making Health Teams Work.* Cambridge, Mass.: Ballinger, 1974.

Wohlking, W. "Organizational Conflict and Its Solution." *Supervisory Nurse* 1, no.10 (1969):17–18.

Wolfe, Joseph, and Moe, Barbara L. "An Experimental Evaluation of a Hospital Supervisory Training Program." *Hospital Administration* 18, no.4(Fall 1973):65–77.

Wyatt, Janice, and Galski, Thomas. "The Psychological Impact of Hospital Expansion." *Health Care Management Review* 2, no.3(Summer 1977): 51–56.

Yanda, Roman L. *Doctors As Managers of Health Teams: A Career Guide for Hospital-based Physicians.* New York: American Management Association, 1977.

Zeleznik, Carter, and Gonnella, Joseph S. "Jefferson Medical College Student Model Utilization Review Committee." *Journal of Medical Education* 54(1979):848–51.

Index

Beds, demand for, 138, 152, 169–170
Beds, supply of, 138, 152
Beer, Michael, 260, 261
Behavioral expert, 165. *See also* Experts
Belgium, 402
Bell, Cecil H., 236
Bennis, Warren G., 40, 235, 236, 260
Bernstein, Marilyn, 90
Biggart, Nicole Woolsey, 99–100
Blackler, Frank, 461
Blake, Robert R., 256, 384, 456
Blood, Milton R., 455
Blue Cross, 50
Blue Cross of Michigan (BCM), 114, 115, 122, 123, 126.
Blue Shield, 141, 145
Board of Trustees. *See* Trustees
Boundary-spanning subsystem, 42, 56–57
Bowers, David, 252, 334, 335, 336, 337, 468
Brandenburg, Robert G., 92
Braybrooke, David, 463
Breadth of interest, 436, 437, 440, 452
Bronx, New York City, 285, 319
Brown, Colin A., 461
Bucher, Rue, 130
Budgets, 60, 80, 117–119, 123, 274, 282, 283
Bureau of Hospital Administration team, 135–197 passim
Bureaucracy, 132, 230, 268, 373, 397, 456, 463, 467
Burns, Tom, 60, 76, 454
Business Week, 453

Caine, Thomas M., 451–452, 472
California hospitals, HMOs, 132, 345
Camman, Cortlandt, 455
Campbell, Donald T., 386, 426, 442, 448, 495
Campbell, John P., 249, 384, 386
Case mix, 121, 124
Casey, David, 473
Cash flow, 116, 118
Catering, dietetics, 76, 127, 136, 410, 494, 499
Causal variables, 334
Center for Interpersonal Development, 387
Centralization-decentralization, 467; and contingency theory, 44, 49, 50, 51, 76, 493; interventions, 231, 261, 467; and program change, 89, 93–97; and medical-surgical wards, 432. *See also* Authority
Central supplies, requisitioning, 413

Central team, 404, 410, 415, 416, 435, 440, 445, 446, 473; role of the, 404, 406, 436, 459
Change agent. *See* Consultants
Charns, Martin P., 77, 272, 275
Chicago hospitals, 131
Child, John, 455
Christman, Luther, 14, 20
CIVs. *See* Cost-influencing variables
Clayton, Peter S., 372, 378, 466
Clayton's tests, 426–430, 443–446, 448, 449
Climate, organizational and group, 250, 251, 252, 315–316, 340–341, 345–346, 348–350, 414, 456–457
Clinics, group practice medical, 11, 39, 44, 52–53, 55–59.
Closed/open systems, 40, 41, 67
Coan, Richard W., 454
Cognitive change, 231, 254–255
Cohen, Arthur R., 387
Cohen, B.S., 425
Collage exercise, 314
Commitment of top management, 102
Committees, 178
Communication, 402; in emergency room, 385, 386; improvement in, 388, 390, 391; organizational, 91, 384, 385, 387, 388, 402, 440; and length of stay, 402, 425–426; problems of, 212, 350, 351, 407–411, 440; training to improve, 385–391, 403; in work team, 286, 288, 294, 295–296, 297, 312–313, 324. *See also* Openness
Communication-feedback exercise, 312–313
Comparison of data, 328
Complexity: and action/understanding systems, 395, 431, 432, 491, 493; and change, 2, 78, 88–89, 93, 94, 95, 96; of organizational technology, 2, 42, 44, 46, 48. *See also* Heterogeneity of staff; Specialization
Comprehensive health care. *See* Team, primary care
Computer problems, 141–142
Conflict resolution, 297–298
Confrontation, 253–254, 262, 336
Congruence of intervention and target, 397, 398, 455–457
Conservative-liberal attitudes, 432, 457, 473
Construction of facilities, 445
Consultant's dilemma, 259–260
Consultants, OD, 6, 101, 102, 266, 387, 468, 473; as experts, 176, 237, 255, 302, 333, 336, 377, 397; inside or outside role of, 101, 236, 354–355, 377; intervention by, defined, 304; legitimacy of, 301, 377; and MBO/ward teams, 369, 370, 377, 378, 379, 383; power

Perrow, Charles, 22, 44, 45, 46, 48, 49, 75, 129, 456

Pharmacy, 127, 132, 136, 378, 416, 417

Phases of change, 100–108, 178, 199, 210, 217–226, 243–247, 299–304, 325, 341, 347–349, 358. *See also* Unfreezing-changing-refreezing

Physical arrangements changed, 97

Physical therapy, 127, 378, 425, 426

Physicians: acceptance/rejection of change, 188, 231, 232, 233, 366; and administrators, 19, 58–60, 76–78, 120–123, 129, 133, 160–161, 193–194, 275, 281–283, 350, 373, 485; and admissions scheduling, 141, 143, 144–145, 172–173, 177, 179, 186; autonomy of, 15, 215, 216, 229–232, 267, 275, 485–486, 487; conflict among, 85, 215, 216; and controls, 48, 79, 130, 131, 276, 277, 373, 482; and costs, 117, 120–127, 180, 283, 500; education of, 21–22, 214, 217–223, 225, 269, 270, 273, 418, 446, 465, 487; and HIC Project, 396, 399, 403, 408–410, 413, 414, 422–424, 441, 442; identity of, 269, 276–278; individualism of, 130, 267; management by, 81, 129–134, 277, 282, 485–486; and MBO, 232, 370, 372, 377, 378, 381–382, 482, 485; and medical center change, 229–233, 281–283, 488, 489; and nurses, 144, 146–148, 152, 160–161, 193, 280, 321, 372, 402, 432; and organizational technology, 42, 47, 76–78, 431–432, 468, 500; and patients, 15, 62; personality of, 276, 432, 448, 500; power of, 15, 50, 59, 60, 81, 85, 130, 185, 188, 231, 397, 398, 485; on primary care team, 231, 292, 312–313, 321–324; recruitment of, 50, 57, 124, 147, 217; and survey research, 136, 348, 350, 351, 488–489; and systems intervention, 214–225; and team-building, 230–232, 312–315, 322, 324, 488, 489. *See also specific medical specialties*

Pilot studies, 103, 105, 153, 180, 202–203, 208, 378, 415–416, 421

Placement vs. training, 67–68

Plans, 22, 23, 27, 28, 29, 106, 107

Plaut, Thomas F., 319–325

Plop effect, 295

Political attitudes, 432, 451, 457, 473. *See also* Values

Political skills, 65, 66, 67, 282

Postal Service (USPS), 99–100

Posteriorities, 31

Power: based on knowledge, 171; to control costs, 124–127; for implementation, 60, 78, 89, 97, 99, 102; ploys, 211; *See also* Centralization; Physicians, power of; Administrators, power of; Consultants, power over clients

PR. *See* Prospective reimbursement

Prahalad, Coimbatore K., 85

Preadmission diagnostic testing, 81

Pressure for change. *See* Stress

Prices of inputs, 123

Primary relations, 17–18

Priorities, 31–32, 272–273

Problem orientation, 216, 434, 436, 440. *See also* Action/understanding orientation

Problem solving, 1, 2, 3, 78, 80, 101, 235, 378–381, 401, 433–434, 440, 457, 493. *See also* Managerial action; Action/understanding systems

Process consultation, 236–238, 252, 336, 460

Process evaluation, 433

Processes in groups, 292–298, 306, 317

Process of change. *See* Phases of change

Process of management, 79–80. *See also* Managerial action

Production emphasis, 91, 94, 95

Production subsystem, 42, 52, 57–58, 67

Productivity. *See* Efficiency

Professional dominance, 130

Professionals, 2, 4, 18–20, 88–89, 94, 269, 270, 272, 395, 431, 463. *See also* Internal/external controls

Program change, 78, 87–96

Prospective reimbursement (PR), 80, 113–128, 482

Protection of system members, 179–180

Psychiatry, 138, 323

Psychological approach to change, 1–3, 229, 395, 486–487, 491, 492, 494. *See also* Action/understanding intervention; Action/understanding orientations; Organization development

Psychological change, 229, 486, 487; contrasted with managerial action and structural change, 1–6, 79, 84, 395–396, 467–469, 474, 490–492, 494; in HIC Project, 399, 434–440, 461, 469, 474, 490–492, 494. *See also* Organization development; Attitude change

Psychological characteristics. *See* People

Psychological forces, 238, 239

Psychotherapy, 451

QMH. *See* Lawrence Quigley Memorial Hospital

Quality emphasis, 91–95

Quality of medical care, 60, 120–121, 126, 131, 132, 274, 464–465. *See also* Patient care

Quasi-stationary equilibrium of behavior, 239, 240, 242

ABOUT THE EDITOR

George Wieland is the co-author of three books, most recently ORGANIZA-
TION THEORY AND DESIGN. He is currently a consultant on evaluation
research in Ann Arbor, Michigan, where he has been associate research
scientist at the School of Public Health at the University of Michigan. He
received his Ph.D. in social psychology from the University of Michigan and
spent three years in England studying the National Health Service.